D1060474

Occupational Asthma

Torben Sigsgaard
Dick Heederik

Editors

Birkhäuser

Editors

Torben Sigsgaard
School of Public Health
Dept. of Environmental and Occupational Medicine
Aarhus University
Bartholin Allé 2
8000 Århus C
Denmark

Dick Heederik
Institute for Risk Assessment Sciences
Division of Environmental and Occupational Health
Utrecht University
Yalelaan 2
3508 TD Utrecht
Netherlands

Library of Congress Control Number: 2009943448

Bibliographic information published by Die Deutsche Bibliothek
Die Deutsche Bibliothek lists this publication in the Deutsche Nationalbibliografie;
detailed bibliographic data is available in the internet at http://dnb.ddb.de

ISBN 978-3-7643-8555-2

P.O. Box 133, CH-4010 Basel, Switzerland
Part of Springer Science+Business Media
Printed on acid-free paper produced from chlorine-free pulp. TCF ∞
Cover design: Markus Etterich, Basel
Cover illustration: see p. 192, with friendly permission by Dick Heederik
Printed in Germany
ISBN 978-3-7643-8555-2
9 8 7 6 5 4 3 2 1

e-ISBN 978-3-7643-8556-9
www.birkhauser.ch

Contents

List of contributors

Xaver Baur, Ordinariat und Zentralinstitut für Arbeitsmedizin und Maritime Medizin, Universität Hamburg, Seewartenstrasse 10, 20459 Hamburg, Germany; e-mail: baur@uke.uni-hamburg.de

Paul D. Blanc, Division of Occupational and Environmental Medicine, University of California San Francisco, San Francisco, California, USA

Sherwood Burge, Heart of England NHS Foundation Trust, Birmingham Heartlands Hospital, Bordesley Green East, Birmingham B9 5SS, UK; e-mail: sherwood.burge@heartofengland.nhs.uk

André Cartier, University of Montreal, Department of Medicine, Hôpital du Sacré-Coeur de Montréal, 5400 Boul. Gouin Ouest, Montréal, P.Q., Canada, H4J 1C5

Francesc Castro-Giner, Centre for Research in Environmental Epidemiology (CREAL), Barcelona, Spain; e-mail: fcastro@creal.cat

Paul Cullinan, Department of Occupational and Environmental Medicine, National Heart and Lung Institute, Imperial College, 1b Manresa Road, London SW3 6LR, UK; e-mail: p.cullinan@imperial.ac.uk

Vinciane D'Alpaos, Service de Pneumologie, Cliniques de Mont-Godinne, Université Catholique de Louvain, B-5530, Yvoir, Belgium; e-mail: vinciane.dalpaos@uclouvain.be

Vanessa De Vooght, O&N 1, Research Unit for Lung Toxicology (Pneumology), Herestraat 49 bus 706, 3000 Leuven, Belgium; e-mail: vanessa.devooght@med.kuleuven.be

Gert Doekes, Division of Environmental Epidemiology, Institute for Risk Assessment Sciences, Utrecht University, PO Box 80178, 3508 TD Utrecht, The Netherlands; e-mail: g.doekes@uu.nl

Denyse Gautrin, Axe de recherche en santé respiratoire, Hôpital du Sacré-Coeur de Montréal, 5400 Gouin Blvd West, Montreal, Canada H4J 1C5; e-mail: d.gautrin@umontreal.ca

Dick Heederik, Division of Environmental Epidemiology, Institute for Risk Assessment Sciences, University of Utrecht, PO Box 80178, 3508 TD Utrecht, The Netherlands; e-mail: d.heederik@uu.nl

Paul K. Henneberger, National Institute for Occupational Safety and Health, Centers for Disease Control and Prevention, MS H2800, 1095 Willowdale Road , Morgantown, WV 26505, USA; e-mail: pkh0@cdc.gov

Valérie Hox, O&N 1, Research Unit for Lung Toxicology (Pneumology), Herestraat 49 bus 706, 3000 Leuven, Belgium; e-mail: valerie.hox@med.kuleuven.be

Hayley L. Jeal, Department of Occupational and Environmental Medicine, National Heart and Lung Institute, Imperial College, 1b Manresa Road, London SW3 6LR, UK; e-mail: hayley.jeal@imperial.ac.uk

Meinir G. Jones, Department of Occupational and Environmental Medicine, National Heart and Lung Institute, Imperial College, 1b Manresa Road, London SW3 6LR, UK; e-mail: meinir.jones@imperial.ac.uk

Francine Kauffmann, Inserm, U780 – Epidemiology and Biostatistics, Villejuif, France; e-mail: francine.kauffmann@inserm.fr

Manolis Kogevinas, Centre for Research in Environmental Epidemiology (CREAL), Barcelona, Spain; e-mail: kogevinas@creal.cat

Kathleen Kreiss, National Institute for Occupational Safety and Health, 1095 Willowdale Rd., MS-H 2800, Morgantown, WV, 26505, USA; e-mail: kkreiss@cdc.gov

Jean-Luc Malo, Axe de recherche en santé respiratoire, Hôpital du Sacré-Coeur de Montréal, 5400 Gouin Blvd West, Montreal, Canada H4J 1C5; e-mail: malojl@med-dir.umontreal.ca

Rachel Nadif, Inserm, U780 – Epidemiology and Biostatistics, Villejuif, France; e-mail: rachel.nadif@inserm.fr

Evert Meijer, IRAS, Institute for Risk Assessment Sciences, Division Environmental and Occupational Health, Utrecht University, 3508 TD, Utrecht, Netherlands

Benoit Nemery, O&N 1, Research Unit for Lung Toxicology (Pneumology), Herestraat 49 bus 706, 3000 Leuven, Belgium; e-mail: ben.nemery@med.kuleuven.be

Anthony Newman-Taylor, Faculty of Medicine, Imperial College, London, UK

Henrik Nordman, Finnish Institute of Occupational Health, Topeliuksenkatu 41 aA, 00250 Helsinki, Finland; e-mail: henrik.nordman@ttl.fi

Dennis Nowak, Institute and Outpatient Clinic for Occupational, Social and Environmental Medicine, Clinical Centre, Ludwig Maximilian University, Ziemssenstr. 1, 80336 München, Germany; e-mail: dennis.nowak@med.lmu.de

Øyvind Omland, School of Public Health, Department of Environmental and Occupational Medicine, Aarhus University, Denmark

Carrie A. Redlich , Occupational and Environmental Medicine and Pulmonary & Critical Care Medicine, Yale University School of Medicine, 135 College Street, 3rd Floor, New Haven, Connecticut 06510, USA; e-mail: carrie.redlich@yale.edu

Vivi Schlünssen, School of Public Health, Department of Environmental and Occupational Medicine, Aarhus University, Bartholin Allé 2, 8000 Århus C, Denmark; e-mail: vs@mil.au.dk

Torben Sigsgaard, School of Public Health, Department of Environmental and Occupational Medicine, Aarhus University, Bartholin Allé 2, 8000 Århus C, Denmark; e-mail: ts@mil.au.dk

Lidwien A.M. Smit, Inserm, U780 – Epidemiology and Biostatistics, Villejuif, France; e-mail: l.a.smit@uu.nl

Peter S. Thorne, Environmental Health Sciences Research Center, University of Iowa, Iowa City, USA

Kjell Torén, Department of Occupational and Environmental Medicine, Sahlgrenska University Hospital, Box 414, 405 30 Göteborg, Sweden; e-mail: kjell.toren@amm.gu.se

Olivier Vandenplas, Service de Pneumologie, Cliniques de Mont-Godinne, Université Catholique de Louvain, B-5530, Yvoir, Belgium; e-mail: olivier.vandenplas@uclouvain.be

Jeroen A.J. Vanoirbeek, O&N 1, Research Unit for Lung Toxicology (Pneumology), Herestraat 49 bus 706, 3000 Leuven, Belgium; e-mail: jeroen.vanoirbeek@med.kuleuven.be

Preface

This issue of "Progress in Inflammation Research" is dedicated to the different aspects of Occupational Asthma from the natural history and risk factors to the preventive strategies and management of the disease.

Now that heavy industry in the Western world has been regulated and reduced in size, mainly during the last part of the 20th Century, occupational asthma (OA) has become one of the leading causes of occupational respiratory diseases [1]. From meta-analyses and systematic reviews, it has been estimated that the attributable fraction for occupational exposures for the burden of asthma is approximately 15%. Considering the increasing background prevalence of child- and adult-onset asthma in the Western world, this is a substantial proportion of the disease spectrum.

One of the challenges of modern research into OA is the possibility of characterizing different phenotypes of asthma. In a recent editorial in the Lancet it was pointed out that the time has come to accept that asthma is not one entity, but a construct with different underlying phenotypes [2]. Two phenotypes in particular have been discussed in the literature in recent years, but more are likely to exist. These two phenotypes are the allergic and the irritative phenotype, caused by IgE-mediated sensitizers and irritants, respectively. The occupational setting offers a great opportunity to study different asthma phenotypes because high concentrations of single compounds occur, and therefore the risk for developing asthma is high. Traditionally OA has been divided into two entities, one immunologically and the other irritant induced, the latter being characterized by increased bronchial hyperresponsiveness. The immunological type of OA is divided into the IgE-mediated form and the non-IgE-mediated form. A third entity is emerging from occupations with exposure to organic dust, and is characterized by neutrophil influx to the airways and asthma symptoms without IgE-mediated sensitization.

This is a theme in several of the chapters, and it will be an issue for research, not only in OA but in asthma research in general for the decades to come. Related to asthma phenotypes is the distinction between asthma, asthma-like symptoms and chronic obstructive pulmonary disease (COPD). This is especially an issue in the farm environment, where different types of inflammatory diseases of the airways occur in parallel. Here it is quite difficult to distinguish between the different phenotypes, which is also true for other industrial settings with organic dust exposure. The newer studies in this area clearly point towards a distinction between the wheezy and the allergic phenotypes. The wheezy phenotype increases, whereas the allergic phenotype decreases, with increasing organic dust exposure [3, 4].

The prevalences of atopy and asthma have reached new levels in the general population of the industrialized world. This challenges the prevention of OA. As these birth cohorts, more of whom are atopic than ever in the past, enter the labor market, an increased pressure is put on the employers to create an occupational environment that can accommodate more susceptible people than previously. Paradoxically, people susceptible for developing asthma will be exposed longer to lower concentrations of pollutants than ever in the post-industrial era. The reason is that, earlier, the exposure levels encountered would cause immediate problems in the susceptible people, forcing them to leave the work within a short period of time; this is no longer the case with the improvements seen in modern work environments.

Sensitization has generally been considered not to be associated to exposure in a classical dose-response-like manner. The latest results from studies with good exposure assessment and quantitative analyses of sensitization have clearly shown that this was a misconception since dose-response associations have been seen for atopics as well as for non-atopics, sparking the discussion of primary prevention of asthma by preventing sensitization in the workforce [5].

Individual susceptibility will become a more important area of research in the coming years. A driving force for this research is the technological development in the field of genomics and application of these techniques in epidemiological studies. Genetic studies involving gene environment interactions in occupational settings are a promising path, which will hopefully lead to more insight into the basic mechanisms driving responses to environmental exposures. A whole section of this issue is related to the semi-experimental studies of apprentice workers entering the working environment, and their unique findings of the initial sensitization and subsequent symptoms in bakers. However, the findings from some of these studies do not seem to directly convey the allergic march deducted from cross-sectional studies [6], and the symptoms experienced during apprenticeship diminishes after ceasing exposure [7], meaning that future studies will have to focus on the whole population of workers exposed to high-molecular-weight allergens and not only the fraction of workers with a specific sensitization towards an allergen.

So far only a few studies have been able to find a relationship between specific polymorphisms and OA, e.g., CD14 and wheezing in those exposed to organic dust, and α-1-antitrypsin and bronchial hyperresponsiveness in farming students [8]. Likewise isocyanate-exposed workers have shown differences in susceptibility according to Balboni et al. [9]. Not all studies on susceptibility will involve genetic characterization. Other approaches to characterize different phenotypes may also find an application. A recent example is separation of populations into low and high responders to endotoxin on the basis of whole blood assays (WBA) [10]. In this study a clear exposure-response relationship was found between endotoxin exposure and wheezing only in high responders. These observations can be brought to the next level by investigating, in a WBA assay, the genes that make a person a high or a low responder. Novel biomedical technology will open avenues for new research, but will without doubt also raise ethical questions, especially in the work environment.

January 2010

Torben Sigsgaard
Dick Heederik

References

1 Sigsgaard T, Nowak D, Annesi-Maesano I, Nemery B, Toren K, Viegi G, Radon K, Burge PS, Heederik D (2010) ERS Position paper on: Work related respiratory diseases in the EU. *Eur Respir J* 35: 234–238

2 (2006) A plea to abandon asthma as a disease concept. *Lancet* 368: 705

3 Eduard W, Douwes J, Omenaas E, Heederik D (2004) Do farming exposures cause or prevent asthma? Results from a study of adult Norwegian farmers. *Thorax* 59: 381–386

4 Smit LA, Heederik D, Doekes G, Blom C, van Zweden I, Wouters IM (2008) Exposure-response analysis of allergy and respiratory symptoms in endotoxin-exposed adults. *Eur Respir J* 31: 1241–1248

5 Heederik D, Thorne PS, Doekes G (2002) Health-based occupational exposure limits for high molecular weight sensitizers: how long is the road we must travel? *Ann Occup Hyg* 46: 439–446

6 Skjold T, Dahl R, Juhl B, Sigsgaard T (2008) The incidence of respiratory symptoms and sensitization in baker apprentices. *Eur Respir J* 32: 452–459

7 Gautrin D, Ghezzo H, Infante-Rivard C, Magnan M, L'Archeveque J, Suarthana E, Malo JL (2008) Long-term outcomes in a prospective cohort of apprentices exposed to high-molecular-weight agents. *Am J Respir Crit Care Med* 177: 871–879

8 Sigsgaard T, Brandslund I, Omland O,.Hjort C, Lund ED, Pedersen OF, Miller MR (2000) S and Z alpha1-antitrypsin alleles are risk factors for bronchial hyperresponsiveness in young farmers: an example of gene/environment interaction. *Eur Respir J* 16: 50–55

9 Balboni A, Baricordi OR, Fabbri LM, Gandini E, Ciaccia A, Mapp CE (1996) Association between toluene diisocyanate-induced asthma and DQB1 markers: a possible role for aspartic acid at position 57. *Eur Respir J* 9: 207–210

10 Smit LA, Heederik D, Doekes G, Krop EJ, Rijkers GT, Wouters IM (2009) Ex vivo cytokine release reflects sensitivity to occupational endotoxin exposure. *Eur Respir J* 34: 795–802

The history of research on asthma in the workplace – Development, victories and perspectives

Jean-Luc Malo[1] *and Anthony Newman-Taylor*[2]

[1]The Department of Chest Medicine, Hôpital du Sacré-Cœur de Montréal, 5400 West Gouin Bld, Montréal, Canada H4J 1C5
[2]Faculty of Medicine, Imperial College, London, UK

Abstract

Here we review the historical landmarks of occupational asthma (OA). Although there has been suspicion for long that proteins can cause allergic sensitisation and OA, it is only in the last century that evidence that chemicals can cause OA has been published. Acute irritation of the bronchi has also been incriminated in the genesis of OA. Although an IgE-mediated process has been clearly identified in OA caused by proteinaceous material, the mechanism of OA remains unknown for chemicals. Population-based studies, examination of population data bank, sentinel-based studies and prospective interventions in high-risk workplaces have greatly improved our estimates of the frequency of the condition and helped to identify risk factors. Although diagnostic means are more diversified, they are still not used sufficiently. However, characterisation of the occupational environment has become more accurate, and scales for assessing impairment/disability are now available. Estimates of the proportion of asthma cases that can be ascertained as OA are now proposed. In a more general way, OA has been proposed as a model of the onset and persistence of asthma in humans.

Introduction

According to its etymological meaning, asthma refers to a "shallow breathing" as initially proposed by Homer in the 15th song of the Iliad (850 BC), which describes the "terrible suffocation" of Hector lying in the plain. Early literature on asthma has distinguished intrinsic from extrinsic causal factors. The arabic physician Razes (*Abu Bakr Mohammed Ibn Zakaria Al-Razi*) (864–930) was the first to identify allergic asthma followed by his colleague Maimonides (*Abu Imran Musa Ben Maimun Ibn Abd Allah*) (1138–1204), Saladin's physician, who, in the first treatise on asthma "*Maqalah fi Al-Rabw*", comments on the influence of heredity, the wintry exacerbations of asthma and the influence of foods, hygiene and emotion. These extrinsic factors were also reported in Sir John Floyer's (1649–1734) *A Treatise of the Asthma*, in which the author who suffered from asthma reports the improvement due to breathing the fresh air in Oxford. The development of immunology

Occupational Asthma, edited by Torben Sigsgaard and Dick Heederik

and allergy in the beginning of the 20th century allowed identification of the factors related to the intrinsic and extrinsic components and to a formal proposal of classification by the American physician Rackeman in 1947.

Although there had been suspicions that the workplace could cause or increase the severity of asthma before, according to Pepys and Bernstein [1] the Scandinavian monk Olaus Magnus was, in 1555, the first to describe the difficult breathing that could occur in grain handlers and might either represent farmer's lung or asthma. In their section on "Diseases of sifters and measurers of grain" [1], Bernardino Ramazzini, the father of occupational medicine, was also reported to have described the difficult breathing of these workers but his description could also correspond to farmers' lung and not necessarily to asthma. In the 19th century, authors such as Thackrah in England and Patissier in France described the occurrence of what could be interpreted as chronic bronchitis in malsters, coffee roasters, hatters, hairdressers and as byssinosis in flax mill workers. Castor beans, various gums (acacia, tragacanth), metal salts and anhydrides were the first occupational sensitising agents described as formerly causing asthma in reports made early in the 20th century [1]. Interestingly, the agents originally incriminated included both high- and low-molecular-weight agents, in particular isocyanates, a still important cause of occupational asthma (OA) [2]. The development by Pepys, considered by many to be the father of OA, of an experimental method of simulated exposure to agents suspected to cause OA [3] enabled the identification of several causative agents, the description of the temporal patterns of asthmatic reactions and the inhibitory effect of drugs, such as sodium cromoglycate and inhaled steroids, on these reactions.

From occupational asthma to asthma in the workplace

Several conditions can be distinguished under the general heading of asthma in the workplace (Fig. 1). First, the workplace can cause asthma through a known or apparently plausible sensitising process that needs a latency period to induce sensitisation and cause symptoms; until recently this was the main focus of interest. Since the early 20th century it had been known that exposure to products with irritant properties could cause pulmonary oedema and bronchial damages [4], the latter being labelled irritant-induced asthma or reactive airway dysfunction syndrome (acronym: RADS) by Brooks and co-workers in 1985 [5]. In contrast, study of exacerbations of asthma at the workplace [6] has been neglected, so that little was known in this field, although it encompasses socioeconomic consequences that are equivalent to OA [7, 8]. Variants of OA have been described, especially in the aluminium industry, which reached its peak manufacturing activity in the 20th century. Here potroom workers were shown to have an excess of respiratory symptoms that included wheezing [9]. Finally, because induced sputum can now be more readily examined, a condition known as eosinophilic bronchitis has also been identified in recent years [10].

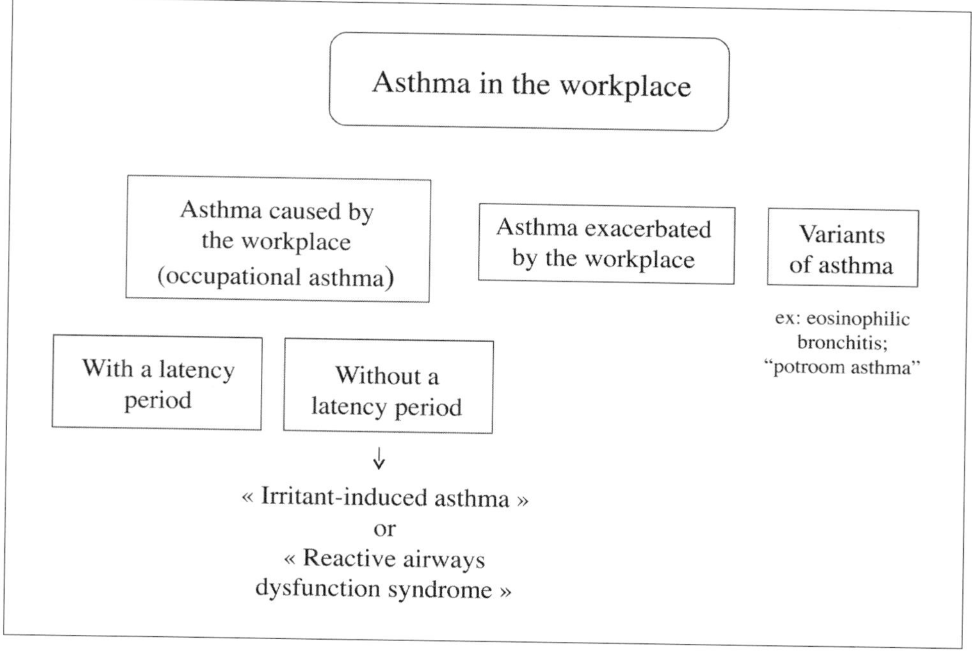

Figure 1.
Different conditions of asthma in the workplace.

Practice guidelines on OA have been issued in the USA [11], Canada [12] and the UK [13].

Suspicion that chemicals and not only proteins can cause "sensitisation"

The capacity of proteins encountered in the workplace, such as those from castor bean, gums acacia and tragacanth, to cause asthma as the manifestation of a hypersensitivity response was recognised by the 1930s and 1940s [14–17]. In each case the development of asthma followed an initial symptom-free period of exposure, with asthma subsequently provoked by levels of exposure to which the individuals themselves were previously, and others continued to be, tolerant, fulfilling the clinical criteria of an acquired hypersensitivity response.

Reports of asthma with similar characteristics caused by low-molecular-weight chemicals encountered at work, such as phthalic anhydride [18] and complex platinum salts [19], followed shortly after. Both of these reports provided evidence for an associated immediate skin test response, implying the presence of reaginic antibody.

Further understanding of the nature and underlying mechanisms of these allergic reactions followed the development of controlled inhalation testing and the discovery of IgE. Inhalation tests demonstrated that similar patterns of immediate, late, dual and nocturnal reactions were provoked by inhalation of proteins encountered both in the general environment (e.g. house dust mite) and at work (enzymes) and by inhalation of low-molecular-weight chemicals [20, 21].

The discovery in the late 1960s of IgE antibodies as the mediators of reaginic or allergic activity by Ishizaka et al. [22] and Johannson [23] led to the understanding of the underlying immunological mechanisms of allergic asthma. It is caused not only by common environmental allergens (e.g. grass pollen, house dust mite) but also by agents inhaled at work, both proteins and some low-molecular-weight chemicals. Specific IgE antibodies were shown to be present to many of the important protein causes of OA, including enzymes [24], flour [25], as well as rat and mouse urine proteins [26]. Specific IgE was also identified to low-molecular-weight chemicals such as acid anhydrides [27, 28] and reactive dyes [29] that were conjugated to human serum albumin. However, no evidence for specific IgE antibody has been reproducibly found in cases of asthma caused by the majority of low-molecular-weight chemicals, such as plicatic acid found in Western red cedar [30] and isocyanates [31, 32]. Although the complex platinum salt ammonium hexachloroplatinate, an essential intermediate in platinum refining, elicits immediate skin prick test responses in the majority of OA cases caused by this salt, no specific IgE has yet been reproducibly found in the sera of these cases. The mechanism of asthma caused by low-molecular-weight chemicals that fulfils the clinical criteria of a hypersensitivity reaction, but where no specific IgE antibody has been reliably found, remains unclear. It remains possible that the appropriate hapten protein conjugate has not been used for specific IgE testing. However, the absence of mRNA for the IgE chain in Th2 lymphocytes from the airways of patients with isocyanate-induced asthma following an inhalation test asthmatic response, argues against this, at least in cases of isocyanate-induced asthma without specific IgE in their sera [32].

Assessment of frequency

Most of the early frequency studies of OA were cross-sectional in design and investigated epidemics of work-related asthma in specific industries where cases had been identified. The potential pitfall of this approach is the healthy survivor bias [33]. More recently, frequency estimates have been obtained by consultation of suitable registries, either from general population data, especially in Scandinavia [34], or from medicolegal statistics, with interest in those available in countries where objective means are routinely applied [35]. Sentinel-based projects have been initiated in several countries and have been fruitful particularly in the USA [36] and the UK [37]. Prospective studies have been more recently carried out in apprentices in high-risk fields, so as to document the natural history of the condition [38, 39]. Finally, large population-based studies like the European Respiratory Health Survey have included key elements that explore the work-relatedness of symptoms with some objective testing [40]. There are current attempts to document the frequency of OA in developing countries where data are still scarce [41].

Occupational asthma as a model for environmental asthma

Asthma caused by allergy to agents inhaled at work has several advantages for investigation over asthma caused by allergy to environmental allergens, for which it has been considered a model. These include: a well-defined population at risk; a well-defined phenotype (both clinical and, for several of its causes, immunological); maximum risk of developing disease within a relatively short period from onset of exposure and, with the development of inhibition immunoassays for specific allergens, the opportunity for well-characterised exposure.

A number of studies have exploited these advantages to investigate, in well-defined workforce cohorts, the determinants of allergy and asthma triggered by several of the different causes of OA, including enzymes used in detergents [42], Western red cedar [43], rat and mouse urine proteins [44], flour and -amylase [45] and acid anhydrides [46]. The strength of some of these studies has been in the follow-up of a proportion of new employees not previously exposed to the relevant allergen or low-molecular-weight chemical, which helps to overcome the problems of survivor bias inherent in cross-sectional surveys, and the ability to relate disease incidence to level of exposure estimated quantitatively by objective measurement of aeroallergen [47–49]. The use of an entirely prospective model has been particularly fruitful in examining apprentices before they enter a training program [39, 50] because this represents an experimental situation in which subjects can be examined before, during and even after stopping exposure, so that the determinants for sensitisation and asthma can be assessed first before any exposure and then before starting to work [51].

Exposure is a more important determinant than personal and genetic factors

Several studies have consistently demonstrated the importance of the level of exposure to airborne allergen (enzyme, flour, α-amylase, detergent enzyme, acid anhydride, Western red cedar) as the major determinant of risk of developing specific IgE allergy and/or asthma. Factors such as atopy and cigarette smoking previously identified as risk factors for some agents (e.g. platinum salts) were found to be of lesser importance than intensity of exposure. The importance of exposure intensity as a determinant of OA and of its reduction in reducing disease incidence is well demonstrated by examining the history of asthma caused by occupational exposures to enzymes in the detergent industry.

Flindt first reported in 1969 [52] that the powdered proteolytic enzyme Alcalase, derived from *Bacillus subtilis*, introduced in 1967 in detergent manufacture could cause allergic reactions, including asthma, in exposed workers. In an accompanying article in the Lancet, Pepys and colleagues [24] described the results of inhalation tests with enzyme extracts in affected workers, which provoked immediate and dual asthmatic reactions, associated with immediate skin prick test responses and specific IgE to the protease in their sera, providing strong evidence that allergy to protease was the cause of their asthma.

By 1970, 80% of soap detergents sold in USA contained enzymes. Cross-sectional studies of factory workforces reported high rates of respiratory symptoms and skin test responses to proteolytic enzymes. In a survey of a UK workforce, Newhouse and colleagues [53] reported allergic symptoms in 47% of the workforce with an association between a skin test response to enzymes and both allergic symptoms and atopy.

The findings of these studies stimulated important advances, in particular the substitution of powdered enzymes by enzymes encapsulated in granules. This, together with major engineering improvements, led to a marked reduction in the levels of airborne enzyme in the workplace [54]. The effectiveness of these interventions in reducing the incidence of asthma and sensitisation was investigated in a 7-year follow up of employees of the enzyme detergents-manufacturing factory where the original cases reported by Flindt had worked [52]. The authors examined the attack rate before and after the introduction of enzyme granulation and improved engineering controls. They found that skin test reactions primarily occurred in the first 2 years of exposure and their incidence was greater in those with higher levels of exposure and among atopics at each level of exposure. Dust concentration fell by more than threefold. In parallel with this, the incidence of skin prick test responses to enzymes and the number of cases transferred from enzyme areas following the development of respiratory symptoms also fell. Whereas 41% of workers employed in 1968/69 developed immediate skin prick test reactions to enzymes, of those employed between 1971 and 1973, 11% developed skin test reactions. Similarly, the number of cases transferred out of the enzyme area with respiratory symptoms fell from 50 between 1968 and 1971 to 1 in each year in 1972–1974 [54]. More recent studies have shown that, while the prevalence of sensitisation to enzymes in the detergent industry can be high, in general the incidence and prevalence of asthma has remained low. This, however, was not the case in detergent-producing factory in NW England, which, despite only using granulated enzymes, was found to have a high prevalence of allergic disease (both rhinitis and asthma) [55]. Of a factory population of 350, 19% had work-related nasal symptoms and 16% work-related asthmatic symptoms together with evidence of specific IgE to protease or amylase or both. The prevalence of disease showed a clear relationship with estimated levels of airborne enzyme. The reasons for this high prevalence of allergic disease (comparable to the reported frequencies in the late 1960s/early 1970s) are not clear, but no other recent studies have reported comparable levels of disease.

The impact of these and other similar studies for disease prevention has stimulated a fundamental shift in focus from the identification and exclusion of a "susceptible" minority of the potential workforce by pre-employment screening, to measures designed to reduce the levels of exposure to the specific agents in the place of work. Recent studies of genetic influences on the development of specific IgE and OA have shown interesting though inconsistent (the number of individuals is generally small) associations with various HLA phenotypes, some having an enhancing and others a protective effect [56]. The interesting and potentially important implication of these observations, if generalisable, is that the more disease incidence is reduced by controlling levels of exposure, the more important genetic susceptibility will become as a determinant of sensitisation and asthma.

Diagnostic means

Originally, the diagnosis of OA was mainly based on the clinical history. The description of OA due to isocyanates, the leading cause of OA, used this approach [2]. Clinical questionnaires generally represent sensitive but not specific tools for making a diagnosis of OA [57]. Skin testing to document possible IgE-mediated sensitisation and spirometry were subsequently used, followed by evaluation of non-specific bronchial responsiveness, for periods at work and away from work. Pepys was the first to experimentally document the occurrence of asthmatic reactions on laboratory exposure to occupational agents [58]. At-work and off-work monitoring of peak expiratory flow rates was subsequently suggested [59], along with the monitoring of non-OA subjects [60]. Other non-invasive means to document airway inflammation, a key element included in recent definitions of asthma [61], have been added to the diagnostic arsenal [62], while attempts to improve the methodology of laboratory challenges have been carried out [63].

Persistence of disease after removal from exposure

For a long time it was naïvely thought that workers with OA would be cured after removal from exposure. Chan-Yeung and co-workers [64] were the first to show that asthma generally persists in workers with OA that had been caused by Western red cedar who were no longer at work. Numerous studies carried out in different populations affected with OA initiated by various agents have subsequently confirmed this original contribution that has enlightened our understanding of the natural history of asthma. OA indeed offers a unique opportunity because workers can be removed from the agent that causes OA, whereas this is not generally feasible for allergic asthma due to ubiquitous allergens. Most often, after cessation of exposure to an agent causing OA, the persistence of asthma is reflected by long-lasting bronchial hyperresponsiveness that improves at a faster rate in the first 2 years after removal from exposure than later on [65]. Even when workers are apparently cured (this occurs in approximately 25% of cases), it has been recently shown that some airway inflammation and remodelling can persist [66].

Impairment and disability

Whereas means and scales for assessing pneumoconiosis had been developed, these tools could not be applied in the case of asthma, a disease characterised by variable airway obstruction. Criteria based on need for medication to control asthma, as well as levels of airway obstruction and hyperresponsiveness, were proposed by the American Thoracic Society in 1993 [67] and endorsed more recently by the American Medical Association [68]. Quality of life and general psychological questionnaires can be used to assess disability [69].

Can we prevent the disease and modify its outcome?

The implication of the cohort studies undertaken in the 1990s is that the incidence of OA could most effectively be diminished by reducing the level of exposure to its specific causes in the workplace. However, while the inference is clear, evidence for the effectiveness of interventions designed to reduce disease incidence can only be provided by well-designed evaluative studies. Studies evaluating the effectiveness of interventions to reduce exposure levels on disease incidence have now been reported for a number of the important causes of OA, including enzymes in the detergent industry, latex in healthcare workers, laboratory animal proteins in a pharmaceutical company and isocyanates in Ontario, Canada. Each of these studies has provided evidence of a reduction in disease incidence following the intervention. Two studies, one of isocyanate-exposed workers [70], the other of healthcare workers exposed to latex proteins [71], both from Ontario, are particularly instructive. In each case the environmental intervention (regulated reduction in isocyanate levels and substitution of non-powdered low-protein latex gloves for powdered high-protein gloves) was accompanied by occupational health measures designed to identify cases at an early stage. In both cases, the institution of occupational health surveillance initially increased the number of identified cases followed by a fall in the number of cases.

Several studies of the outcome of OA have reported a poor prognosis for OA, with the majority of cases having continuing symptoms and evidence of airway hyper-responsiveness 3–5 years after avoidance of exposure. The most consistent factor associated with a poor outcome has been the duration of symptomatic exposure, i.e. the longer a case of symptomatic OA remains exposed to its cause, the less likely recovery with avoidance of exposure becomes [35]. These findings emphasise the need for early recognition of sensitisation and disease and removal of workers from exposure.

Irritant-induced asthma and reactive airways disease syndrome

This condition, which is rarer than OA with its latency period, has received greater publicity as a result of inhalational accidents that affected the civil population in Bhopal [72] and firemen at the site of the World Trade Center [73]. This condition differs from OA, which has a latency period, in that cough is more frequent than wheeze, airway obstruction is less reversible [74] and the degree of bronchial responsiveness to methacholine does not reflect the severity of the clinical status.

Occupational rhinitis

Patients with asthma very often have upper airway symptoms, which has led recently to the proposal of the united airway concept. Better treatment of rhinitis improves asthma and vice versa. The existence of occupational rhinoconjunctivitis has been known for years but its investigation and impact have been neglected. Workers with OA often present rhinoconjunctivitis symptoms, especially in the case of sensitisation to high-molecular-weight agents. Occupational rhinoconjunctivitis is commoner than OA [75]. Objective means, such as rhinometry and nasal lavages, to confirm this condition are being developed [76].

Perspectives

Asthma in the workplace is a condition that has been recognised for centuries, although more so in the 20th century. Recognition of its importance as a public health problem and clinical entity can be dated to the outbreaks of allergy and asthma that occurred in various workplaces in the second part of the 20th. These outbreaks stimulated the application of methods for assessing frequency and risk factors, the development of safe and reproducible clinical and immunological criteria, and the recognition of the psychosocioeconomic impact.

We have to face several challenges in the forthcoming years:

- OA represents only a small proportion of asthma in the workplace, the rest being mostly asthma exacerbated by the workplace. Better characterisation and assessment of this condition is necessary to prevent and manage it.

- The immunological mechanisms of asthma caused by the majority of chemicals still remains puzzling, which is a surprise given the fantastic impulse of immunology in recent years. Immunologists have neglected this important field and this should be corrected.
- Refinement of methods to assess the frequency of the disease should be a priority because this represents the ideal means to know whether frequency and the nature of causal agents vary and whether control efforts are efficient.
- The effectiveness of a reduction in the level of aeroallergen concentration in reducing the incidence of sensitisation and asthma has been demonstrated in large workplaces. The challenge now is to determine the means to effect this more widely in locations, such as small bakeries and body repair shops, that are less amenable to effective intervention than large factories.
- OA should be more widely recognised as a valuable model of adult-onset asthma in particular in examining the complex relationship between genes and the environment.
- Considering the existence of various efficient diagnostic means, it is hard to believe that in developed countries these are seldom applied. General physicians do not routinely ask questions about occupations and readily prefer to mask inflammation by prescribing potent steroid inhalers. This results in delays in diagnosis and maintenance of exposure of the worker with the long-term negative consequences. We have to make general physicians aware of asthma in the workplace, identify accredited referral centres and promote early referrals.
- The medicolegal management of cases is inappropriate even in developed countries. Readaptation programs with retraining and psychosocial interventions should be preferred to allocation of a lump sum. Scales to assess impairment have been proposed but tools to evaluate disability have to be further validated and used.
- The characteristics that differentiate irritant-induced asthma from OA with its latency period should be further identified.
- Occupational rhinitis is frequently associated with OA but this condition, which is even commoner than OA, has not been studied to the same extent. A "united airways" approach should be explored.

References

1 Pepys J, Bernstein IL. Historical aspects of occupational asthma. In: *Asthma in the Workplace*, 3rd edn. Bernstein IL, Chan-Yeung M, Malo JL, Bernstein DI., eds. Taylor & Francis, New York 2006: 9–35

2 Fuchs S, Valade P. Étude clinique et expérimentale sur quelques cas d'intoxication par le Desmodur T (diisocyanate de toluylene 1-2-4 et 1-2-6). *Arch Mal Profess* 1951; 12: 191–196

3 Pepys J, Hutchcroft BJ. Bronchial provocation tests in etiologic diagnosis and analysis of asthma. *Am Rev Respir Dis* 1975; 112: 829–859

4 Das R, Blanc PD. Chlorine gas exposure and the lung: A review. *Toxicol Ind Health* 1993; 9: 439–455

5 Brooks SM, Weiss MA, Bernstein IL. Reactive airways dysfunction syndrome (RADS); Persistent asthma syndrome after high level irritant exposures. *Chest* 1985; 88: 376–384

6 Henneberger PK. Work-exacerbated asthma. *Curr Opin Allergy Clin Immunol* 2007; 7: 146–151

7 Cannon J, Cullinan P, Newman Taylor A. Consequences of occupational asthma. *BMJ* 1995; 311: 602–603

8 Vandenplas O, Toren K, Blanc P. Health and socioeconomic impact of work-related asthma. *Eur Respir J* 2003; 22: 689–697

9 Kongerud J, Boe J, Soyseth V, Naalsund A, Magnus P. Aluminium potroom asthma: The Norwegian experience. *Eur Respir J* 1994; 7: 165–172

10 Quirce S. Eosinophilic bronchitis in the workplace. *Curr Opin Allergy Clin Immunol* 2004; 4: 87–91

11 American Thoracic Society. Guidelines for assessing and managing asthma risk at work, school, and recreation. *Am J Respir Crit Care Med* 2004; 169: 873–881

12 Tarlo SM, Liss FGM. Evidence based guidelines for the prevention, identification and, management of occupational asthma. *Occup Environ Med* 2005; 62: 288–289

13 Newman Taylor AJ, Cullinan P, Burge PS, Nicholson P, Boyle C. BOHRF guidelines for occupational asthma. *Thorax* 2005; 60: 364–366

14 Bernton HS. On occupational sensitisation to the castor bean. *Am J Med Sci* 1923; 165: 196–202

15 Figley KD, Elrod RH. Endemic asthma due to castor bean dust. *JAMA* 1928; 90: 79–82

16 Spielman AD, Baldwin HS. Atopy to acacia (gum arabic). *JAMA* 1933; 101: 444–445

17 Gelfand HH. The allergenic properties of vegetable gums: A case of asthma due to tragacanth. *J Allergy* 1943; 14: 203–219

18 Kern RA. Asthma and allergic rhinitis due to sensitisation to phthalic anhydride. Report of a case. *J Allergy* 1939; 10: 164–165

19 Hunter D, Milton R, Perry KMA. Asthma caused by the complex salts of platinum. *Br J Ind Med* 1945; 2: 92–98

20 Colldahl H. A study of provocation test on patients with bronchial asthma. *Acta Allergol* 1952; 5: 133–142

21 Gelfand HH. Respiratory allergy due to chemical compounds encountered in the rubber, lacquer, shellac, and beauty culture industries. *J Allergy* 1963; 34: 374–381

22 Ishizaka K, Ishizaka T, Hornbrook MM. Physiochemical properties of reaginic antibody. IV. Presence of a unique immunoglobulin as a carrier of reaginic activity. *J Immunol* 1966; 97: 75–85

23 Johansson SGO. Raised levels of a new immunoglobulin class (IgND) in asthma. *Lancet* 1967; 951–953

24 Pepys J, Longbottom JL, Hargreave FE, Faux J. Allergic reactions of the lungs to enzymes of *Bacillus subtilis. Lancet* 1969; 1: 1811–1814

25 Hendrick DJ, Davies RJ, Pepys J. Bakers' asthma. *Clin Allergy* 1976; 6: 241–250

26 Taylor G, Davies GE, Altounyan REC, Brown H Morrow, Frankland AW, Smith J Morrison, Winch R. Allergic reactions to laboratory animals. *Nature* 1976; 260: 280

27 Zeiss CR, Patterson R, Pruzansky JJ, Miller MM, Rosenberg M, Levitz D. Trimellitic anhydride-induced airway syndromes: Clinical and immunologic studies. *J Allergy Clin Immunol* 1977; 60: 96–103

28 Newman Taylor AJ, Venables KM, Durham SR, Graneek BJ, Topping MD. Acid anhydrides and asthma. *Int Arch Allergy Appl Immunol* 1987; 82: 435–439

29 Alanko K, Keskinen H, Byorksten F, Ojanen S. Immediate-type hypersensitivity to reactive dyes. *Clin Allergy* 1978; 8: 25–31

30 Chan-Yeung M. Immunologic and nonimmunologic mechanisms in asthma due to western red cedar (*Thuja plicata*). *J Allergy Clin Immunol* 1982; 70: 32–37

31 Wisnewski A, Redlich CA, Mapp CE, Bernstein DI. Polyisocyanates and Their Prepolymers. In: *Asthma in the Workplace*, 3rd edn. Bernstein IL, Chan-Yeung M, Malo JL, Bernstein DI., eds. Taylor & Francis, New York 2006: 481–504

32 Jones MG, Floyd A, Nouri-Aria K T, Jacobson MR, Durham SR, Newman Taylor A. Is occupational asthma to diisocyanates a non-IgE-mediated disease? *J Allergy Clin Immunol* 2006; 117: 663–669

33 Newman-Taylor A. Non-malignant diseases. 6. Asthma. In: McDonald JC, ed. *Epidemiology of work related diseases.* BMJ Publishing Group, London 1995: 117–142

34 Karjalainen A, Kurppa K, Martikainen R, Karjalainen J, Klaukka T. Exploration of asthma risk by occupation-extended analysis of an incidence study of the Finnish population. *Scand J Work Environ Health* 2002; 28: 49–57

35 Bersntein Il, Keskinen H, Blanc PD, Chan-Yeung M, Malo JL. Medicolegal aspects, compensation aspects, and evaluation of impairment/disability. In: *Asthma in the Workplace*, 3rd edn. Bernstein IL, Chan-Yeung M, Malo JL, Bernstein DI, eds. Taylor & Francis, New York 2006: 319–351

36 Jajosky RA Romero, Harrison R, Reinisch F, Flattery J, Chan J, Tumpowsky C, Davis L, Reilly MJ, Rosenman KD, Kalinowski D, Stanbury M, Schill DP, Wood J. Surveillance of work-related asthma in selected U.S. states using surveillance guidelines for state health departments-California, Massachusetts, Michigan and New Jersey. *MMWR* 1999; 48, SS-3: 1–20

37 McDonald JC, Chen Y, Zekveld C, Cherry NM. Incidence by occupation and industry of acute work related respiratory diseases in the UK, 1992–2001. *Occup Environ Med* 2005; 62: 836–842

38 Nguyen B, Ghezzo H, Malo JL, Gautrin D. Time course of onset of sensitization to common and occupational inhalants in apprentices. *J Allergy Clin Immunol* 2003; 111: 807–812

39 Walusiak J, Hanke W, Gorski P, Palczynski C. Respiratory allergy in apprentice bakers: Do occupational allergies follow the allergic march? *Allergy* 2004; 59: 442–450

40 Kogevinas M, Zock JP, Jarvis D, Kromhout H, Lillienberg L, Plana E, Radon K, Torén K, Alliksoo A, Benke G et al. Exposure to substances in the workplace and new-onset asthma: An international prospective population-based study (ECRHS-II). *Lancet* 2007; 370: 336–341

41 Jeebhay MF, Quirce S. Occupational asthma in the developing and industrialised world: A review. *Int J Tuberc Lung Dis* 2007; 11: 122–133

42 Greenberg M, Milne JF, Watt A. A survey or workers exposed to dusts containing derivatives of *Bacillus subtilis*. *Br Med J* 1970; 2: 629–633

43 Chan-Yeung M, Vedal S, Kus J, Maclean L, Enarson D, Tse KS. Symptoms, pulmonary function, and bronchial hyperreactivity in Western Red Cedar workers compared with those in office workers. *Am Rev Respir Dis* 1984; 130: 1038–1041

44 Hollander A, Van Run P, Spithoven J, Heederik D, Doekes G. Exposure to laboratory animal workers to airborne rat and mouse urinary allergens. *Clin Exp Allergy* 1997; 27: 617–626

45 Houba R, Heederik DJJ, Doekes G, Run PEM van. Exposure-sensitization relationship for a-amylase allergens in the baking industry. *Am J Respir Crit Care Med* 1996; 154: 130–136

46 Barker RD, Tongeren MJA van, Harris JM, Gardiner K, Venables KM, Newman Taylor AJ. Risk factors for sensitisation and respiratory symptoms among workers exposed to acid anhydrides: A cohort study. *Occup Environ Med* 1998; 55: 684–691

47 Nieuwenhuijsen MJ, Heederik D, Doekes G, Venables KM, Newman-Taylor AJ. Exposure-response relations to alpha-amylase sensitisation in British bakeries and flour mills. *Occup Environ Med* 1999; 56: 197–201

48 Cullinan P, Cook A, Gordon S, Nieuwenhuijsen MJ, Tee RD, Venables KM, McDonald JC, Newman Taylor AJ. Allergen exposure, atopy and smoking as determinants of allergy to rats in a cohort of laboratory employees. *Eur Respir J* 1999; 13: 1139–1143

49 Cullinan P, Cook A, Nieuwenhuijsen MJ, Sandiford C, Tee RD, Venables KM, McDonald JC, Newman Taylor AJ. Allergen and dust exposure as determinants of work-related symptoms and sensitization in a cohort of flour-exposed workers; a case-control analysis. *Ann Occup Hyg* 2001; 45: 97–103

50 Gautrin D, Ghezzo H, Infante-Rivard C, Malo JL. Incidence and determinants of IgE-mediated sensitization in apprentices: A prospective study. *Am J Respir Crit Care Med* 2000; 162: 1222–1228

51 Gautrin D, Ghezzo H, Infante-Rivard C, Magnan M, L'Archevêque J, Suarthana E, Malo JL. Long-term outcomes in a prospective cohort of apprentices exposed to high-molecular-weight agents. *Am J Respir Crit Care Med* 2008; 177: 871–879

52 Flindt MLH. Pulmonary disease due to inhalation of derivatives of *Bacillus subtilis* containing proteolytic enzyme. *Lancet* 1969; 1: 1177–1181

53 Newhouse ML, Tagg B, Pocock SJ, McEwan AC. An epidemiological study of workers producing enzyme washing powders. *Lancet* 1970; 1: 689–693

54 Juniper CP, How MJ, Goodwin BFJ. *Bacillus subtilis* enzymes: A 7-year clinical, epidemiological and immunological study of an industrial allergen. *J Soc Occup Med* 1977; 27: 3–12
55 Cullinan P, Harris JM, Newman Taylor AJ, Hole AM, Jones M, Barnes F, Jolliffe G. An outbreak of asthma in a modern detergent factory. *Lancet* 2000; 356: 1899–1900
56 Newman-Taylor AJ, Yucesov B. Genetics and Occupational Asthma. In: *Asthma in the Workplace*, 3rd edn. Bernstein IL, Chan-Yeung M, Malo JL, Bernstein DI eds. Taylor & Francis, New York 2006: 87–108
57 Vandenplas O, Ghezzo H, Munoz X, Moscato G, Perfetti L, Lemière C, Labrecque M, L'Archevêque J, Malo JL. What are the questionnaire items most useful in identifying subjects with occupational asthma? *Eur Respir J* 2005; 26: 1056–1063
58 Pepys J. Inhalation challenge tests in asthma. *New Engl J Med* 1975; 293: 758–759
59 Burge PS, O'Brien IM, Harries MG. Peak flow rate records in the diagnosis of occupational asthma due to isocyanates. *Thorax* 1979; 34: 317–323
60 Turner-Warwick M. Another look at asthma. *Br J Dis Chest* 1977; 71: 73
61 National Institutes of Health National Heart, Lung and Blood Institute. *Global initiative for asthma (GINA). Global strategy for asthma management and prevention. NHLBI/SHO workshop report.* National Institutes of Health publication, no. 95–3659, 1995
62 Lemière C, Biagini RE, Zeiss CR. Immunological and inflammatory assessments. In: *Asthma in the Workplace*, 3rd edn. Bernstein IL, Chan-Yeung M, Malo JL, Bernstein DI eds. Taylor & Francis, New York 2006: 179–197
63 Vandenplas O, Cartier A, Malo JL. Occupational Challenge Tests. In: *Asthma in the Workplace*, 3rd edn. Bernstein IL, Chan-Yeung M, Malo JL, Bernstein DI. Taylor & Francis, New York 2006: 227–252
64 Chan-Yeung M. Fate of occupational asthma. A follow-up study of patients with occupational asthma due to western red cedar (*Thuja plicata*). *Am Rev Respir Dis* 1977; 116: 1023–1029
65 Malo JL, Ghezzo H. Recovery of methacholine responsiveness after end of exposure in occupational asthma. *Am J Respir Crit Care Med* 2004; 169: 1304–1307
66 Sumi Y, Foley S, Daigle S, L'archeveque J, Olivenstein R, Letuve S, Malo JL, Hamid Q. Structural changes and airway remodelling in occupational asthma at a mean interval of 14 years after cessation of exposure. *Clin Exp Allergy* 2007; 37: 1781–1787
67 American Thoracic Society. Guidelines for the evaluation of impairment/disability in patients with asthma. *Am Rev Respir Dis* 1993; 147: 1056–1061
68 American Medical Association. *Guides to the Evaluation of Permanent Impairment*, 5th edn. Cocchiarella L, Andersson GBJ, eds. Chicago, IL 2001
69 Yacoub MR, Lavoie K, Lacoste G, Daigle S, L'Archevêque J, Ghezzo H, Lemière C, Malo JL. Assessment of impairment/disability due to occupational asthma through a multidimensional approach. *Eur Respir J* 2007; 29: 889–896
70 Tarlo SM, Liss GM, Yeung KS. Changes in rates and severity of compensation claims for

asthma due to diisocyanates: A possible effect of medical surveillance measures. *Occup Environ Med* 2002; 59: 58–62

71 Saary MJ, Kanani A, Alghadeer H, Holness DL, Tarlo SM. Changes in rates of natural rubber latex sensitivity among dental school students and staff members after changes in latex gloves. *J Allergy Clin Immunol* 2002; 109: 131–135

72 Cullinan P, Acquilla S, Ramana Dhara V, on behalf of the International Medical Commission. Respiratory morbidity 10 years after the Union Carbide gas leak at Bhopal: A cross sectional survey. *Br Med J* 1997; 314: 338–343

73 Prezant DJ, Weiden M, Banauch GI, McGuinness G, Rom WN, Aldrich TK, Kelly KJ. Cough and bronchial responsiveness in firefighters at the World Trade Center site. *N Engl J Med* 2002; 347: 806–815

74 Gautrin D, Bernstein IL, Brooks SM, Henneberger PK. Reactive airways dysfunction syndrome and irritant-induced asthma. In: *Asthma in the Workplace*, 3rd edn. Bernstein IL, Chan-Yeung M, Malo JL, Bernstein DI eds. Taylor & Francis, New York 2006: 579–627

75 Siracusa A, Desrosiers M, Marabini A. Epidemiology of occupational rhinitis: Prevalence, aetiology and determinants. *Clin Exp Allergy* 2000; 30: 1519–1534

76 Gautrin D, Desrosiers M, Castano R. Occupational rhinitis. *Curr Opin Allergy Clin Immunol* 2006; 6: 677–684

Epidemiology and risk factors of occupational respiratory asthma and occupational sensitization

Dick Heederik[1] *and Torben Sigsgaard*[2]

[1]Division of Environmental Epidemiology, Institute for Risk Assessment Sciences, Utrecht University, The Netherlands
[2]Department Environmental and Occupational Medicine, School of Public Health, Aarhus University, Aarhus, Denmark

Abstract

Information on the occurrence of occupational asthma comes from different sources; disease registries, general population studies and workforce-based studies. Each source has its strengths and weaknesses. For multi-causal diseases such as asthma, reliable information from well-designed epidemiological studies is to be preferred. However, a complication is that occupational asthma is not directly measured (diagnosed) in general population studies and an attributable risk is usually calculated on the basis of crude information about exposure. The exposure information is usually derived from questionnaire responses to questions on exposure to gases, fumes or dusts, or is based on so-called 'job exposure matrices'. Disease registry data, from occupational disease registries, allows direct estimation of the occurrence of occupational asthma. However, the information is often incomplete or difficult to interpret because of diagnostic criteria which vary and can also be dependent on compensation and insurance criteria, more related to severity of disease rather than to occurrence of disease. As a result, registries may give only crude estimates of the occurrence of disease, but at the same time allow evaluation of trends over time. Workforce-based studies have given most information about determinants of work-related asthma and allergy. An important determinant of asthma and allergy is the exposure intensity and for high-molecular-weight sensitizers atopy clearly modifies the risk. It is expected that improved phenotypical characterization of occupational asthma together with genotyping and detailed exposure assessment will give more insight in the occurrence and determinants of disease and prognosis.

General introduction

In Western countries there has been a clear shift observable over the last few decades from pneumoconiosis and cancer due to mineral dust exposures (asbestos and silica) to work-related obstructive diseases such as occupational asthma (OA) and chronic obstructive pulmonary disease (COPD) [1]. In most Western countries, OA is now the most frequently occurring occupational disease. Information about the occurrence of occupational respiratory diseases and their contribution to morbidity and mortality in the general population comes from different sources of varying quality.

Occupational Asthma, edited by Torben Sigsgaard and Dick Heederik

Data from these different sources are not always easily comparable since the quality of the information, and the aims for which they were gathered, differ. Nevertheless, an attempt is made in this chapter to give insight into the associations between occupational exposures to occurrence of OA. Information on determinants of OA mainly comes from workforce-based studies, and these determinants are also briefly discussed.

Occupational asthma in an epidemiological context

OA is usually defined as a disease characterized by variable airway airflow limitation and/or airway hyperresponsiveness due to causes and conditions attributable to a particular workplace environment and not to stimuli encountered outside the workplace [2]. Usually, OA with and without a latency period is distinguished. Asthma with a latency period includes all forms of asthma for which an immunological mechanism has been identified. In most cases an IgE-mediated allergy is the underlying mechanism. Causes of immunological asthma are low- and high-molecular-weight sensitizers of which more than 250 have been identified. High-molecular-weight sensitizers are usually large proteins of more than 5 kDa such as enzymes like fungal α-amylase derived from *Aspergillus oryzae*, or more heterogeneous natural substances such as latex and cereals like wheat. Most high-molecular-weight sensitizers induce the development of specific IgE antibodies. The reaction between antibody and allergen leads to an allergic inflammatory response in the airways. Few population studies exist that focus on the changes shortly after sensitization, but a small longitudinal study in laboratory animal workers suggests that bronchial hyperresponsiveness and symptoms develop soon after sensitization, and accelerated decline in lung function becomes measurable [3].

For many other substances the mechanism by which inflammation develops is often at least partially unknown. Specific antibodies against isocyanates for instance have been found in a minority of the sensitized workers, but the role of these antibodies is not completely clear, and the mechanism does not seems to be IgE mediated in all isocyanate-sensitized workers [4, 5]. Irritants induce asthma by non-immunological mechanisms and no latency period is observed in most cases. An example of OA without a latency period is the reactive airways dysfunction syndrome (RADS), which develops after exceptionally high concentrations of an irritant agent. Small work shift changes in lung function, without persistent bronchial hyperresponsiveness and eosinophilia are usually not referred to as OA, but as OA-like disorders. A typical example of an asthma-like disorder is Monday morning airway obstruction associated with endotoxin exposure in agricultural workers [6], although some nowadays may refer to this as non-allergic asthma [7, 8].

There is no consensus on the best way to identify OA in epidemiological studies. A provocation test with the suspected causal agent is generally accepted as the gold standard, but this approach cannot be applied in large scale surveys of industry-based studies or the general population. Questionnaires form an important survey tool and many have modified these questionnaires for their own purposes by adding questions on work relatedness of symptoms [9]. Other relevant tests that can be applied in surveys are bronchial hyperresponsiveness testing, spirometry, serology and skin prick testing for evaluation of sensitization in case of immunological asthma. Records of peak expiratory flow (PEF) measurements over longer periods have been commonly used for establishing a clinical diagnosis. Unfortunately, few examples can be found of application in epidemiological studies, and the response rate for repeated PEF testing in population surveys is usually low [10].

Incidence data from monitoring systems

Considerable attention has been given to disease monitoring systems for asthma across the world since the mid-1990s when it became apparent that OA had replaced the pneumoconiosis as the leading occupational disease. A major source of information included disease registries for compensation purposes, since these also give an impression of the burden on society of OA. Point estimates from occupational disease registries indicated an incidence between 2 and 15 cases per 100 000 (Tab. 1). Differences are, among other factors, associated with differences in industrial structure between countries, differences in definition of work-related (and compensable) asthma, differences in case finding methods, and changes over time in asthma incidence. Through the voluntary Surveillance of Work Related and

Table 1. Reported occupational asthma incidence by different asthma monitoring programs and some occupational disease registries.

Reference	Country	Incidence/100 000	Range
[11, 13, 15, 17]	UK	2.0-4.3	1–183 [17]
[12]	USA	2.9	0–17
[14]	Finland	3.6	5–30
[16]	Germany	4.2	
[18]	Canada (Quebec)	6.3	
[19]	Sweden	8.1-19.1	1–77
[20, 21, 23–25]	Finland	8.1	
[22]	Canada (Br. Columbia)	9.2	
[26]	USA		5.8–20.4*

*Estimates based on capture-recapture method

Ocupational Respiratory Disease (SWORD) reporting system in the UK, occupational physicians, lung specialists and allergists voluntarily reported 3000–4500 cases of respiratory diseases. More than a quarter of the cases involved OA, which makes OA the most reported work-related respiratory disease. Diisocyanates, which are low-molecular-weight sensitizers, and high-molecular-weight allergens from animals, flour and grain appear the most important sensitizers. In Germany, only 1500 of the 5600 suspected cases could be confirmed as OA [16]. Of these, another 400 were rejected because they were not in accordance with additional clinical or non-medical criteria. In a study from the USA, OA cases reported through different disease registries in one state were evaluated using the capture-recapture method, a statistical technique that used the overlap between sources of information to obtain an estimate of the 'true' rate [26]. Reports from physicians, hospital discharge records and worker compensation claims were used, and the incidence of new onset OA was estimated between 5.8 and 20.4 cases/100 000 individuals per year, clearly higher than the directly observed incidence of 2.7 cases/100 000 individuals per year, but in range with the data from registries in other countries. Some disease registries have been able to show strong changing trends in numbers of reported cases reported, like for latex-associated respiratory allergy in Germany [27]. A strong drop in cases was associated with a targeted reduction of exposure to powdered high-protein latex gloves. Similarly, in Ontario, Canada, a program to reduce exposure to diisocyanates and to introduce medical surveillance was associated with earlier diagnosis and fewer cases in a compensation population [28].

Occurrence in general population studies

General population studies were more often explored as a means to estimate the population attributable risk for both asthma and COPD since the late-1970s and mid-1980s [29–46]. This design became popular because it was believed that general population studies were less sensitive to the healthy worker effect. A general population sample was considered superior compared to a workforce-based population sample from which workers who had developed disease had already left. General population studies allowed evaluation of associations between job title and asthma not only for the present but also for previous jobs [47]. This made a more direct evaluation of the healthy worker effect possible. In addition, introduction of so-called 'Job Exposure Matrices' – expert systems that cross-link job titles with specific occupational exposures in a qualitative or semi-quantitative way – made characterization of exposure possible in these studies. A strength of these general population studies is that exposures have been identified that were outside the classical basic high-risk industries. An example is the identification of cleaning agents as a cause of OA [48].

The early general population studies made use of self-reported exposure and some may have been affected to some extent by misclassification of exposure in the form of recall bias. Most studies were cross-sectional and used prevalence data. The studies included information on respiratory symptoms associated with asthma, lung function or bronchial hyperresponsiveness testing, and allowed calculation of the risk for developing asthma for individuals with a certain exposure. This allowed the calculation of the contribution of occupational exposures to the prevalence of asthma, the etiological fraction. Most studies estimate contributions as being between a few percent and 20%.

An important example is the large prospective one among 6837 participants from 13 countries who previously took part in the European Community Respiratory Health Survey (1990–1995) [49]. The individuals included did not report respiratory symptoms or a history of asthma at baseline. Asthma was assessed by methacholine challenge test and by questionnaire-registered asthma symptoms. Exposures were defined by high-risk occupations, an asthma-specific job exposure matrix with additional expert judgment, and through self-report of acute inhalation events. A significant excess asthma risk was seen after exposure to substances known to cause OA [relative risk (RR), 1.6; 95% CI 1.1–2.3]. Risks were highest for asthma defined by bronchial hyperreactivity in addition to symptoms (RR, 2.4; 95% CI 1.3–4.6). Asthma risk was increased in participants who reported an acute symptomatic inhalation event (fire, mixing cleaning products, chemical spill) (RR, 3.3; 95% CI 1.0–11.1). The population-attributable risk for adult asthma due to occupational exposures ranged from 10% to 25%. This is equivalent to an incidence of new-onset OA of 250–300 cases per million people per year. Although this study is among the larger general population studies, it shows some specific limitations of general population studies. Risk estimates for specific occupational groups are sometimes based on small sample sizes, leading to instability in the risk estimates for specific occupational titles or exposures. Intermediary endpoints such as specific work-related sensitization have up to now not been included in general population studies and this makes it difficult to link results to workforce-based studies. A future challenge for all general population study is adequate exposure assessment. People move more frequently from job to job and the exposure is more diffusely spread through the population in modern service economies without large basic industries. This makes characterization of the exposure on the basis of job title information more challenging and probably more detailed techniques will be required.

Occurrence of occupational asthma in workforce-based studies

Important information also comes from studies in specific workforces. For instance studies in bakers suggest sensitization rates of 5–25% for several work-related allergens [50], which is in most cases accompanied by symptoms. Similar figures are available for workers exposure to a range of high- and low-molecular-weight allergens. Typically, workforce-based studies have a cross-sectional or cohort design and include between 100 and 1000 workers. Given the incidence of OA, these studies are usually too small to directly study the occurrence of clinically relevant OA. Therefore, asthma is defined on the basis of questionnaire responses and intermediate effects such as sensitization or hyperresponsiveness are considered as endpoints in the analysis.

The discrepancies in the magnitude of the hazard estimated by different information sources (general population studies, disease registries, and studies in specific occupational groups) is most likely due to differences in (the definition of) endpoints considered, the diagnosis, and severity of what is considered OA, and selection out of the workforce. Most evidence on determinants and modifiers of risk for OA comes from workforce-based studies. Modern workforce-based studies often involve a quantitative exposure assessment component. Phenotypical evaluation of the workers is often more detailed and specifically chosen for the type of asthma resulting from the exposure than in general population studies. The information that is generated by this type of study contributes to risk assessment and prevention.

Exposure

Allergen exposure level is a clear determinant of risk of occupational allergy and asthma. Exposure-response relationships have been shown for both high- and low-molecular-weight sensitizers. Some recent studies in specific occupational groups illustrated the existence of exposure sensitization relationships for some high-molecular-weight sensitizers. In particular, a series of European studies in bakers and laboratory animal workers shed new light on some aspects of the development of occupational allergic asthma and rhinitis due to exposure to high-molecular-weight sensitizers. A more complete overview can be found elsewhere [51–56]. A small retrospective cohort study among laboratory animal workers, who underwent a pre-employment medical examination, indicated that the time until development of symptoms was dependent on both exposure intensity and atopy [57]. The risk for developing sensitization and allergy is measurable directly after start of exposure and remains high with ongoing exposure. A follow-up study showed that the 12-year incidence rates of symptoms among workers from laboratories exposed to rodents were 2.26 (95% CI 1.61–2.91) and 1.32 (95% CI 0.76–1.87) per 100 person-years, respectively. Higher relative risks were seen with increasing hours of exposure to tasks that involved working with animal cages or with many animals at one time. The most common symptoms were related to rhinitis rather than to asthma. Incidence might be reduced by limiting exposure through reducing the number of hours per week of exposure to laboratory animals [58, 59].

Atopy

Atopy is usually defined as either specific IgE against a series of common allergens or a positive skin prick test response to the same panel of allergens. Usually, tree pollen, grass pollen, house dust mite, cat and dog allergens are considered common allergens in occupational studies. Atopy is a strong risk modifier for high-molecular-weight sensitization. This is most clearly illustrated by a large pooled European study in 650 Laboratory Animal Workers [56]. Atopic workers were at higher risk for having work-related sensitization compared to non-atopic workers. The atopic workers already had a clearly increased risk at the lowest exposure levels and there was no evidence of an exposure threshold. For non-atopic workers a steadily increasing exposure-response relationship was found. Atopy is the most important risk modifier of work-related sensitization high-molecular-weight sensitizers. There is no clear evidence that atopy is a modifier of the risk for work-related sensitization and asthma in case of low-molecular-weight sensitizers.

Atopy was until recently seen as an individual susceptibility factor with presumably a genetic background. However, atopy has no perfect penetration and cannot only be interpreted as a factor solely determined by individual susceptibility. It seems also associated with environmental factors. There is increasing evidence that farm exposures throughout life are protective against atopy, allergic rhinitis, and atopic asthma [60]. Several studies have observed a strongly decreased prevalence of allergic sensitization [61–63], hay fever [64, 65], and asthma [8] among adults with childhood and current farm exposures. According to the hygiene hypothesis, bacterial and viral infections, and environmental exposures to microbial compounds may protect from the development of allergic disease by influencing immune responses. Farmers, and children growing up on farms, are exposed to high levels of microbial pathogens causing zoonoses, and proinflammatory agents such as bacterial endotoxin and fungal $\beta(1\rightarrow3)$-glucans. It has been hypothesized that exposure to such agents may induce a shift from atopic Th2 responses to Th1 responses through stimulation of the innate immune system and regulatory T cells [66]. Protective effects of house dust endotoxin on the development of atopy and asthma have been shown in children [67–69], and more recently, studies among adults have shown similar inverse relationships between endotoxin exposure and atopic asthma [8], allergic sensitization [65, 70, 71], and hay fever [64]. Thus, the more recent studies among occupationally exposed populations have shown that, in accordance with the hygiene hypothesis, effects of early exposures can be long-lasting. However, some of these studies also suggest that immune deviation from Th2 to Th1 responses may take place throughout life, and exposure in adulthood to endotoxin and other microbial compounds seem been associated with a lower prevalence of allergy or allergic asthma. Most evidence is still based on cross-sectional studies, and longitudinal studies are needed to observe reversal of atopic status under the influence of high microbial exposures directly.

Since endotoxin and other microbial agents are potent proinflammatory agents, the downside of increased exposure can be an elevated risk of non-allergic or non-atopic asthma [72–74]. Only a few studies have explicitly reported the Janus-faced nature of endotoxin – a protective effect on atopic disease, paralleled by an increased risk of non-atopic asthma and non-specific airway hyperresponsiveness – in the same population sample. There also appears to be a clear difference in susceptibility for endotoxin exposure, measurable at the population level [75] (Fig. 1).

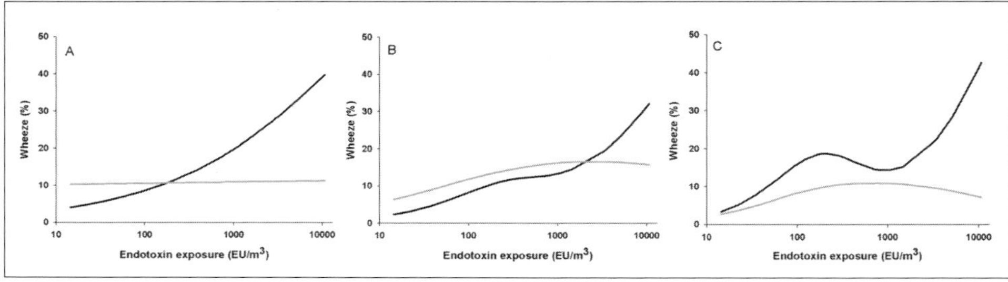

Figure 1.
Different exposure-response relationships for endotoxin exposure and wheeze for low and high responders in a whole blood stimulation assay. Low (gray line) and high (black line) responders defined on their tumor necrosis factor-α (A), interleukin-1β (B), and interleukin-10 responses (C). Exposure expressed in endotoxin units (EU) (with permission from [75]).

Smoking

One study identified smoking of cigarettes as a risk factor of work-related sensitization for high-molecular-weight sensitizers [76]. Smokers seemed at higher risk to have work-related sensitization in especially one of the three subsamples than non-smokers in this cross-sectional study. However, this finding has not been reproduced in many larger and better controlled studies [55, 56, 77]. Most evidence available at present for high-molecular-weight sensitizers indicates that smoking is not an effect modifier for the association between allergen exposure, sensitization and allergic asthma. Interesting results have recently been published for other sensitizing agents such as platinum salts. For low-molecular-weight sensitizers, such as platinum salts, smoking is an effect modifier [78–80]. The incidence of platinum salt sensitization depended on the solubility of the platinum salt, after correction for smoking habits at median levels below 0.5 $\mu g/m^3$ [79].

Genetic markers

Studies on the role of genetic markers have traditionally been conducted on relatively small samples of OA cases or within industrial cohorts, especially considering workers with exposure to specific agents such as isocyanates and red cedar wood dust. The genes associated so far with OA are HLA class II genes, genes involved in antioxidant protection, α-1-antitrypsin, and genes regulating the native immune pathways (see for review [81]). Few interactions have been demonstrated as yet but large-scale genetic studies of asthma that are now underway will likely change the situation. A first genome-wide association study (GWAS) including large working populations will be published soon, but yielded little important information on top of GWAS studies among adult asthmatics not specifically focused on occupational exposures. It is expected that a new generation of studies based on specific hypotheses (candidate interactions) in combination with improved phenotypical and environmental characterization will create more useful evidence on gene environment interactions. There is awareness about the potential use of genetic information in, for instance, pre-employment testing and asthma surveillance [82]. However, the associations between genetic markers and asthma or sensitization are based on cross-sectional analyses and usually relatively weak. Prediction of future occurrence of disease is practically not possible at the moment and present information indicates that predictions will be imprecise. A study among laboratory animal workers for instance showed that HLA-DR7 was associated with sensitization [odds ratio (OR), 1.82; CI, 1.12–2.97], respiratory symptoms at work (OR, 2.96; CI, 1.64–5.37) and, most strongly, sensitization with symptoms (OR, 3.81; CI, 1.90–7.65) [83]. HLA-DR3 was protective against sensitization (OR, 0.55; CI, 0.31–0.97). Atopy defined phenotypically, on the basis of an immunological evaluation, was more strongly associated with work-related sensitization than any of the phenotypical markers.

Prognosis

A limited number of epidemiological studies focused on the prognosis of OA [84–88]. The available studies suggest that symptoms can still be present up to 12 years after exposure cessation [84, 85]. One study describes results from an interview 6 years after diagnosis of a group of 79 individuals with OA [86]. Most had the impression that symptoms had improved, although 72% still used medication and 33% were still unemployed. Others found indications that symptoms can still worsen after exposure is terminated [24, 89]. Some have argued that exposure reduction is associated with a poorer prognosis than complete removal from exposure [90]. However, the studies underlying this statement involved a limited number of asthma cases and were poorly controlled in terms of the exposure [91, 92]. The changes in exposure were only monitored qualitatively, and it is not known if any exposure reduction occurred objectively or that the exposure reduction was sufficiently large to have any effect.

Prevention

Information on exposure-response relationships can be used for risk assessments and will be the input of standard setting procedures in different countries. For instance, the American Conference of Governmental Industrial Hygienists and the Dutch Health Council are among the first to use data on exposure-response relationships for bio-aerosols, such as wheat allergens, to propose a standard for wheat dust levels in the air [93, 94]. It is expected that similar standards will be developed for some other high-molecular-weight sensitizers because the principles for risk assessment for sensitizing agents have recently been described [95]. Standards do exist for several low-molecular-weight sensitizers, such as toluene diisocyanate (TDI) and platinum salts, but it not the rule that these standards take into account the risk for sensitization. In addition, some of these standards were derived several decades ago, and it is not always certain what the scientific basis was for these standards and if they truly protect the workers.

Future developments

Over the last few years, new technologies have become available to measure inflammatory markers in nasal and bronchial lavage samples. Less invasive technologies are expected to become available such as exhaled nitric oxide (eNO) and measurements based on exhaled breath condensate samples or exhaled air. These developments will give more insight into the heterogeneity in phenotypes and will improve phenotyping in epidemiological studies. Some examples of this development do already exist, but usually refer to patient data and seldom come from open population studies.

References

1 Sigsgaard T, Nowak D, Annesi-Maesano I, Nemery B, Torén K, Viegi G, Radon K, Burge S, Heederik D and the European Respiratory Societies "Environmental and Occupational Health Group" (2010) ERS Position paper on: Work related respiratory diseases in EU. *European Respiratory Journal, in press*

2 Bernstein IL, Chan-Yeung M, Malo J-L, Bernstein DI (1993) Definition and Classifica-

tion of Asthma. In: Bernstein IL, Chan-Yeung M, Malo J-L, Bernstein DI (eds), *Asthma in the Workplace*, 1st edn. Marcel Dekker, New York

3 Renström A, Malmberg P, Larsson K, Larsson PH, Sundblad BM (1995) Allergic sensitization is associated with increased bronchial responsiveness: A prospective study of allergy to laboratory animals. *Eur Respir J* 8: 1514–1519

4 Bernstein, JA (1996) Overview of diisocyanate occupational asthma. *Toxicology* 111: 181–189

5 Liu Q, Wisnewski AV (2003) Recent developments in diisocyanate asthma. *Ann Allergy Asthma Immunol* 90: 35–41

6 Schenker MB, Christiani D, Dimich-Ward H, Doekes G, Dosman J, Douwes J, Dowling K, Enarson D, Green F, Heederik D et al (1998) Respiratory health in agriculture. *Am J Respir Crit Care Med* 158: s1–s76

7 Dalphin JC (2007) In the agricultural environment there is asthma and asthma... or the paradox of agricultural asthma. *Rev Mal Respir* 24: 1083–1086

8 Eduard W, Douwes J, Omenaas E, Heederik D (2004) Do farming exposures cause or prevent asthma? Results from a study of adult Norwegian farmers. *Thorax* 59: 381–386

9 Rylander RR, Peterson Y, Donham KJ (1990) Questionnaire evaluating organic dust exposure. *Am J Ind Med* 17: 121–126

10 Hollander A, Heederik D, Brunekreef B (1998) Work related changes in peak expiratory flow among laboratory animal workers. *Eur Respir J* 11: 929–936

11 Meredith, S (1993) Reported incidence of occupational asthma in the United Kingdom, 1989–90. *J Epidemiol Community Health* 47: 459–463

12 Rosenman KD, Reilly MJ, Kalinowski DJ (1997) A State-Based Surveillance System for Work-Related Asthma. *J Occup Environ Med* 39: 415–425

13 Gannon PFG, Burge PS (1991) A preliminary report of a surveillance scheme of occupational asthma in the West Midlands. *Br J Ind Med* 48: 579–582

14 Keskinen H, Alanko K, Saarinen L (1978) Occupational asthma in Finland. *Clin Allergy* 8: 569–579

15 Meredith S, Nordman H (1996)) Occupational asthma: Measures of frequency from four countries. *Thorax* 51: 435–440

16 Baur X, Degens P, Weber K (1998) Occupational obstructive airway diseases in Germany. *Am J Ind Med* 33: 454–462

17 Gannon PFG, Burge PS (1993) The SHIELD scheme in the West Midlands Region, United Kingdom. *Br J Ind Med* 50: 791–796

18 Provencher S, Labrèche FP, De Guire L (1997) Physician based surveillance system for occupational respiratory diseases: The experience of PROPULSE, Québec, Canada. *Occup Environ Med* 54: 272–276

19 Torén K (1996) Self reported rate of occupational asthma in Sweden 1990–2. *Occup Environ Med* 53: 757–761

20 Vaaranen V, Vasama M, Alho J (1985) *Occupational diseases in Finland in 1984*. Institute of Occupational Health, Helsinki

21 Vaaranen, V (1995) *Occupational diseases in Finland in 1994*. Institute of Occupational Health, Helsinki

22 Contreras GR, Rousseau R, Chan-Yeung M (1994) Occupational respiratory diseases in British Columbia, Canada in 1991. *Occup Environ Med* 51: 710–712

23 Kanerva L, Jolanki R, Toikkanen J (1994) Frequencies of occupational allergic diseases and gender differences in Finland. *Int Arch Occup Environ Health* 66: 111–116

24 Nordman H (1994) Occupational asthma – time for prevention. *Scand J Work Environ Health* 20: 108–115

25 Reijula K, Haahtela T, Klaukka T, Rantanen J (1996) Incidence of occupational asthma and persistent asthma in young adults has increased in Finland. *Chest* 110: 58–61

26 Henneberger PK, Kreiss K, Rosenman KD, Reilly MJ, Chang Y-F, Geidenberger CA (1999) An evaluation of the incidence of work-related asthma in the United States. *Int J Occup Environ Health* 5: 1–8

27 Latza U, Haamann F, Baur X (2005) Effectiveness of a nationwide interdisciplinary preventive programme for latex allergy. *Int Arch Occup Environ Health* 78: 394–402

28 Tarlo SM (2007) Prevention of occupational asthma in Ontario. *Can J Physiol Pharmacol* 85: 167–172

29 Fishwick D, Pearce N, D'Souza W, Lewis S, Town I, Armstrong R, Kogevinas M, Crane J (1997) Occupational asthma in New Zealanders: A population based study. *Occup Environ Med* 54: 301–306

30 Fishwick D, Bradshaw LM, D'Souza W, Town I, Armstrong R, Pearce N, Crane J (1997) Chronic bronchitis, shortness of breath, and airway obstruction by occupation in New Zealand. *Am J Respir Crit Care Med* 156: 1440–1446

31 Heederik D, Pouwels H, Kromhout H, Kromhout D (1989) Chronic non-specific lung disease and occupational exposures estimated by means of a job exposure matrix: The Zutphen study. *Int J Epidemiol* 18: 382–388

32 Heederik D, Kromhout H, Kromhout D, Burema J, Biersteker K (1992) Relations between occupation, smoking, lung function, and incidence and mortality of chronic non-specific lung disease: The Zutphen Study. *Br J Ind Med* 49: 299–308

33 Kauffmann F, Drouet D, Lellouch J, Brille D (1982) Occupational exposure and 12-year spirometric changes among Paris area workers. *Br J Ind Med* 39: 221–232

34 Kivity S, Shochat Z, Bressler R, Wiener M, Lerman Y (1985) The characteristics of bronchial asthma among a young adult population. *Chest* 108: 24–27

35 Korn RJ, Dockery DW, Speizer FE, Ware JW, Ferris BG (1987) Occupational exposures and chronic respiratory symptoms – A population based study. *Am Rev Respir Dis* 136: 296–304

36 Kogevinas M, Anto JM, Soriano JB, Tobias A, Burney P (1996) The risk of asthma attributable to occupational exposures. A population-based study in Spain. Spanish Group of the European Asthma Study. *Am J Respir Crit Care Med* 154: 137–143

37 Kogevinas M, Anto JM, Sunyer J, Tobias A, Kromhout H, Burney P (1999) Occupational asthma in Europe and other industrialised areas: A population-based study. European Community Respiratory Health Survey Study Group. *Lancet* 353: 1750–1754

38 Krzyzanowski M, Kauffmann F (1988) The relation of respiratory symptoms and ventilatory function to moderate occupational exposure in a general population. Results from the French PAARC study among 16000 adults. *Int J Epidemiol* 17: 397–406

39 Krzyzanowski M, Jedrychowski W, Wysocki M (1986) Factors associated with the change in ventilatory function and the development of chronic obstructive pulmonary disease in a 13-year follow-up of the Cracow study. *Am Rev Respir Dis* 134: 1011–1019

40 Krzyzanowski M, Jedrychowski W, Wysocki M (1988) Occupational exposures and changes in pulmonary function over 13 years among residents of Cracow. *Br J Ind Med* 45: 747–754

41 McWorther, WP, Polis, MA, Kaslow, RA (1989) Occurrence, predictors, and consequences of adult asthma in NHANES I and follow-up survey. *Am Rev Respir Dis* 139: 721–724

42 Milton DK, Solomon GM, Rosiello RA, Herrick RF (1998) Risk and incidence of asthma attributable to occupational exposure among HMO members. *Am J Ind Med* 33: 1–10

43 Ng TP, Hong CY, Goh LG, Wong ML, Chung Koh KT, Ling SL (1994) Risks of asthma associated with occupations in a community based case control study. *Am J Ind Med* 25: 709–718

44 Sunyer J, Kogevinas M, Kromhout H, Anto J, Roca J, Tobias A, Vermeulen R, Payo F, Maldonado JA, Martinez-Moratalla J, Muniozguren N et al (1998) Pulmonary ventilation defects and occupational exposures in a population-based study in Spain. *Am J Respir Crit Care Med* 157: 512–517

45 Viegi G, Prediletto R, Paoletti P, Carrozzi L, Di Pede F, Vellutini M, Di Pede C, Giuntini C, Lebowitz MD (1991) Respiratory effects of occupational exposure in a general population sample in north Italy. *Am Rev Respir Dis* 143: 510–515

46 Yunginger J-W, Reed, CE, O'Connel EJ, Melton LJ 3rd, O'Fallon WM, Silverstein, MD (1992) A community-based study of the epidemiology of asthma. Incidence rates, 1964–1983. *Am Rev Respir Dis* 146: 888–894

47 Post WK, Heederik D, Kromhout H, Kromhout D (1994) Occupational exposures estimated by a population specific job exposure matrix and 25 year incidence rate of chronic nonspecific lung disease (CNSLD): The Zutphen Study. *Eur Respir J* 7: 1048–1055

48 Zock JP, Kogevinas M, Sunyer J, Jarvis D, Torén K, Antó JM (2002) European Community Respiratory Health Survey. Asthma characteristics in cleaning workers, workers in other risk jobs and office workers. *Eur Respir J* 20: 679–685

49 Kogevinas M, Zock JP, Jarvis D, Kromhout H, Lillienberg L, Plana E, Radon K, Torén K, Alliksoo A, Benke G et al (2007) Exposure to substances in the workplace and new-onset asthma: An international prospective population-based study (ECRHS-II). *Lancet* 370: 336–341

50 Houba R, Doekes G, Heederik D (1998) Occupational respiratory allergy in bakery workers: A review of the literature. *Am J Ind Med* 34: 529–546

51 Houba R, D Heederik, G Doekes (1998) Wheat sensitization and work related symp-

toms in the baking industry are preventable: An epidemiological study. *Am J Respir Crit Care Med* 158: 1499–1503

52 Cullinan P, Lowson D, Nieuwenhuijsen MJ, Gordon S, Tee RD, Venables KM, McDonald JC, Newman-Taylor AJ (1994) Work related symptoms, sensitisation, and estimated exposure in workers not previously exposed to laboratory rats. *Occup Environ Med* 51: 589–592

53 Cullinan P, Lowson D, Nieuwenhuijsen MJ, Sandiford C, Tee RD, Venables KM, McDonald JC, Newman Taylor AJ (1994) Work related symptoms, sensitisation, and estimated exposure in workers not previously exposed to flour. *Occup Environ Med* 51: 579–583

54 Houba R, D Heederik, G Doekes, P van Run (1996) Exposure-sensitization relationship for α-amylase allergens in the baking industry. *Am J Respir Crit Care Med* 154: 130–136

55 Hollander A, Heederik D, Doekes G (1997) Respiratory allergy to rats: Exposure-response relationships in laboratory animal workers. *Am J Respir Crit Care Med* 155: 562–567

56 Heederik D, Venables K, Malmberg P, Hollander A, Karlsson A-S, Renström A, Doekes G, Nieuwenhuijsen M (1999) Exposure-response relationships for occupational respiratory sensitizers: Results from an European study in laboratory animal workers. *J Allergy Clin Immunol* 103: 678–684

57 Kruize H, Post W, Heederik D, Martens B, Hollander A, van der Beek E (1997) Respiratory allergy in laboratory animal workers: A retrospective cohort study using pre-employment screening data. *Occup Environ Med* 11: 830–835

58 Elliott L, Heederik D, Marshall S, Peden D, Loomis D (2005) Incidence of allergy and allergy symptoms among workers exposed to laboratory animals. *Occup Environ Med* 62: 766–771

59 Elliott L, Heederik D, Marshall S, Peden D, Loomis D (2005) Progression of self-reported symptoms in laboratory animal allergy. *J Allergy Clin Immunol* 116: 127–132

60 Heederik D, Sigsgaard T (2005) Respiratory allergy in agricultural workers: Recent developments. *Curr Opin Allergy Clin Immunol* 5: 129–134

61 Koskela HO, Happonen KK, Remes ST, Pekkanen J (2005) Effect of farming environment on sensitisation to allergens continues after childhood. *Occup Environ Med* 62: 607–611

62 Portengen L, Sigsgaard T, Omland O, Hjort C, Heederik D, Doekes G (2002) Low prevalence of atopy in young Danish farmers and farming students born and raised on a farm. *Clin Exp Allergy* 32: 247–253

63 Radon K, Schulze A, Nowak D (2006) Inverse association between farm animal contact and respiratory allergies in adulthood: Protection, underreporting or selection? *Allergy* 61: 443–446

64 Smit LAM, Zuurbier M, Doekes G, Wouters IM, Heederik D, Douwes J (2007) Hay fever and asthma symptoms in conventional and organic farmers in the Netherlands. *Occup Environ Med* 64: 101–107

65 Smit LAM, Heederik D, Doekes G, Lammers JWJ, Wouters IM (2009) Occupational endotoxin exposure reduces the risk of atopy in adults without a farm childhood. *Int Arch Allergy Immunol* 152: 151–158

66 Romagnani S (2004) Immunologic influences on allergy and the TH1/TH2 balance. *J Allergy Clin Immunol* 113: 395–400

67 Braun-Fahrlander C, Riedler J, Herz U, Eder W, Waser M, Grize L, Maisch S, Carr D, Gerlach F, Bufe A et al (2002) Environmental exposure to endotoxin and its relation to asthma in school-age children. *N Engl J Med* 347: 869–877

68 Douwes J, van Strien R, Doekes G, Smit J, Kerkhof M, Gerritsen J, Postma D, de Jongste J, Travier N, Brunekreef B (2006) Does early indoor microbial exposure reduce the risk of asthma? The Prevention and Incidence of Asthma and Mite Allergy birth cohort study. *J Allergy Clin Immunol* 117: 1067–73

69 Gereda JE, Leung DY, Thatayatikom A, Streib JE, Price MR, Klinnert MD, Liu AH (2000) Relation between house-dust endotoxin exposure, type 1 T-cell development, and allergen sensitisation in infants at high risk of asthma. *Lancet* 355: 1680–1683

70 Portengen L, Preller L, Tielen M, Doekes G, Heederik D (2005) Endotoxin exposure and atopic sensitization in adult pig farmers. *J Allergy Clin Immunol* 115: 797–802

71 Gehring U, Bischof W, Fahlbusch B, Wichmann HE, Heinrich J (2002) House dust endotoxin and allergic sensitization in children. *Am J Respir Crit Care Med* 166: 939–944

72 Liu AH (2002) Endotoxin exposure in allergy and asthma: Reconciling a paradox. *J Allergy Clin Immunol* 109: 379–392

73 Park JH, Spiegelman DL, Burge HA, Gold DR, Chew GL, Milton DK (2000) Longitudinal study of dust and airborne endotoxin in the home. *Environ Health Perspect* 108: 1023–1028

74 Thorne PS, Kulhankova K, Yin M, Cohn R, Arbes SJ Jr, Zeldin DC (2005) Endotoxin exposure is a risk factor for asthma: The national survey of endotoxin in United States housing. *Am J Respir Crit Care Med* 172: 1371–1377

75 Smit LAM, Heederik D, Doekes G, Krop EJM, Rijkers GT, Wouters IM (2009) Ex vivo cytokine release reflects sensitivity to occupational endotoxin exposure. *Eur Respir J* 34: 795–802

76 Venables KM, Upton JL, Hawkins ER, Tee RD, Longbottom JL, Newman Taylor AJ (1988) Smoking, atopy and laboratory animal allergy. *Br J Ind Med* 45: 667–671

77 Das R, Tager IB, Gamsky T, Schenker MB, Royce S, Balmes JR (1992) Atopy and airways reactivity in animal health technicians. A pilot study. *J Occup Med* 34: 53–60

78 Calvery AE, Rees D, Dowdeswell RJ, Linnett PJ, Kielkowski D (1995) Platinum salt sensitivity in refinery workers: Incidence and effects of smoking and exposure. *Occup Environ Med* 52: 661–666

79 Linnett PJ, Hughes EG (1999) 20 years of medical surveillance on exposure to allergenic and non allergenic platinum compounds: The importance of chemical speciation. *Occup Environ Med* 56: 191–196

80 Venables KM, Dally MB, Nunn AJ, Stevens JF, Stephens R, Farrer N, Hunter JV, Stewart

M, Hughes EG, Newman Taylor AJ (1989) Smoking and occupational allergy in workers in a platinum refinery. *BMJ* 299: 939–942

81 Castro-Giner F, Kauffmann F, Cid R de, Kogevinas M (2006) Gene–environment interactions in asthma. *Occup Environ Med* 63: 776–786

82 Vineis P, Ahsan H, Parker M (2005) Genetic screening and occupational and environmental exposures. *Occup Environ Med* 62: 657–662

83 Jeal H, Draper A, Jones M, Harris J, Welsh K, Taylor AN, Cullinan P (2003) HLA associations with occupational sensitization to rat lipocalin allergens: A model for other animal allergies? *J Allergy Clin Immunol* 111: 795–799

84 Barker RD, Harris JM, Welch JA, Venables KM, Newman Taylor AJ (1998) Occupational asthma caused by tetrachlorophthalic anhydride: A 12-year follow-up. *J Allergy Clin Immunol* 101: 717–719

85 Marabini A, Dimich-Ward H, Kwan SYL, Kennedy SM, Waxler-Morrison N, Chan-Yeung M (1993) Clinical and socioeconomic features of subjects with red cedar asthma. *Chest* 104: 821–824

86 Merget R, Reineke M, Rueckmann A, Bergmann EM, Schultze-Werninghaus G (1994) Non-specific and specific bronchial responsiveness in occupational asthma caused by platinum salts after allergen avoidance. *Am J Respir Crit Care Med* 150: 1146–1149

87 Paggiaro PL, Vagaggini B, Bacci E, Bancalari L, Carrara M, Di Franco A, Giannini D, Dente FL, Giuntini C (1994) Prognosis of occupational asthma. *Eur Respir J* 7: 761–767

88 Venables KM, Davison AG, Newman Taylor AJ (1989) Consequences of occupational asthma. *Respir Med* 83: 437–440

89 Paggiaro PL, Bacci E, Paoletti P, Bernard P, Dente FL, Marchetti G, Talini D, Menconi GF, Giuntini C (1990) Bronchoalveolar lavage and morphology of the airways after cessation of exposure in asthmatic subjects sensitized to toluene diisocyanate. *Chest* 98: 536–542

90 Vandenplas O, Toren K, Blanc PD (2003) Health and socioeconomic impact of work-related asthma. *Eur Respir J* 22: 689–697

91 Heederik D, van Rooy F (2008) Exposure assessment should be integrated in studies on the prevention and management of occupational asthma. *Occup Environ Med* 65: 149–150

92 Cullinan P (2008) Occupational asthma. *Occup Environ Med* 65: 151

93 ACGIH. American Conference of Governmental Industrial Hygienists (1999) *Flour dust TLV documentation*. ACGIH, Cincinnati, USA

94 DECOS (1999) *Health based recommended occupational exposure limit for flour dust*. Dutch Expert Committee on Occupational Standards, The Hague, The Netherlands

95 Rijnkels JM, Smid T, Van den Aker EC, Burdorf A, van Wijk RG, Heederik DJ, Houben GF, Van Loveren H, Pal TM, Van Rooy FG et al (2008) Prevention of work-related airway allergies; summary of the advice from the Health Council of the Netherlands. *Allergy* 93: 1593–1596

Epidemiology of laboratory animal allergy

Hayley L. Jeal, Meinir G. Jones and Paul Cullinan

Department of Occupational and Environmental Medicine, National Heart and Lung Institute, Imperial College, 1b Manresa Road, London SW3 6LR, UK

Abstract

Laboratory animal allergy is common and an important occupational health issue for the research, pharmaceutical and toxicological sectors. In most settings where there is regular contact with laboratory animals – chiefly small mammals – the prevalence of specific sensitisation is around 15% and the prevalence of clinical allergy around 10%. These figures probably underestimate the true risk of disease since epidemiological studies of the disease have been beset by response and survivor biases. Allergen exposure appears to be the most important modifiable risk factor, but the effects of such exposure seem to be modified importantly by individual susceptibility. Laboratory animal research shows no signs of becoming less common, and an increasingly susceptible (atopic) population is likely to be recruited into such work. Future studies should be designed to take into account the inherent biases of occupational epidemiology, to study in detail the immunological mechanisms that underlie sensitisation and tolerance, and to identify early biomarkers of each.

Introduction

Human allergy to furred animals has a history, presumably, that is as long as that of the domestication of wild beasts. With a general increase in atopy it is probably more common now than it has ever been. Animal allergy in an occupational, laboratory setting on the other hand is a far more recent phenomenon, reflecting the development of vivisection as a means of studying human biology and responses to toxins and pharmaceuticals.

Early descriptions of laboratory animal allergy were in case report form only and are reviewed by Hunskaar and Fosse [1]. An interesting example is given by Sorrell and Gottesman [2] who in 1957 reported a single case of mouse allergy in a female research worker after she developed rhinitis at work. She was treated by specific immunotherapy with an autogenous extract, after which she was able to continue working with mice for up to 4 h at a time.

In 1961 Rakja identified, on the basis of skin and exposure tests, ten cases of laboratory animal allergy at the Karolinska Hospital in Sweden [3] and suggested that

Occupational Asthma, edited by Torben Sigsgaard and Dick Heederik

hypersensitivity to laboratory animals was not as uncommon in research laboratory workers as might previously have been thought. It was not until the 1970s, however, that proper epidemiological studies of laboratory animal workers were carried out and a better idea of the scale of the occupational problem was determined. Over the subsequent 35 years laboratory animal allergy has been the subject of extensive epidemiological study and is now universally recognised as an important occupational health issue. With the possible exception of baker's asthma, it is the best understood of all the occupational respiratory allergies.

Causes, species and allergens

The contemporary use of animals for research purposes is dominated by the pharmaceutical, toxicological and academic sectors. In 2007, for example, just over 3.2 million scientific procedures were carried out on animals in the United Kingdom; 83% included rodents. The total number was a 6% rise over the previous year, due mainly to an increase in the use of genetically modified mice in scientific experiments.

A bewildering variety of animal species are used in laboratory-based research (Tab. 1). Most procedures use mammalian species and, as the figures above suggest, most of these now involve mice because of the relative ease of genetic manipulation in that species. Other commonly used mammals include rats, guinea pigs, hamsters and ferrets, cats and dogs, pigs, sheep and goats. Non-human primate research is far less common; interestingly human allergy to other primates appears to be very rare.

Commonly used non-mammalian species include insects, amphibians and fish; allergic responses to the last two of these appear to be extremely rare. A wide variety of species of insects have been identified as causing occupational allergy: fruit flies, cockroaches, locusts, grasshoppers, bumblebees, mites, spiders and chironomid midges. Birds are occasionally used in research, chiefly in behavioural studies.

Table 1 lists commonly used species and their associated allergens. The majority of the major mammalian allergens belong to a family of proteins known as lipocalins [4]. The sequence identity of lipocalin allergens often falls below 20% but they have a similar three-dimensional structure and contain between one and three structurally conserved regions [5]. Lipocalins also share biological functions that predominantly relate to the transport of small hydrophobic ligands such as vitamins and pheromones. Interestingly, lipocalins share a sequence homology with schistosome proteins and it is possible that molecular mimicry may be responsible for the high rates of sensitisation to lipocalin allergens in the workplace.

Laboratory animal workers may also be exposed to other types of allergen in the workplace. These include allergens in animal or fish food (such as mealworms or corn cob), natural rubber latex (gloves), moulds, pollens, enzymes, antibiotics and several sensitising chemicals

Table 1. Animal species (and associated allergens) commonly used in laboratory research

Species	Allergens	Mol. mass (kDa)	Source
Mammalian			
Mouse (*Mus musculus*)	Mus m 1 (prealbumin) Mus m 2 Albumin	19 16 68	Hair, dander, urine Hair, dander, urine Serum
Rat (*Rattus norvegicus*)	Rat n 1 Rat n 2 (α_{2u}globulin) Albumin	21 17 67	Hair, dander, urine Hair, dander, urine Serum
Guinea pig (*Cavia porcellus*)	Cav p 1 Cav p 2	20 17	Hair, dander, urine Hair, dander, urine
Hamster (*Cricetus cricetus*)	Unknown	-	-
Ferret (*Mustela putorius furo*)	Unknown	-	-
Rabbit (*Oryctolagus cuniculus*)	Ory c 1 Ory c 2	17 21	Hair, dander, saliva Hair, dander, urine
Cat (*Felis domesticus*)	Fel d 1 Fel d 4 Albumin	38 19.7 65–69	Hair, dander, saliva Saliva Serum, dander, saliva
Dog (*Canis familaris*)	Can f 1 Can f 2 Albumin	25 19 67	Hair, dander, saliva Hair, dander, saliva Serum
Pig (*Sus domesticus*)	Unknown	-	-
Sheep (*Ovis aries*)	Unknown	-	-
Goat (*Capra hircus*)	Unknown	-	-
Other			
Fruit fly (*Drosophila melanogaster*)	Unknown	-	-
Locust (several species)	Unknown	-	-
Cockroach (several species)	Bla g 2 Bla g 4 Bla g 5	36 21 23	Faeces, saliva and body of cockroach

Clinical characteristics of laboratory animal allergy

Laboratory animal allergy has clinical characteristics typical of an immediate-type hypersensitivity to a protein aeroallergen. Symptoms develop after a latent period of exposure that is generally between 3 and 24 months. Upper respiratory symptoms of rhinitis and itchy eyes are almost universal and may be accompanied by asthma and by urticarial skin responses to animal scratches or abrasions. In the early stages of disease there is noticeable improvement when away from the workplace. With continuing exposure a hypersensitive state tends to develop with symptoms provoked by increasingly smaller exposures [6] and any improvement away from work becoming less apparent. Under these conditions standard treatments for asthma and rhinitis are relatively ineffective. Conversely, the avoidance of exposure to the causative allergen generally results in considerable – or complete – improvement.

As with its symptomatology, the immunopathology of laboratory animal allergy is typical of a type 1 allergic response. The development of sensitisation is complex and involves interaction of antigen-presenting cells and Th2 lymphocytes, which secrete IL-4, IL-5, IL-9 and IL-13 cytokines leading to an allergic response, with associated specific IgE response that may be detected by serum assay or skin prick testing. With appropriate test methods for all relevant allergens the detection of an IgE response is almost wholly sensitive. Thus, the false-negative rate is very low, and a negative result to both skin prick testing and serum assay effectively rules out the diagnosis.

Disease frequency

There are several ways in which the prevalence or incidence of laboratory animal allergy may be estimated. Each has particular drawbacks but all probably underestimate the true frequency of disease. The reasons for this include:

- Specific sensitisation to animal proteins may be clinically unapparent and thus detectable only through skin prick testing or by the measurement of serum-specific IgE antibodies. Survey methods that do not include such techniques will lead to an underestimation of the true frequency of sensitisation.
- The tools – generally self-completed questionnaires – that are used to determine the frequency of laboratory animal allergy in clinical or workplace populations may be insensitive; either intrinsically as they may not include all relevant questions or because participants may be reluctant to disclose full information. While high sensitivity is desirable in obtaining a true estimate of disease prevalence, specificity is also important, particularly in deriving unbiased estimates of exposure-response relationships [7].

- Epidemiological methods that do not include all or a very high proportion of the eligible population are likely to suffer from a responder bias. The direction of this bias in the context of laboratory animal allergy is not known but it is the experience of the authors that symptomatic workers are less likely to participate in surveys.
- The use of cross-sectional survey to measure the prevalence of laboratory animal allergy probably incurs a risk of survivor bias, an example of a healthy worker effect. Employees who have developed laboratory animal allergy may be more likely than others to seek alternative employment or, within the workplace, to move to jobs that entail less (or no) exposure to the allergens that incite their symptoms [8]. The first process (selection out of the workforce) will result in a cross-sectional population whose disease experience is healthier than is truly the case; the second (selection within the workplace) may lead to erroneous estimates of exposure-response relationships.

If conducted carefully, cohort studies provide not only a measure of the incidence of laboratory animal allergy but potentially also an account of any (internal) selection, and thus an unbiased estimate of exposure-response relationships. In practice they have rarely if ever been entirely successful in these respects; they are certainly far less common than cross-sectional designs.

As with the case of potential responder bias, the size of any 'healthy worker' effect in the animal laboratory setting is unknown. There are several probable determinants that include the relatively short latency period for the induction of laboratory animal allergy and, once disease has developed, the very brief interval between exposure and the elicitation of symptoms. Once established and under conditions of continuing exposure, laboratory animal allergy displays other characteristics of an immediate-type hypersensitivity, in particular the incitement of symptoms at increasingly low concentrations of allergen exposure. Each of these factors permits an obvious relationship between exposures at work and the manifestations of disease and together they are likely to have an important influence on employment behaviour. More individual factors that are likely also to impact on retention within a job or a workplace include the severity of symptoms – which appears to be variable – and the attitudes of employers. For the most part, those who employ laboratory animal workers have a more enlightened view of occupational disease among their employees than is generally the case. Thus, many laboratory animal workers with a specific occupational allergy are afforded an unusual degree of flexibility in their work.

Cross-sectional surveys

The most common approach to measuring the frequency of laboratory animal allergy is to estimate its prevalence through the use of a cross-sectional survey of a workforce. Table 2 provides a comprehensive but succinct summary of published results from 29 such surveys. The numbers of employees included range from 62 to over 5500; where information is available response rates between 61% and, in some cases, 100% are reported.

The reported prevalences of 'allergic symptoms' vary widely from around 10% ('any symptoms') to over 50%. There is similar if less pronounced variability in the estimated prevalences of specific sensitisation. Such variation has at least three sources: true variation reflecting differences in site- or population-specific risk factors; between-study inconsistency in the definition and measurement of 'allergy'; and variation in the study populations reflecting, as above, different survival patterns.

Perhaps the most important of these is the second. Very few published cross-sectional surveys provide sufficient information on the constitution of their surveyed population; even the most basic information, such as on the duration of employment, is frequently lacking. Thus, it is generally very difficult to judge to what extent the reported findings reflect true disease incidence rather than the effects of important survival processes. Even the apparently consistent – and certainly plausible – observation that upper respiratory symptoms (rhinitis) are more common than symptoms of asthma may in part be a result of employees with asthma re-locating at a greater frequency than those with rhinitis alone.

Few cross-sectional surveys have attempted to address this problem. Exceptions include a study of research workers in the United Kingdom [8] in which analyses were restricted to those who had not had exposure to laboratory animals prior to their current employment, and surveys by Hollander et al. [27] and Heederik et al. [28] in which analysis was confined to employees with less than 4 years exposure to laboratory animals. Although imperfect, these techniques probably lessen the impact of any healthy worker effect and may lead to associations that approximate those observed in cohort studies.

A recent ecological examination of prevalence estimates from 15 cross-sectional surveys concluded that the prevalence of occupational asthma – but not of occupational rhinitis – among laboratory workers had declined by about 50% between 1976 and 2001 [34]. This decline was not, however, evident in those studies where workers were exposed to rats, mice, rabbits or guinea pigs. Comparisons such as these should be viewed cautiously since, as above, studies in this field rarely share a common methodology. Thus, it is not possible to account for the several biases inherent in cross-sectional epidemiology, particularly perhaps those that relate to survival pressures.

Cohort studies

Cohort ('longitudinal') studies circumvent many of the difficulties associated with cross-sectional surveys. In particular, if they are carried out carefully, they have

Table 2. Prevalence studies from cross-sectional surveys (English language publications).

						Prevalence of allergic symptoms (%)			Prevalence of sensitisation: SPT or IgE (%)		
Study/year	**Country**	**Facility**	**Species***	**N (% response)**	**Average duration of exposure**	**Any**	**Chest**	**Eye/ nose**	**Mouse**	**Rat**	**Any/other**
Lincoln 1974 [9]	US	Research	M, R, Rb, Gp, H	238 (NA)	NA	11%	5%	9%	NA	NA	10% (SPT)
Lutsky 1975 [10]	US	Mixed	M, R, Rb, Gp, C, D, H	1293 (NA)	NA	15%	10%	15%	NA	NA	NA
Taylor 1976 [11]	UK	Research, pharma	LA	474 (NA)	NA	23%	9%	17%	NA	NA	NA
Gross 1980 [12]	US	Research	M, R, Rb, Gp	399 (100%)	NA	15%	8%	15%	NA	NA	NA
Cockcroft 1981 [13]	UK	Research	M, R, Gp, Rb, S	179 (61%)	NA	27%	12%	25%	NA	NA	16% (SPT)
Davies 1981 [14]	UK	Research, pharma	LA	585 (NA)	NA	20%	3%	11%	NA	NA	NA
Schumacher 1981 [15]	Australia	Research	M	121 (82%)	3 years	32%	4%	24%	33%	-	-
Slovak 1981 [16]	UK	Pharma	LA	146 (NA)	NA	30%	10%	23%	NA	NA	15% (SPT)
Beeson 1983 [17]	UK	Pharma	M, R, Gp, Rb	62 (83%)	NA	24%	5%	21%	5%?	11%	32% (IgE)?

Table 2 (continued)

						Prevalence of allergic symptoms (%)			Prevalence of sensitisation: SPT or IgE (%)		
Study/year	**Country**	**Facility**	**Species***	**N (% response)**	**Average duration of exposure**	**Any**	**Chest**	**Eye/ nose**	**Mouse**	**Rat**	**Any/other**
Agrup 1986 [18]	Sweden	Research	M, R, Rb, Gp, H, C	101 (100%)	NA	30%	20%	10%	18%?	18%	any:19% (SPT+IgE): Rb: 11%, Gp: 26%, C: 31%
Bland 1986 [19]	US	Research	R, Rb, Gp, C	549 (93%)	NA	24%	NA	NA	NA	NA	NA
Lutsky 1986 [20]	Israel	Research	R, M, Rb, Gp	90 (NA)	9 years	7%	4%	7%	NA	NA	NA
Platts-Mills 1987 [21]	UK	Research	R	213 (NA)	NA	17%	10%	7%	-	12% (SPT)	-
Venables 1988 [22]	UK	Pharma	R, M, Rb, Gp	138 (87%)	9 years	44%	11%	37%	NA	NA	26%
Venables 1988 [23]	UK	Mixed	R, M, Rb, Gp	296 (NA)	8 years	47%	13%	NA	NA	NA	17% (SPT)
Aoyama 1992 [24]	Japan	Research, breeding	R, M, Gp, Rb, H, C, D, P, Mn	5641 (64%)	NA	23%	6%	18%	NA	NA	NA
Cullinan 1994 [8]	UK	Research	R	323 (88%)	21 months	31%	10%	22%	-	10% (SPT)	-
Bryant 1995 [25]	Australia	Research	LA	130 (NA)	NA	56%	22%	NA	NA	NA	NA

Hollander 1996 [26]	Netherlands	Research, pharma,	R	458 (77%)	11years	19%	6%	17%	-	18% (SPT)	-
Hollander 1996 [26]	Netherlands	Research, pharma,	M	377 (77%)	10years	10%	3%	9%	10% (SPT)	-	-
Hollander 1997 [27]	Netherlands	Research, pharma	R	398 (77%)	NA	20%	NA	NA	-	17% (SPT)	-
Heederik 1999 [28]	Sweden	Research, training	R	74 (82%)	<4 years	-	3%	12%	-	5%	-
Heederik 1999 [28]	Netherlands	Research, pharma, training	R	219 (77%)	<4years	-	5%	15%	-	8%	-
Heederik 1999 [28]	UK	Research, pharma	R	357 (88%)	<4 years	-	9 (3%)	10%	-	4%	-
Lieutier-Colas 2002 [29]	France	Research	R	113 (100%)	NA	39%	4%	34%	-	12%	-
Ruoppi 2004 [30]	Finland	Research	R, M	156 (61%)	6 years	47%	26%	42%	NA	NA	NA
Jeal 2006 [31]	UK	Research	R	689 (96%)	8 years	22%	NA	NA	-	11%	-
Krakowiak 2007 [32]	Poland	Vets	R, M, H, Rb, Gp	200 (NA)	NA	NA	10%	14%	16% (SPT)	17% (SPT)	H: 6%, Gp: 13%, Rb: 5%
Hewitt 2008 [33]	New Zealand	Research	LA	50 (NA)	11 years	22%	4%	18%	4%	2%	Gp: 2%

* M, mouse; R, rat; Rb, rabbit; Gp, guinea pig; H, hamster; D, dog; C, cat; S, sheep; Mn, monkey; LA, laboratory animals unspecified; SPT, skin prick test.
NA, not available.

the ability to examine the determinants of employees' movements within or out of a workforce. Furthermore (see below), they allow the measurement of relevant workplace exposures, a particular advantage in an immunological disease such as laboratory animal allergy where it is probably the case that very early exposures determine the risk of sensitisation.

However, cohort studies are far more difficult to conduct well, and tend to be far more expensive, than cross-sectional surveys. Probably for these reasons they have been far fewer in number. Occasionally (e.g. [35, 36]) cohort studies are embedded within routine surveillance schemes, potentially a far more efficient approach – and certainly one that is underused.

Eleven published cohort studies are summarised in Table 3 with estimates of disease and sensitisation incidence rates where these are available. As with the cross-sectional surveys described earlier, the response rates for several are low – a serious problem with any cohort design.

Some studies have been of very short duration and probably have produced underestimates of true incidence rates. A further important limitation of many studies is that they incorporate participants with previous occupational exposure to laboratory animals. This effectively negates much if not all of the advantage of a longitudinal approach over the cross-sectional survey. Some [35, 43] have restricted analyses to, or included analysis of, newly exposed employees and so gained valuable insights. In a longitudinal study of pharmacological research employees in the United States for example [35], the estimated incidence rate of laboratory animal allergy was about 2.3 per 100 person years. In an analysis confined to employees without prior exposure to laboratory animals, however, the estimated incidence rate was about twice as high, suggesting an important degree of 'selection out' in that workforce.

A note of further caution in relation to estimated incidence rates for laboratory animal allergy in warranted. The immunological nature of this short-latency condition is reflected in a high incidence of disease shortly after first exposure – and probably a diminishing risk thereafter, under conditions of continuing similar exposure. If this is true then rates derived across a longitudinal survey may hide differential annual rates; few, if any, studies have been large enough to examine this in any detail.

Surveillance schemes

Alternative methods of measuring the frequency of laboratory animal allergy depend on routine surveillance statistics. Several countries – notably Finland, the UK and France but also South Africa and parts of Spain, Canada and Australia – have established surveillance schemes for occupational asthma. Each measures disease that is newly recognised and reported by specialised physicians, usually in occupational

Table 3. Estimated incidence rates of laboratory animal allergy from longitudinal studies.

Study/year	Country	Facility	Species*	n (% of eligible population)	Duration of follow-up	Estimated incidence of allergic symptoms per 100 person years: Any	Chest	Eye/nose	Estimated incidence of sensitisation (SPT or IgE) per 100 person years
Davies 1983 [37]	UK	Pharma	M, R, Rb, Gp	148 (100%)	1 year	15	2	NA	NA
Botham 1987 [36]	UK	Pharma	R, M, Gp, Rb	383 (NA)	Variable	12–37	NA	NA	NA
Kibby 1989 [38]	US	Research	LA	169 (70%)	2 years	6.5	NA	NA	NA
Das 1992 [39]	US	Training	LA	29 (55%)	7 months	0	0	0	NA
Renstrom 1995 [40]	Sweden	Training	M, R, Rb, H, Ho, P, Ch	38 (100%)	18 months	6	2	5	5
Kruize 1997 [41]	US	Pharma	LA	99 (44%)	10 years	1.9	0.8	1.4	NA
Fisher 1998 [42]	US	Pharma	LA	159 (NA)	≤5 years	0–10	NA	NA	NA
Cullinan 1999 [43]	UK	Research	R	342 (80%)	7 years	–	3.5	7.3	4.1
Gautrin 2001 [44]	Canada	Training	M, R, Rb	373 (89%)	44 months	–	2.7	–	NA
Rodier 2003 [45]				387 (93%)			–	9.6	
De Meer 2003 [46]	Netherlands	Research	M, R, Rb, Gp,	105 (NA)	2 years	6	NA	NA	NA
Elliot 2005 [35]	US	Pharma	LA	495 (82%)	12 years	2.3		3	1.32

* M, mouse; R, rat; Rb, rabbit; Gp, guinea pig; H, hamster; D, dog; C, cat; S, sheep; Ho, horse; P, pig; Ch, chicken; LA, laboratory animals unspecified; SPT, skin prick test.
NA, not available.

or respiratory medical practice; in some instances the schemes are closely linked to compensation claims. They are of course entirely dependent on the presentation of disease by an employee and its recognition and reporting by an appropriate specialist. Surveillance in this manner certainly leads to an underestimate of the true incidence of occupational asthma; in the case of laboratory animal allergy this is enhanced by the omission of cases without overt asthma.

Some surveillance schemes can be linked to national workforce denominators to estimate occupation-specific incidence rates (Tab. 4). Such denominators are rarely, if ever, specific to laboratory animal workers. Hence the rates from which they are derived are a further underestimate of the true job-specific incidence. In the UK, for example, the annual incidence rate of occupational asthma among 'laboratory assistants and technicians' was estimated to be 0.24/1000, based on a workforce of 127478. A subsequent exercise to establish a more specific estimate of the size of the laboratory animal-exposed workforce produced a figure of between 12000 and 17300 employees working with small mammals. From these were derived new estimates of annual disease incidence of 1.26/1000 and 2.54/1000 for occupational asthma and occupational rhinitis, respectively [47].

Analysis of reports from surveillance schemes in different countries also affords the possibility of international comparisons (Tab. 4). Where they are available (but see above), estimated annual incidence rates vary between 17 and 79 cases per

Table 4. Numbers of total cases of occupational asthma and laboratory animal asthma with estimated annual incidence rates per million workers from surveillance schemes in seven different countries.

	All occupational asthma		Laboratory animal asthma		Laboratory animal asthma as a proportion of all cases
Scheme	**No. of cases**	**Annual incidence**	**No. of cases**	**Annual incidence**	
UK (1989–1990) [48]	1985	20	50	188	2.5%
France (1996–1999) [49]	2178	24	27	NA	1.2%
Finland (1989–1995) [50]	2602	17	52	116	2.0%
South Africa (1997–1999) [51]	324	18	3	NA	0.9%
Quebec (1992–1993) [52]	287	42–79	19*	329**	7%
Catalonia, Spain (2002) [53]	174	NA	7	NA	4%
Australia† (1997–2001) [54]	170	NA	4	NA	2.4%

*Occupational asthma to 'laboratory and farm animals' in **'agricultural and related service industries'
† Victoria and Tasmania
NA = not available

million workers; the last (highest) figure, however, also includes agricultural workers. The proportions of all registered cases of occupational asthma that are attributed to laboratory animal exposures are remarkably consistent between approximately 1% and 7%, the lowest figure being for three provinces in South Africa.

Aside from the professional surveillance schemes above, estimates of the incidence of laboratory animal allergy may be made from counts of claims for statutory compensation or, through the courts, for personal injury. The obvious weaknesses in each of these is likely to compound the problems of under-ascertainment described above.

Risk factors

The imperative to reduce the incidence of laboratory animal allergy has produced a focus on the study of modifiable risk factors. The most important of these is believed to be allergen exposure within the workplace. Most allergen exposure-response studies have, like those of disease frequency, been carried out in cross-sectional occupational populations. A summary of these ($n = 18$) together with the findings of five cohort studies is displayed in Table 5. In addition, where it is available, information on disease latency is provided. The evidence that laboratory animal allergy is usually a condition of short latency is both consistent and strong.

Allergen exposure

'Exposure' has, in most cases, been assessed by job title and only occasionally by direct measurement of airborne allergen. The use of 'zoning' techniques whereby employees in different jobs are grouped by their likely exposures (e.g. into 'scientist', 'animal technician' and 'other') allows job title to be a good, albeit broad, proxy of direct measurement [55]. Where proxies are used as the main indicator of exposure, it is helpful if they are supplemented by quantitative exposure information. Neither approach, however, has proved to be a good indicator of the variability in exposure 'quality'; the exposure of animal technicians, for example, who carry out the day-to-day care of animals, is likely to be more consistent than that of scientists whose experimental protocols generally cause a far more variable exposure pattern.

In general it has been more difficult in cross-sectional surveys to demonstrate any relationship between allergen exposure – however defined – and disease risk. The reasons for this have been discussed above and probably relate primarily to survival processes including those that determine survival within a particular job within a workplace. In a survey of UK research workers [8], no relationship between disease prevalence and current exposure was observed; however, such was evident when exposure at the time of onset of disease was examined, suggesting that employees

Table 5. Cross-sectional and cohort studies of the relationship between exposure and the risk of laboratory animal allergy.

Study/year	Species*	*n*	Exposure measurement	Latency	Exposure-response
Cross-sectional surveys					
Taylor 1976 [11]	Mixed	474	ND	"No increase in incidence of LAA after 2 years"	ND
Gross 1980 [12]	Mixed	399	Frequency of entry into animal house	Average 11 months. "LAA most likely to occur within 6 m and rarely >2–3 years"	ND
Cockcroft 1981 [13]	Mixed	179	Job category	High exposed groups < medium exposed	ND
Schumacher 1981 [15]	M	121	Frequency/ duration of exposure	usually <1 year	Neither frequency nor duration of exposure significantly related to sensitisation or symptoms.
Slovak 1981 [16]	Mixed	146	Job category	Asthma: 66% ≤3 years	Asthma cases confined to high exposure group
Beeson 1983 [17]	Mixed	62	Duration of exposure	ND	No significant difference in duration of exposure between LAA and non-LAA cases
Bland 1986 [19]	Mixed	549	Job category, frequency	ND	Dose effect for frequency in low/moderate but not in high exposure group. No. of species handled is a risk factor for LAA
Platts-Mills 1987 [21]	R	213	Job categories	Mean 2.5 years	Sensitisation: 0% (low exposure), 6% (medium), 20% (high). Duration is less important than exposure
Venables 1988a [22]	Mixed	138	Job category, duration of exposure	ND	Non-significant inverse trend by duration of exposure for prevalence of LAA
Aoyama 1992 [24]	Mixed	5641	Job category, frequency, # species	33% ≤1 year, 70% ≤3 years	Prevalence of LAA increased with higher frequency of exposure and with increasing # species handled. No significant association with job categories

Cullinan 1994 [8]	R	323	Aeroallergen measurement	ND	Prevalence of LAA symptoms related to intensity of exposure. Stronger in atopic subjects
Hollander 1997 [27]	R	398	Aeroallergen measurement	ND	In those exposed <4 years – prevalence of sensitisation in low, medium and high exposure groups were 4.1, 5.0 and 7.2 times higher than control group. Exposure –response relationship steeper in atopics
Fisher 1998 [42]	Mixed	159	Intensity of exposure	ND	High exposure not a significant predictor of LAA
Heederik 1999 [28]	R	650	Aeroallergen measurement	ND	Risk of sensitisation increased with exposure intensity. Atopics had elevated risk of sensitisation at low allergen exposures.
Lieutier-Colas 2002 [29]	R	113	Aeroallergen measurement	ND	No relationship between rat exposure and development of sensitisation or symptoms
Ruoppi 2004 [30]	R, m	156	Frequency of handling	ND	Exposure-response relationship between intensity of exposure and development of respiratory disease.
Jeal 2006 [31]	R	689	Job category, # rats handled	ND	High-exposure attenuation of exposure–response relationship for sensitisation and symptoms
Krakowiak 2007 [32]	Mixed	200	Frequency	ND	Exposure-response relationship for symptoms (OR 50.2; 95% CI, 2.84; 884.99)
Cohort studies					
Davies 1983 [37]	R	142	ND	Symptoms within 0.5–12 years – rhinitis preceded asthma	ND
Kibby 1989 [38]	Mixed	450	Aeroallergen measurement	ND	Duration unrelated to LAA Positive association between LAA and intensity of exposure (PR = 1.75; 95% CI, 1.06–2.39; p = 0.03) Positive association between LAA and weighted job exposure (PR = 1.58; 95% CI 1.00–2.50)

Table 5 (continued)

Study/year	Species*	n	Exposure measurement	Latency	Exposure-response
Cullinan 1999 [43]			Aeroallergen measurement	Median: skin, eye/nose 12 months, chest 18 months	In those exposed <2 years, exposure related to development of symptoms – but attenuated at highest exposure. Relationship stronger in atopics.
Rodier 2003 [45]	Mixed	417	Time in contact	ND	Contact time associated with the incidence of rhinoconjuctivitis in dose-dependent manner
Eliott 2005 [35]	Mixed	495	Frequency of handling	ND	Risk of LAA increased with duration of exposure to animals and work in animal-related tasks

LAA, laboratory animal allergy

with symptoms had moved away from jobs of higher exposure. Similar factors presumably explain why duration of exposure appears irrelevant [38] – or even inversely related to risk [22].

Many cohort studies of laboratory animal employees have been set up to examine exposure-response relationships and thus have done so with greater attention to detail. Some [43] have had this aim as primary, others [36, 42] in order to examine changes in disease incidence in relation to primary preventive programmes. Broadly, their findings suggest that higher allergen exposure intensities are related to the risk of laboratory animal allergy – with some important modifying influences (see below). What is far less clear is the detail of such a relationship and in particular the existence – and level – of any threshold of exposure below which there is no measurable risk. This is a problem common to any immunological outcome, reflecting in part the wide range of individual susceptibility. Arguably this is an issue that will not be amenable to further epidemiological study.

A recent and interesting observation is that the relationship between exposure intensity and risk, which is almost certainly non-linear, may also not be monotonic. Thus, there is some evidence [31, 43] that at highest exposures there is a degree of attenuation in risk; this may reflect qualitative differences in exposure (e.g. 'constant' vs 'intermittent'), differences in exposure route or even a phenomenon of high-dose 'immunotolerance'. The last of course – if established with certainty – would have interesting implications for occupational health practice.

Atopy

Atopy, the tendency to develop immediate-type immune responses to environmental aeroallergens, is a well-documented risk factor for the development of laboratory animal allergy [8, 13, 19, 27], its relative risk being of the order of 3.0–4.0 [8, 13, 19, 27, 41]. Cross-sectional studies generally report higher risk estimates than do those of longitudinal design, perhaps a reflection of co-sensitisation. In addition, atopic employees are more likely to develop occupational asthma as a result of exposure [13, 41], and are more likely to be absent from work or transferred to another job because of symptoms of laboratory animal allergy [41]. Indeed, the latter observation suggests that survival is further influenced by atopic status, in which case its true relative risk may be higher than is commonly measured. The onset of symptoms from laboratory animals following first exposure is probably shorter in atopic employees than it is in those who are not atopic [36, 41]. For example, Kruize et al. [41] reported that the mean latency for laboratory animal allergy was significantly shorter in atopics (45 months) than in non-atopics (109 months).

Furthermore, atopy may confer quantitative differences in the response to allergen exposure in the laboratory. Several studies suggest a stronger exposure response for the development of laboratory animal allergy in atopic than non-atopic workers

[8, 27, 28, 41, 43], although this is not an entirely consistent observation and probably dependent on both exposure levels and any definition of atopy. Differences may also reflect lower outcome rates – and thus less statistical power in non-atopic subgroups. Kruize et al. [41] reported similar exposure-response patterns in atopic and non-atopic groups, but a stronger relationship in those who were atopic. Similarly, other studies suggest interactions between allergen exposure and atopy whereby, in general, exposure-response relationships are steeper for workers with atopy-associated risk factors [8, 27]. Heederik et al. [28], on the other hand, reported a flatter association in atopic workers; this finding probably reflects exposures above an important threshold for atopic workers who, at the lowest level of exposure, had a more than threefold increase in risk of allergy.

Clearly atopy is a strong risk factor in the development of laboratory animal allergy and the question arises as to whether it could be used as a predictive tool. In their longitudinal study of pharmaceutical research workers, Botham et al. [36] observed that laboratory animal workers who developed symptoms during their first year of exposure were mainly atopic, but that the majority of atopic subjects remained non-symptomatic during the first year of exposure. The number of atopics becoming symptomatic in the second and third year of exposure was small with an increasing proportion of non-atopics developing laboratory animal allergy. Similarly, Slovak and Hill [56] in an examination of several different methods of defining 'atopy' concluded that none had sufficiently high predictive sensitivity or specificity. A more recent study has essentially confirmed these findings [57]; although atopy is strongly associated with the development of laboratory animal allergy, its predictive value is low and most employees with atopy – currently a high proportion of laboratory animal workers – will not develop a specific sensitisation. Thus, the exclusion of atopic people from working with laboratory animals seems to be insufficiently discriminatory as a factor to be considered as a means of screening for susceptible individuals.

Human leucocyte antigen

There have been few studies investigating the association of HLA genes and laboratory animal allergy. The first of two relatively small studies found statistically significant associations with HLA-B15, -DR4 and (inversely) -B16 and sensitisation to rat urine [58]. The second reported an excess of HLA-DR4, -DR11 and -DRw17 in human T lymphocyte responses to the major mouse allergen, Mus m 1 [59].

In a relatively large case ($n = 109$) referent ($n = 397$) analysis of a cross-sectional survey of pharmaceutical researchers, HLA-DR7 was associated with sensitisation, respiratory symptoms at work and most strongly with the combination of sensitisation and symptoms [60]. HLA-DR3 was found to be protective against sensitisation. Furthermore, amino acid analyses of HLA-DR7 and -DR3 indicated a biologically plausible explanation for the associations found. There was no evidence of any modification by exposure of the association between HLA-DR7 and sensitisation to rat urinary protein, or respiratory symptoms at work.

In the same study, the risk estimate of being sensitised to rat urinary protein was almost doubled in the presence of HLA-DR7; this risk was lower than those associated with atopy (fivefold) or a crude estimate of exposure (fourfold). These figures suggested that approximately 40% of occupational asthma in that population study could be attributed to HLA-DR7; in comparison, attributable proportions for atopy and daily work in animal house were 58% and 74%, respectively.

Conclusion

Laboratory animal allergy is common and an important occupational health issue for the research, pharmaceutical and toxicological sectors. In most settings where there is regular contact with laboratory animals – chiefly small mammals – the prevalence of specific sensitisation is around 15% and the prevalence of clinical allergy around 10%. These figures probably underestimate the true risk of disease since epidemiological studies of the disease have been beset by response and survivor biases. Allergen exposure appears to be the most important modifiable risk factor; however, the effects of such exposure seem to be modified importantly by individual susceptibility. Laboratory animal research shows no signs of becoming less common and an increasingly susceptible (atopic) population is likely to be recruited into such work. Future studies should be designed to take into account the inherent biases of occupational epidemiology, to study in detail the immunological mechanisms that underlie sensitisation and tolerance, and to identify early biomarkers of each.

References

1 Hunskaar, S. and R. T. Fosse. 1990. Allergy to laboratory mice and rats: A review of the pathophysiology, epidemiology and clinical aspects. *Lab Anim* 24: 358–374

2 Sorrel, A. H. and J. Gottesman. 1957. Mouse allergy: Case report. *Ann Allergy* 15: 662–663

3 Rajka, G. 1961. Ten cases of occupational hypersensitivity to laboratory animals. *Acta Allergol* 15: 168–176

4 Virtanen, T. 2001. Lipocalin allergens. *Allergy* 56 (Suppl 67): 48–51

5 Flower, D. R., A. C. Nrth, and T. K. Attwood. 1993. Structure and sequence relationships in the lipocalins and related proteins. *Protein Sci* 2: 753–761

6 Eggleston, P. A., A. A. Ansari, N. F. Adkinson, Jr., and R. A. Wood. 1995. Environmental challenge studies in laboratory animal allergy. Effect of different airborne allergen concentrations. *Am J Respir Crit Care Med* 151: 640–646

7 Armstrong, B. 2008. Measurement error,. In: D. Baker and M. J. Nieuwenhuijsen (eds.): *Environmental Epidemiology: Study Methods and Application*. OUP, Oxford, 93–112

8 Cullinan, P., D. Lowson, M. J. Nieuwenhuijsen, S. Gordon, R. D. Tee, K. M. Venables, J. C. McDonald, and A. J. Newman Taylor. 1994. Work related symptoms, sensitisation, and estimated exposure in workers not previously exposed to laboratory rats. *Occup Environ Med* 51: 589–592

9 Lincoln, T. A., N. E. Bolton, and A. S. Garrett, Jr. 1974. Occupational allergy to animal dander and sera. *J Occup Med* 16: 465–469

10 Lutsky, I. I. and I. Neuman. 1975. Laboratory animal dander allergy: I. An occupational disease. *Ann Allergy* 35: 201–205

11 Taylor G, Davies GE, Altounyan REC, Morrow Brown H, Frankalnd AW, Morrison Smith J, and Winch R. Allergic reactions to laboratory animals. *Nature* 260, 280. 1976

12 Gross, N. J. 1980. Allergy to laboratory animals: Epidemiologic, clinical, and physiologic aspects, and a trial of cromolyn in its management. *J Allergy Clin Immunol* 66: 158–165

13 Cockcroft, A., J. Edwards, P. McCarthy, and N. Andersson. 1981. Allergy in laboratory animal workers. *Lancet* 1: 827–830

14 Davies, G. E. and L. A. McArdle. 1981. Allergy to laboratory animals: A survey by questionnaire. *Int Arch Allergy Appl Immunol* 64: 302–307

15 Schumacher, M. J., B. D. Tait, and M. C. Holmes. 1981. Allergy to murine antigens in a biological research institute. *J Allergy Clin Immunol* 68: 310–318

16 Slovak, A. J. and R. N. Hill. 1981. Laboratory animal allergy: A clinical survey of an exposed population. *Br J Ind Med* 38: 38–41

17 Beeson, M. F., J. M. Dewdney, R. G. Edwards, D. Lee, and R. G. Orr. 1983. Prevalence and diagnosis of laboratory animal allergy. *Clin Allergy* 13: 433–442

18 Agrup, G., L. Belin, L. Sjostedt, and S. Skerfving. 1986. Allergy to laboratory animals in laboratory technicians and animal keepers. *Br J Ind Med* 43: 192–198

19 Bland, S. M., M. S. Levine, P. D. Wilson, N. L. Fox, and J. C. Rivera. 1986. Occupational allergy to laboratory animals: An epidemiologic study. *J Occup Med* 28: 1151–1157

20 Lutsky, I. I., G. L. Baum, H. Teichtahl, A. Mazar, F. Aizer, and S. Bar-Sela. 1986. Respiratory disease in animal house workers. *Eur J Respir Dis* 69: 29–35

21 Platts-Mills, T. A., J. Longbottom, J. Edwards, A. Cockroft, and S. Wilkins. 1987. Occupational asthma and rhinitis related to laboratory rats: Serum IgG and IgE antibodies to the rat urinary allergen. *J Allergy Clin Immunol* 79: 505–515

22 Venables, K. M., R. D. Tee, E. R. Hawkins, D. J. Gordon, C. J. Wale, N. M. Farrer, T. H. Lam, P. J. Baxter, and A. J. Newman Taylor. 1988. Laboratory animal allergy in a pharmaceutical company. *Br J Ind Med* 45: 660–666

23 Venables, K. M., J. L. Upton, E. R. Hawkins, R. D. Tee, J. L. Longbottom, and A. J. Newman Taylor. 1988. Smoking, atopy, and laboratory animal allergy. *Br J Ind Med* 45: 667–671

24 Aoyama, K., A. Ueda, F. Manda, T. Matsushita, T. Ueda, and C. Yamauchi. 1992. Allergy to laboratory animals: An epidemiological study. *Br J Ind Med* 49: 41–47

25 Bryant, D. H., L. M. Boscato, P. N. Mboloi, and M. C. Stuart. 1995. Allergy to laboratory animals among animal handlers. *Med J Aust* 163: 415–418

26 Hollander, A., G. Doekes, and D. Heederik. 1996. Cat and dog allergy and total IgE as risk factors of laboratory animal allergy. *J Allergy Clin Immunol* 98: 545–554

27 Hollander, A., P. Van Run, J. Spithoven, D. Heederik, and G. Doekes. 1997. Exposure of laboratory animal workers to airborne rat and mouse urinary allergens. *Clin Exp Allergy* 27: 617–626

28 Heederik, D., K. M. Venables, P. Malmberg, A. Hollander, A. S. Karlsson, A. Renstrom, G. Doekes, M. Nieuwenhijsen, and S. Gordon. 1999. Exposure-response relationships for work-related sensitization in workers exposed to rat urinary allergens: Results from a pooled study. *J Allergy Clin Immunol* 103: 678–684

29 Lieutier-Colas, F., P. Meyer, F. Pons, G. Hedelin, P. Larsson, P. Malmberg, G. Pauli, and F. De Blay. 2002. Prevalence of symptoms, sensitization to rats, and airborne exposure to major rat allergen (Rat n 1) and to endotoxin in rat-exposed workers: A cross-sectional study. *Clin Exp Allergy* 32: 1424–1429

30 Ruoppi, P., T. Koistinen, P. Susitaival, J. Honkanen, and H. Soininen. 2004. Frequency of allergic rhinitis to laboratory animals in university employees as confirmed by chamber challenges. *Allergy* 59: 295–301

31 Jeal, H., A. Draper, J. Harris, A. N. Taylor, P. Cullinan, and M. Jones. 2006. Modified Th2 responses at high-dose exposures to allergen: Using an occupational model. *Am J Respir Crit Care Med* 174: 21–25

32 Krakowiak, A., M. Wiszniewska, P. Krawczyk, B. Szulc, T. Wittczak, J. Walusiak, and C. Palczynski. 2007. Risk factors associated with airway allergic diseases from exposure to laboratory animal allergens among veterinarians. *Int Arch Occup Environ Health* 80: 465–475

33 Hewitt, R. S., A. D. Smith, J. O. Cowan, J. C. Schofield, G. P. Herbison, and D. R. Taylor. 2008. Serial exhaled nitric oxide measurements in the assessment of laboratory animal allergy. *J Asthma* 45: 101–107

34 Folletti, I., A. Forcina, A. Marabini, A. Bussetti, and A. Siracusa. 2008. Have the prevalence and incidence of occupational asthma and rhinitis because of laboratory animals declined in the last 25 years? *Allergy* 63: 834–841

35 Elliott, L., D. Heederik, S. Marshall, D. Peden, and D. Loomis. 2005. Incidence of allergy and allergy symptoms among workers exposed to laboratory animals. *Occup Environ Med* 62: 766–771

36 Botham, P. A., G. E. Davies, and E. L. Teasdale. 1987. Allergy to laboratory animals: A prospective study of its incidence and of the influence of atopy on its development. *Br J Ind Med* 44: 627–632

37 Davies, G. E., A. V. Thompson, Z. Niewola, G. E. Burrows, E. L. Teasdale, D. J. Bird, and D. A. Phillips. 1983. Allergy to laboratory animals: A retrospective and a prospective study. *Br J Ind Med* 40: 442–449

38 Kibby, T., G. Powell, and J. Cromer. 1989. Allergy to laboratory animals: A prospective and cross-sectional study. *J Occup Med* 31: 842–846

39 Das, R., I. B. Tager, T. Gamsky, M. B. Schenker, S. Royce, and J. R. Balmes. 1992. Atopy and airways reactivity in animal health technicians. A pilot study. *J Occup Med* 34: 53–60

40 Renstrom, A., P. Malmberg, K. Larsson, P. H. Larsson, and B. M. Sundblad. 1995. Allergic sensitization is associated with increased bronchial responsiveness: A prospective study of allergy to laboratory animals. *Eur Respir J* 8: 1514–1519

41 Kruize, H., W. Post, D. Heederik, B. Martens, A. Hollander, and B. E. van der. 1997. Respiratory allergy in laboratory animal workers: A retrospective cohort study using pre-employment screening data. *Occup Environ Med* 54: 830–835

42 Fisher, R., W. B. Saunders, S. J. Murray, and G. M. Stave. 1998. Prevention of laboratory animal allergy. *J Occup Environ Med* 40: 609–613

43 Cullinan, P., A. Cook, S. Gordon, M. J. Nieuwenhuijsen, R. D. Tee, K. M. Venables, J. C. McDonald, and A. J. Taylor. 1999. Allergen exposure, atopy and smoking as determinants of allergy to rats in a cohort of laboratory employees. *Eur Respir J* 13: 1139–1143

44 Gautrin, D., C. Infante-Rivard, H. Ghezzo, and J. L. Malo. 2001. Incidence and host determinants of probable occupational asthma in apprentices exposed to laboratory animals. *Am J Respir Crit Care Med* 163: 899–904

45 Rodier, F., D. Gautrin, H. Ghezzo, and J. L. Malo. 2003. Incidence of occupational rhinoconjunctivitis and risk factors in animal-health apprentices. *J Allergy Clin Immunol* 112: 1105–1111

46 de, M. G., D. S. Postma, and D. Heederik. 2003. Bronchial responsiveness to adenosine-5'-monophosphate and methacholine as predictors for nasal symptoms due to newly introduced allergens. A follow-up study among laboratory animal workers and bakery apprentices. *Clin Exp Allergy* 33: 789–794

47 Draper, A., T. A. Newman, and P. Cullinan. 2003. Estimating the incidence of occupational asthma and rhinitis from laboratory animal allergens in the UK, 1999–2000. *Occup Environ Med* 60: 604–605

48 McDonald, J. C., H. L. Keynes, and S. K. Meredith. 2000. Reported incidence of occupational asthma in the United Kingdom, 1989–97. *Occup Environ Med* 57: 823–829

49 Ameille, J., G. Pauli, A. Calastreng-Crinquand, D. Vervloet, Y. Iwatsubo, E. Popin, M. C. Bayeux-Dunglas, and M. C. Kopferschmitt-Kubler. 2003. Reported incidence of occupational asthma in France, 1996–99: The ONAP programme. *Occup Environ Med* 60: 136–141

50 Karjalainen, A., K. Kurppa, S. Virtanen, H. Keskinen, and H. Nordman. 2000. Incidence of occupational asthma by occupation and industry in Finland. *Am J Ind Med* 37: 451–458

51 Esterhuizen, T. M., E. Hnizdo, D. Rees, U. G. Lalloo, D. Kielkowski, E. M. van Schalkwyk, N. White, F. C. Smith, B. Hoggins, and T. Curtis. 2001. Occupational respiratory diseases in South Africa--results from SORDSA, 1997–1999. *S Afr Med J* 91: 502–508

52 Provencher, S., F. P. Labreche, and L. De Guire. 1997. Physician based surveillance system for occupational respiratory diseases: The experience of PROPULSE, Quebec, Canada. *Occup Environ Med* 54: 272–276

53 Orriols, R., R. Costa, M. Albanell, C. Alberti, J. Castejon, E. Monso, R. Panades, N. Rubira, and J. P. Zock. 2006. Reported occupational respiratory diseases in Catalonia. *Occup Environ Med* 63: 255–260

54 Elder, D., M. Abramson, D. Fish, A. Johnson, D. McKenzie, and M. Sim. 2004. Surveillance of Australian workplace Based Respiratory Events (SABRE): Notifications for the first 3.5 years and validation of occupational asthma cases. *Occup Med (Lond)* 54: 395–399

55 Nieuwenhuijsen, M. J., S. Gordon, J. M. Harris, R. D. Tee, K. M. Venables, and A. J. Newman Taylor. 1995. Variation in rat urinary aeroallergen levels explained by differences in site, task and exposure group. *Ann Occup Hyg* 39: 819–825

56 Slovak, A. J. and R. N. Hill. 1987. Does atopy have any predictive value for laboratory animal allergy? A comparison of different concepts of atopy. *Br J Ind Med* 44: 129–132

57 Meijer, E., D. E. Grobbee, and D. Heederik. 2004. A strategy for health surveillance in laboratory animal workers exposed to high molecular weight allergens. *Occup Environ Med* 61: 831–837

58 Low, B., L. Sjostedt, and S. Willers. 1988. Laboratory animal allergy – Possible association with HLA B15 and DR4. *Tissue Antigens* 31: 224–226

59 Kerwin, E. M., J. H. Freed, J. K. Dresback, and L. J. Rosenwasser. 1993. HLA DR4,DRw11(5), and DR17(3) function as restriction elements for Mus m1 allergic human t cells. *J Allergy Clin Immunol* 91: 235

60 Jeal, H., A. Draper, M. Jones, J. Harris, K. Welsh, A. N. Taylor, and P. Cullinan. 2003. HLA associations with occupational sensitization to rat lipocalin allergens: A model for other animal allergies? *J Allergy Clin Immunol* 111: 795–799

Population-attributable fraction for occupation and asthma

Kjell Torén[1] *and Paul D. Blanc*[2]

[1]Department of Occupational and Environmental Medicine, Sahlgrenska University Hospital, Göteborg, Sweden
[2]Division of Occupational and Environmental Medicine, University of California San Francisco, San Francisco, California, USA

Abstract

Here we review the use of the concept of population-attributable risk (PAR) of asthma associated with occupation and give the context for its interpretation. For asthma there is major interest in delineating the "burden of disease", because such assessments can inform health care priorities, intervention policies, and assessment of impact once such steps are implemented. For asthma, the burden of disease from occupational factors is of particular relevance because asthma is a common disease that affects persons of working age and because asthma can be associated with major morbidity and economic cost. In 1999, we carried out a systematic review of the published literature relevant to the occupational PAR in asthma. Of 23 published PAR estimates identified, the median value was 9%, but among those, the 10 estimates based on population-based studies yielded a median PAR estimate of 15%. A few years later a task force of the American Thoracic Society (ATS) summarized the general population-based studies in this field, ending up with a median value of 15%. We have summarized data from publications that have appeared since 2000 and the median value from these publications is 14.4% (range 6–31%).

We show in this analysis that 3 in 20 cases of asthma among adults are likely to be linked to occupational factors. Longitudinal incidence-based estimates, which should be the most reliable, suggest that, if anything, the actual PAR may even be higher. Other measures such as impaired quality of life and economic disadvantage are also important, but are not addressed in this review as there is lack of studies. This points to future research needs to address this knowledge gap in the field of work-related asthma. In the meantime, the consistency of the PAR data that we do have certainly underscores the importance of workplace factors in the overall burden of asthma.

Introduction

The aim of this chapter on the population-attributable risk (PAR) of asthma associated with occupation is to provide both the data germane to this topic and a context for its interpretation. For chronic conditions generally, there is major interest in delineating the "burden of disease", because such assessments can inform health care priorities, intervention policies, and assessment of impact once such steps are implemented. For asthma, estimating the burden of disease from occupational

Occupational Asthma, edited by Torben Sigsgaard and Dick Heederik

factors is of particular relevance because asthma is a common disease that affects persons of working age and because asthma can be associated with major morbidity and economic cost. Moreover, certain agents have long been recognized to cause new-onset asthma among persons exposed at work, making occupational asthma a widely recognized medical entity. Because of these factors, there is considerable accumulated evidence pertinent to the population burden of asthma attributable to occupation. In this chapter, we first address general epidemiological aspects of attributable risk estimation. We then review the body of evidence that yields such attributable risk estimates, summarizing previous systematic reviews of the literature and presenting data from key analyses that have appeared in the last 10 years. Finally, we place these data in their public health context.

Estimating PAR

The relative risk (RR) and the odds ratio (OR), the two risk measures most widely familiar to non-epidemiologists, compare the likelihoods of disease among exposed as opposed to non-exposed groups. The measure "population-attributable risk", PAR, is a less familiar construct and, to a certain extent, a less intuitive one. The PAR takes into account both comparative risk (RR or OR) and the frequency of exposure in the population studied. Based on these two components, or risk and exposure, the PAR estimates the proportion of the disease burden among exposed people that is likely to have been caused by the exposure of interest. The PAR is commonly interpreted as the amount of disease that would be prevented (the reduced burden) were the risk factor in question to be removed altogether.

A synonymous term, "population-attributable fraction" (PAF) is preferred by some authors; the expanded term PAR percent also is frequently used. In addition to a lack of familiarity with the construct and inconsistencies in terminology (PAR, PAR%, PAF) that can lead to unnecessary confusion, PAR estimates have other attributes that further complicate their interpretation. As noted above, the PAR estimation can utilize either an RR or OR value in its calculation, but the exposure prevalence (which is a major driver in the ultimate value derived) also has two variants: either the proportion of cases exposed or the overall population exposure rate. Provided that either the RR or OR and that either the case exposure rate or overall exposure proportion has been provided, then the PAR can be estimated *post hoc* from a published study, even if it failed to include an explicit PAR calculation. If the RR or OR used is derived from a multivariate predictive model, then the point estimate of the PAR does reflect the role of any confounding variables included in the model. *Post hoc* calculations without access to the original data set, however, cannot take into account the variance of such covariates, and thus cannot estimate confidence intervals (CI) around PAR estimates derived from published risk and exposure values.

A key attribute of the PAR metric is that, for any given outcome with multiple risk factors, the sum of the estimated risk factors derived form a multivariate model can add up to more the 100% of the risk [1]. This phenomenon is consistent with the effects of risk factors that are inter-related in a more than additive fashion. Although there are no established examples of this in the case of occupational asthma, such a relationship could be possible in the example of estimates for the PAR for chronic obstructive pulmonary disease (COPD) associated with occupation and smoking [2]. There are also other conceptual as well as computational nuances to the estimation and interpretation of attributable risk that are beyond the scope of this chapter; these issues are addressed in a seminal paper by Greenland and Robbins, as well as in a recent review by Benichou [3, 4].

It should also be kept in view that estimates of proportional attribution can be arrived at by other means, although the limitations of such approaches have to be taken into consideration. This is particularly relevant to the occupational asthma literature where incident occupational asthma may be estimated based on a clinically cased attribution, and the "numerator" so generated is divided by the general incidence of asthma from all causes. This proportion can be approached as one form of attributable risk estimate, bearing in mind the limitations of under-diagnosis or over-attribution. Using occupational asthma surveillance data for the numerator in such an exercise (taking the denominator from age-equivalent population incidence) is especially fraught with limitations of under-diagnosis (under-reporting).

Previous systematic reviews of occupationally associated PAR for asthma

In 1999, we carried out a systematic review of the published biomedical literature dating back to 1966 relevant to the occupational PAR in asthma [5]. This review applied very generous inclusion criteria that captured full publications including PAR estimates and those that only provide data that allowed *post hoc* calculation, as well as published letters and abstracts and even consensus-based estimates in reviews. Of 23 published PAR estimates identified the median values was 9%, but among those, the 10 estimates based on population-based studies yielded a median PAR estimate of 15%. A series of estimates derived *post hoc* from 8 other population-based studies yielded a somewhat higher median PAR value of 20%. Because of the heterogeneity of the data set, we also applied a quality rating schema to the publications. This yield a weighted mean PAR of 15% ($n=28$ values, excluding 3 non-data-based estimates); the median PAR value among the 12 studies that scored highest in quality was also 15%. Finally, we also extrapolated PAR estimates based on surveillance data for occupational data from 12 systems and presuming an adult general incidence of 1 per 1000 per year. The median PAR extrapolation using that approach was 5%. Of note, in that subset, Finish surveillance-based data yield an extrapolation close to overall central tendency of the data, in the 14–17% range.

Shortly after that systematic review appeared, a task force of the ATS embarked on a similar data synthesis intended to summarize the general population-based studies in this field. This eventually led to the formal adoption (2002) of a statement, *Occupational Contribution to the Burden of Airway Disease* [6]. The ATS systematic review used stricter selection criteria, excluding consensus estimates, letters, and abstracts. Many, but not all of the publications in the ATS review also had been included in the previous review. Even with this different approach, however, the PAR estimates for asthma summarized in the ATS statement also yielded a median value of 15%.

The ATS estimate of 15% was based on 21 different publications. Of these, 7 were asthma cohorts or case series in which the estimated occupational contribution was not based on an epidemiological estimate, but rather the proportion of occupationally attributed cases to all asthma cases. The remaining 14 studies were all population-based and either reported a PAR estimate or provided data from which a PAR estimate could be calculated for the purposes of the ATS review. Table 1 lists the findings from those 14 studies, many of which were quite large in size [7–20]. One study was based on an analyses of the European Community Respiratory Health Survey (ECRHS I), including 22 countries from three continents [7]. The range of the PAR was wide from 5% to 51%, with a mean value of 19.5%.

Table 1. The occupational contribution to the burden of asthma. General population studies reviewed in the ATS document

Endpoints	**Number of studies**	**PAR median**	**PAR range**	**Reference**
Bronchial hyperreactivity and symptoms	1	10%	NA	[7]
Clinical diagnosis	6	34.5%	5–51%	[8–13]
Self-reported asthma, including physician-diagnosed	7	19%	15–29%	[14–20]
Total	14	19.5%	5–51%	[7–20]

Recent longitudinal studies of PAR

The variability in previous PAR estimates, even with a central tendency in the 15–20% range (depending on the study range included) underscores the value in evaluating additional relevant studies that have appeared in the interim. Because we have the benefit of such a rich data set of previously analyzed material, the field has sufficiently evolved so that more restricted analysis is appropriate. To that end, we emphasize here estimates derived from general population sampling. Moreover, we highlight in particular data obtained through longitudinal follow-up, as opposed to cross-sectional analyses.

Table 2 summarizes the data from 12 publications relevant to occupational risk for asthma based on general population studies or other systematic recruitment that have appeared since 2000 [21–32]. Overall, the studies summarized in Table 2 support and amplify the findings of the earlier ATS statement. In total, these studies represent 51 294 subjects, excluding the large longitudinal cohort study from Finland, which included 829 351 additional subjects [25]. For the data shown in Table 2, we derived all of the PAR estimates, based either on the published PAR value or by calculating the PAR using the published risk estimates and exposure proportions according to the same methods that were also used in the ATS statement [6].

Three of the studies (Tab. 2) are prospective longitudinal investigations, based on follow-up of previous general population samples [21, 24, 25]. The Norwegian study represents a follow-up of a general population sample of 3886 subjects investigated in 1985 [21]. The age at study baseline in 1985 ranged from 15 to 70 years. The study participants were investigated 10 years later, 1996, with a new questionnaire that was completed by 2819 subjects (89% of the baseline group). Asthma at follow-up was defined as an affirmative answer to "having been hospitalized or treated by a physician for asthma". The occupational exposure was defined by the self-report questionnaire item "Have you ever had a workplace with much dust or fumes in the air?" The exposure prevalence was 28%, with a considerable difference between males (44%) and females (13%). The risk for incident asthma during follow-up in relation to ever exposed to dust or fumes was analyzed using logistic regression models, yielding a 60% increased odds of disease associated with exposure (OR 1.6, 95% CI 1.01–2.5). The PAR associated with dust or fumes and incident asthma, presented in the published paper, was 14.4% (95% CI 1.2–27.6). Risk estimates stratified by sex were not included. Strengths of this study, over and above its relatively large, population-based cohort, include the longitudinal design, thus assessing incident asthma, the high subject retention rate, mitigating selection effects, and the provision of a PAR estimates that includes 95% CI values. Because the exposure and incident asthma occurred over the follow-up period is not analyzed in terms of specific time points, a potential study weakness lies in lack of a temporal anchor (i.e., in some cases exposure might have followed disease onset). Because of job stability and the low likelihood that persons with asthma will migrate from low exposure to high exposure jobs this concern is more theoretical than practical. In addition, risk estimates stratified by sex were not provided. Other weaknesses include the lack of sex-stratified risk estimates and the reliance on a single exposure metric.

The second study with high quality is the follow-up analysis of the European Respiratory Health Survey (ECRHS II) [24]. The ECRHS is an international cross-

Table 2. The occupational contribution to the burden of asthma: Population-based studies published since 2000

Ref.	N	Design	Country	Asthma definition	Occupational exposure	PAR
21	2819	Longi-tudinal cohort	Norway	Self report of physician-diagnosed asthma	Self-reported exposure to much dust or fumes	14.4%
22	13826	Cross-sectional cohort	South Africa	Self report of physician or nurse diagnosed asthma	Ever regularly exposed to smoke, dust, fumes or strong smells or worked underground in a mine	13.6%
23	1922	Cross-sectional cohort	Brazil	BHR and work-related asthma symptoms	Self-reported exposure to vapor, gas, fumes, chemical products, paints and humidity	22.9%
24	6837 (3994, BHR tested subset)	Longi-tudinal cohort	Inter-national	Asthma symptoms or asthma medication; above definition + BHR	Job Exposure Matrix defined occupational risk	11% 23% Med = 17%
25	892351	Longi-tudinal cohort of all employed Finns	Finland	Physician diagnosis based on asthma symptoms and at least one criteria of airway reversibility	Occupations a priori classified as exposed	29% (Males) 17% (Females) Weighted = 22%
26	5331	Cross-sectional cohort	New Zealand	Self-report of physician-diagnosed, adult-onset asthma	Occupations a priori classified as exposed	9.5%
27	14151	Cross-sectional cohort	France	Dyspnea with wheezing or asthma attacks; asthma onset after start of current job	Self reported exposure; occupations a priori classified as exposed using a JEM	9%, 14%; 1%; 3% Med = 6%
28	376	Cross-sectional case control	France	Specialist physician diagnosis	Occupations a priori classified as exposed using a JEM	10%
29, 30	6827	Cross-sectional cohort	USA	Self-report of physician-diagnosed asthma and work-related symptoms	Industries a priori classified as exposed; Occupations a priori classified as exposed	36.5%; 26% Med = 31%

Table 2 (continued)

Ref.	N	Design	Country	Asthma definition	Occupational exposure	PAR
31	566	Cross-sectional case control	Sweden	General MD diagnosis	Occupations a priori classified as exposed	18%
32	1482	Cross-sectional cohort	USA	Self-report of MD diagnosis	Self-report of exposure; Occupations a priori classified as exposed using a JEM	17%; 5% Med = 11%

BHR, Bronchial hyperreactivity measured by methacholine challenge; JEM, job exposure matrix; Med, midpoint or median value

sectional investigation drawing on data from 28 centers in 13 countries. At baseline data collection (1990–1995), each center mailed a questionnaire to 3000 randomly selected subjects aged 20–44 years of age. From the responders there was further selection of a random smaller sample and a sample enriched with subjects with asthma and asthma symptoms. At baseline, a cross-sectional analysis was performed observing increased risks for asthma among farmers, painters and cleaners, and this was included in the ATS review [6]. Ten years later, follow-up was performed in which the participants completed extensive questionnaires including detailed occupational histories covering interval job duties and potential exposures. Subjects with asthma, wheezing and dyspnea at baseline were excluded from the analysis in order to study incident disease. Asthma during follow-up was defined in several ways, but the most restrictive definition used reporting an asthma attack or having used asthma medication in the 12 months preceding the follow-up interview, in combination with a positive methacholine-challenge test at the follow-up visit. Work-related exposure was assessed by linking the occupations held during follow-up to an asthma-specific job-exposure matrix (JEM) used in the previous cross-sectional analyses. A second measure of risk was based on broadly classified "high-risk" occupations. The reported PAR of the JEM-classified occupational exposure for new-onset asthma was 23% (95% CI 1–40%). The broader occupational risk definition yielded a slightly higher PAR estimate of 26%. Using a less strict definition of asthma that did not include methacholine responsiveness, the estimated PAR (JEM-based exposures) was 11% (95% CI 1–20%). This analysis allowed utilization of a larger study number (6788 vs 3994). The strengths of this study, in addition to its large, international scope and its longitudinal design, include the multiple measures of exposure and the conservative (as well as more liberal) definitions of disease. One limitation in the ECRHS is its low overall follow-up successful response rate of 58%, and the further loss of subjects in the methacholine-based analyses. In addition, CIs for the PAR estimates were not provided nor was PAR estimated for sex-specific strata.

The Finnish study included in Table 2 was based on follow-up of three cohorts of employed Finns aged 25–59 years at baseline [25]. The cohorts were defined 1985, 1990 and 1995 and followed for 5 years each. Hence, by design these cohorts do not overlap in time. Onset of asthma during follow-up was obtained from a National Register for Reimbursement, based on asthma medication cost coverage. To be qualified for reimbursement, a physician must certify a valid diagnosis of asthma including objective documentation of variable airway obstruction or hyperresponsiveness (reversible FEV_1, serial peak flow measurements, or a positive methacholine-challenge test) and the presence of symptoms consistent with disease. Subjects with asthma at baseline were excluded from the analysis. Work-related exposure was defined on the basis of certain occupations held at baseline and considered *a priori* to carry increased risk of causing asthma. Incidence rates of asthma in each occupation were estimated, and incidence ratios using log-linear models adjusting for age were calculated. The PAR for occupational exposure and new-onset asthma, provided in the published study results, was 29% (95% CI 25–33%) for men and 17% (95% CI 15–19%) for women. This study has high internal and external validity, utilizing national registry data. One weakness is that the study is biased towards more severe asthma, given that only cases reimbursed for medication are included. This is counter-balanced by a reduction in classification error for disease in the direction of non-asthmatics being classified as ill. In addition, the broad, occupation-based exposure is a fairly crude metric. Finally, although the study provides sex-stratified PAR estimates with accompanying CIs, no calculation of attributable risk is provided for males and females combined. A weighted PAR value of 22% can be derived from the data.

Taking the three studies above as yielding the highest quality PAR estimates, the summary values to be considered are: 14%, 11–23% (depending on the asthma definition, the mid-point is 17%) and 22%.

Cross-sectional studies

All of the remaining nine studies whose results are summarized in Table 2 are cross-sectional rather than longitudinal [22, 23, 26–31]. Some yielded multiple PAR estimates using differing measures of exposure or asthma outcome or both, including two published analyses of the same national survey data, one based on industry and one based on occupation [27, 29, 30, 32]. Where multiple PAR values were presented, Table 2 also provides a mid-point (median) value. All but two studies explicitly presented a PAR estimate; the values were calculated for these [23, 28].

The eight summary PAR values yielded by these nine cross-sectional studies range from 6% to 31%, with a median of 12.4%. The heterogeneity in results is not surprising. The definitions of asthma differed considerably. Of particular note, the highest PAR estimate was derived from a study that defined asthma as both the report of a physician's diagnosis and self-report of work-related symptoms; this is treated by the authors as a measure of "work-related asthma" [29, 30]. In general, JEM-based PAR estimates were lower than those based on self-report: 1–3% compared to 9–14% in one study and 5% compared to 17% in another [27, 32].

One the studies shown did not provide risk and exposure data to yield a classic PAR estimate, but rather attributable risk based on the number cases of adult onset asthma with work-related symptoms asthma symptoms and onset of new asthma on that job [23]. The 22.9% PAR in that series is the second highest estimate among the cross-sectional studies. This study is special interest, however, because it represents one of only two estimates from studies in developing economies, the other being a PAR of 13.6% from South Africa [22].

Cross-sectional studies of asthma broadly defined to include onset at any age may be at risk of under-estimating occupational risk. To the extent that persons with life-long asthma either manifest no association with workplace factors or self-select into lower exposure jobs, this will bias to the null or even a negative occupational association. Even limited to adult-onset asthma, cross-sectional analyses ascertaining current occupations rather than the job held at the onset of disease run the risk of survivor bias towards the null. Cross-sectional studies may also face reporting biases if they depend on self-report of exposure, although this phenomenon may be less important that sometimes presumed [33].

If all 11 summary PAR estimates from Table 2 are considered together, the median value is 14.4% (range 6–31%). Once again, this wholly in line with previous ATS estimate.

Other data sources

There are also a few additional reports not included in Table 2 that, nonetheless, should be mentioned. An analysis of the Singapore Chinese Health Study included 52 325 subjects [34]. Although this study does not provide PAR estimates, it does include risk estimates for adult-onset asthma for three categories or workplace exposures; dusts, smokes, and vapors. Although these three exposure categories yield PAR estimates of 2.7,%,1.7% and 4.2%, respectively, it is not clear to what extent the exposure categories overlap and only for vapors does the 95% CI for the OR exclude 1.0.

There have also been two recent U.S. studies of asthma incidence in which an attribution of work-relatedness was made. In one study of incident adult asthma in a large health maintenance organization (HMO) data set (203 701 person years of observation) concluded that 33% of incident asthma (which could include "recurrent" asthma previously in remission) was work-related [35]. Another large HMO study (109 125 person years of observation) found that 24% of the cases had at least moderate evidence of an occupational trigger [36]. These studies have limitations due to subject participation in the structured interviews forming the basis of attribution, a selection effect that may in part account for the relatively high proportional attributions.

Finally, it should be noted that occupational disease registries continue to provide estimates of occupational asthma incidence, which can be used to extrapolate an attributable fraction as a proportion of incidence among all persons of working age. Our 1999 extrapolations used registry and other surveillance data from Canada (British Columbia and Quebec), the U.S. (California and Michigan), the United Kingdom (including Shield and Sword), Finland, Sweden, and Germany [5]. Since that time, surveillance-based data (annual rates per 100000 workers) have been reported from Norway (10.1), France (2.4), Belgium (2.4), Italy (Piedmont region, 2.4), Spain (Catalonia, 7.7), Australia (3.1), New Zealand (3.1), and South Africa (1.3 overall; 3.8 from the Western Cape) [37–44]. Even assuming a relatively low general asthma incidence of 100 per 100000 in adults of working age, these rates would equate to an attributable proportion of only 1–10%. It is well recognized, however, that such registry data fail to capture the majority of true cases. For example, data from Finland indicate that, even after excluding officially recognized occupational asthma cases, excess risk of disease was still evident on epidemiological grounds; the remaining risk was consistent with under-detection of one half to two-thirds of cases proportionally, even for well-recognized risk groups such as bakers, fur workers, and painters [45]. Consistent with this, survey data from three U.S. states found that, although 5.8% to 6.1% of adults with asthma had been told that by a physician that their condition was work related, the total increased to 7.4–9.7% if the respondents own assessment was included, an incremental increase proportionally of up to two-thirds greater prevalence [46]. Thus, it should be presumed that any PAR value extrapolated from registry sources would be a woeful underestimate.

Conclusion

Prior systematic reviews of the literature identified a wide range of estimates for the PAR for occupational exposures in asthma, but with a central tendency close to 15% [5, 6]. As we have shown, emerging data continue to support the estimation that 3 in 20 cases of asthma among adults are likely to be linked to occupational factors. Moreover, longitudinal incidence-based estimates that should be the most reliable suggest that, if anything, the actual PAR may even be higher.

Certain limitations of this analysis should also be borne in mind. First of all, we have not addressed the burden of work-aggravated asthma, i.e., pre-existing asthma made worse by work. Epidemiological analysis of this complex problem is challenging and far beyond the scope of this review. It has been suggested that PAR estimates of exacerbation of chronic disease (e.g., work-aggravated asthma) may also need to take causation into account so that the burden of disease is not underestimated [47].

Beyond this, use of the PAR as a measure of risk itself has been questioned. It is important to remember that a basic assumption is that the relative risk upon which the PAR is based must accurately reflect exposure effects in the target population [3, 48]. Another assumption is that the dichotomous classification of exposure into two levels, exposed and unexposed, yields an unbiased estimate of the PAF when there is non-differential misclassification of exposure, an assumption that has been challenged [49].

Finally, the burden of disease, which the PAR attempts to capture, may transcend simplistic notions of the presence or absence of a diagnosis. One alternative measure of burden is 'disability adjusted life years' (DALYS). To apply this to a specific health condition, such as occupationally related asthma, requires an assumption of the proportional risk. In other words, the PAR as conceptualized above is intrinsically linked to such an exercise. For example, Driscoll et al. [50] presumed an occupational PAF of 21% to estimate a global burden of occupationally associated asthma DALYS of 1 621 000.

Beyond DALYS, which address disability, other manifestations of the burden of disease, such as impaired quality of life and economic disadvantage, are by no means trivial. This points the way to future research, which needs to address this knowledge gap in the field of work-related asthma. In the meantime, the consistency of the PAR data that we do have certainly underscores the importance of workplace factors in the overall burden of asthma.

References

1 Rowe AK, Powell KE, Flanders D. Why population attributable fractions can sum to more than one. *Am J Prev Med* 2004; 26: 243–9

2 Blanc PD, Toren K. Occupation in COPD and chronic bronchitis: An update. *Int J Tuberc Lung Dis* 2007; 11: 251–7

3 Greenland S, Robins JM. Conceptual problems in the definition and interpretation of attributable fractions. *Am J Epidemiol* 1988; 128: 1185–97

4 Benichou J. Biostatistics and epidemiology: Measuring the risk attributable to an environmental or genetic factor. *C R Biologies* 2007; 220: 281–98

5 Blanc PD, Torén K. How much adult asthma can be attributed to occupational factors? *Am J Med* 1999; 107: 580–587

6 Balmes J, Becklake M, Blanc P, Henneberger P, Kreiss K, Mapp C, Milton D, Schwartz D, Torén K, Viegi G. American Thoracic Society Statement: Occupational contribution to the burden of airway disease. *Am J Respir Crit Care Med* 2003; 167: 787–797

7 Kogevinas M, Antó JM, Sunyer J, Tobias A, Kromhout H, Burney P. A population-based study on occupational asthma in Europe and other industrialised countries. *Lancet* 1999; 353: 1750–1754

8 Ng TP, Hong CY, Koh KTC, Ling SL. Risk of asthma associated with occupation in a community-based case-control study. *Am J Ind Med* 1994; 25: 709–718

9 Isoaho R, Puolijoki H, Huhti E, Kivelä SL, Tala E. Prevalence of asthma in elderly Finns. *J Clin Epidemiol* 1994; 47: 1109–1118

10 Flodin U, Ziegler J, Jönsson P, Axelson O. Bronchial asthma and air pollution at workplaces. *Scand J Work Environ Health* 1996; 22: 451–456

11 Reijula K, Haahtela T, Klaukka T, Rantanen J. Incidence of occupational asthma and persistent asthma in young adults has increased in Finland. *Chest* 1996; 110: 50–61

12 Torén K, Balder B, Brisman J, Lindholm N, Löwhagen O, Palmqvist M, Tunsäter A. The risk of asthma in relation to occupational exposures: A case-control study. *Eur Respir J* 1999; 13: 496–501

13 Katz I, Moshe I, Sosna J. The occurrence, recrudescence and worsening of asthma in a population of young adults. *Chest* 1999; 116: 614–618

14 Blanc PD. Occupational asthma in a national disability survey. *Chest* 1987; 92: 613–617

15 Viegi G, Prediletto R, Paoletti P, Carozzi L, di Pede F, Vellutini M, di Pede C, Giuntini C, Lebowitz M. Respiratory effects of occupational exposure in a general population sample in North Italy. *Am Rev Respir Dis* 1991; 143: 510–515

16 Bakke P, Eide GE, Hanoa G, Gulsvik A. Occupational dust or gas exposure and the prevalences of respiratory symptoms and asthma in the general population. *Eur Respir J* 1991; 4: 273–278

17 Xu X, Christiani D. Occupational exposures and physician-diagnosed asthma. *Chest* 1993; 104: 1364–1370

18 Neijari C, Tessier JF, Letenneur L, Datigues JF, Salamon R. Prevalence of self-reported asthma symptoms in a French elderly sample. *Respir Med* 1996; 90: 401–408

19 Monso E, Munoz-Rino F, Izquierdo J, Roca J, Masia N, Rosell A, Morera J. Occupational asthma in the community: Risk factors in a western Mediterranean population. *Arch Environ Health* 1998; 53: 93–98

20 Forastiere F, Balmes J, Scarinci M, Tager IB. Occupations, asthma and chronic respiratory symptoms in a community sample of older women. *Am J Respir Crit Care Med* 1998; 157: 1864–1870

21 Eagan T, Gulsvik A, Eide GE, Bakke PS. Occupational airborne exposure and the incidence of respiratory symptoms and asthma. *Am J Respir Crit Care Med* 2002; 166: 933–938

22 Ehrlich RI, White N, Norman R, Laubscher R, Steyn K, Lombard C, Bradshaw D. Wheeze, asthma diagnosis and medication use: A national adult survey in a developing country. *Thorax* 2005; 60: 895–901

23 Caldeira RD, Bettiol H, Barboeri MA, Terra-Filho J, Garcia CA, Vianna EO. Prevalence

and risk factors for work related asthma in young adults. *Occup Environ Med* 2006; 63: 694–699

24 Kogevinas M, Zock J-P, Jarvis D, Kromhout H, Lillienberg L, Plana E, Radon K, Torén K, Allikso A, Benke G, et al. Exposure to substances in the workplace and new-onset asthma: An international prospective population-based study (ECRHS-II). *Lancet* 2007; 370: 336–341

25 Karjalainen A, Kurppa K, Martikainen R, Klaukka T, Karjalainen K. Work is related to a substantial portion of adult-onset asthma incidence in the Finnish population. *Am J Respir Crit Care Med* 2001; 164: 565–568

26 Johnson A, Toelle BG, Yates D, Belousova E, Ng K, Corbett S, Marks G. Occupational asthma in New South Wales (NSW): A population-based study. *Occup Med* 2006; 56: 258–262

27 Le Moual N, Kennedy SM, Kauffmann F. Occupational exposures and asthma in 14,000 adults from the general population. *Am J Epidemiol* 2004; 160: 1108–1116

28 Kennedy SM, Le Moual N, Choudat D, Kauffmann F. Development of an asthma specific job exposure matrix and its application in the epidemiological study of genetic and environment in asthma (EGEA). *Occup Environ Med* 2000; 57: 635–41

29 Arif AA, Whitehead LW, Delclos GL, Tortolero SR, Lee ES. Prevalence and risk factors of work-related asthma by industry among united Sates workers: Data from the third national health and nutrition examination survey (1988–94). *Occup Environ Med* 2002; 59: 505–511

30 Arif AA, Delclos GL, Whitehead LW, Tortolero SR, Lee ES. Occupational exposures associated with work-related asthma and wheezing among U.S. workers. *Am J Ind Med* 2003; 44: 368–76

31 Flodin U, Jönsson P. Non-sensitizing air pollution at workplaces and adult-onset asthma. *Int Arch Occup Environ Health* 2004; 77: 17–22

32 Blanc PD, Eisner MD, Balmes JR, Trupin L, Yelin EH, Katz PP. Exposure to vapours, gas, dust or fumes: Assessment by a single survey item compared to a detailed exposure battery and a job exposure matrix. *Am J Ind Med* 2005; 48: 110–117

33 Quinlan PJ., Earnest G, Eisner MD, Yelin EH, Katz PP, Balmes JR, Blanc PD. Performance of self-reported occupational exposure compared to a job exposure matrix approach in asthma and chronic rhinitis. *Occup Environ Med* 2009; 66: 154–160

34 LeVan TD, Koh W-P, Lee H-P, Koh D, Yu MC, London SJ. Vapor, dust, and smoke exposure in relation to adult-onset asthma and chronic respiratory symptoms. *Am J Epidemiol* 2006; 163: 1118–28

35 Vollmer WM, Heumann MA, Breen VR, Henneberger PK, O'Connor EA, Villnave JM, Frazier EA, Buist AS. Incidence of work-related asthma in members of a health maintenance organization. *J Occup Environ Med* 2005; 47: 1292–97

36 Sama SR, Milton DK, Hunt PR, Houseman EA, Henneberger PK, Rosiello RA. Case-by-case assessment of adult-onset asthma attributable to occupational exposures among members of a health maintenance organization. *J Occup Environ Med* 2006; 48: 400–407

37 Leira HL, Bratt U, Slåstad S. Notified cases of occupational asthma in Norway: Exposure and health consequences for health and income. *Am J Ind Med* 2005; 48: 359–64

38 Amielle J, Pauli G, Calastren-Crinquand A, Vervloët D, Iwatsubo Y, Popin E, et al. Reported incidence of occupational asthma in France, 1996–99: The ONAP program. *Occup Environ Med* 2003; 60: 136–41

39 Vandenplas O, Larbanois A, Bugli C, Kempeneers E, Nemery B. Épidémiologie de l'asthme professionel en Belgique. *Rev Mal Respir* 2005; 22: 421–30

40 Bena A, D'Errico A, Mirabelli D. Un sistema di rilevazione atriva dell'asma bronchiale professionale: I resultati di due anni di attività del programma PRiOR. *Med Lav* 1999; 90: 4: 556–571

41 Orriols R, Costa R, Albanell M, Alberti C, Castejon J, Monso E, et al. Reported occupational respiratory diseases in Catalonia. *Occup Environ Med* 2006; 63: 255–260

42 Elder D, Abramson M, Fish D, Johnson A., McKenzie D, Sim M. Surveillance of Australian workplace Based Respiratory Events (SABRE): Notifications for the first 3.5 years and validation of occupational asthma cases. *Occup Med* 2004; 54: 395–00

43 Walls C, Crane J, Gillies J, Wilsher M, Wong C. Occupational asthma cases notified to OSH from 1996 to 1999. *N Z Med J* 2000; 113: 491–2

44 Hnizdo E, Esterhuizen TM, Rees D, Lalloo UG. Occupational asthma as identified by the Surveillance of Work-related and Occupational Respiratory Diseases programme in South Africa. *Clin Expir Allergy* 2001; 31: 32–9

45 Karjalainen A, Kurppa K, Martikainen R, Karjalainen J, Klaukka T. Exploration of asthma risk by occupation – Extended analysis of an incidence study of the Finnish population. *Scand J Work Environ Health* 2002; 28: 49–57

46 Flattery J, Davis L, Roseman KD, Harrison R, Lyon-Callo S, Filios M. The proportion of self-reported asthma associated with work in three states: California, Massachusetts, and Michigan, 2001. *J Asthma* 2006; 43: 213–8

47 Kunzli N, Perez L, Lurmann F, Hricko A, Penfld B, McConnell R. An attributable risk model for exposures assumed to cause both chronic disease and its exacerbations. *Epidemiology* 2008; 19: 179–85

48 Greenland S. Attributable fractions: Bias from broad definition of exposure. *Epidemiology* 2001; 12: 518–520

49 Wacholder S, Benichou J, Heineman EF, Hartge P, Hoover RN. Attributable risk: Advantages of a broad definition of exposure. *Am J Epidemiol* 1994; 140: 303–309

50 Driscoll T, Nelson DI, Steenland K, Leigh J, Concha-Barrientos M, Fingerhut M, Prüss-Üstün A. The global burden of non-malignant respiratory disease due to occupational airborne exposures. *Am J Ind Med* 2005; 48; 432–45

Definition and diagnosis of occupational asthma

André Cartier

University of Montreal, Department of Medicine, Hôpital du Sacré-Coeur de Montréal, 5400 Boul. Gouin Ouest, Montréal, Canada

Abstract

Occupational asthma is a disease characterized by variable airflow limitation and/or hyperresponsiveness and/or inflammation due to causes and conditions attributable to a particular occupational environment and not to stimuli encountered outside the workplace. Two types of occupational asthma are distinguished based on their appearance after a latency period or not: the classical occupational asthma requiring a period of sensitization and irritant-induced asthma occurring after acute exposure to high concentrations of irritants. The diagnosis of occupational asthma should be based on objective means and cannot rely only on history (which is, although very sensitive, not sufficiently specific) or even on confirming the presence of asthma with positive skin tests to the relevant allergen/agent found at work. Inquiring about direct or indirect exposure to known sensitizers should be part of the questionnaire of any adult with new onset asthma. Monitoring of peak expiratory flows at and off work is a useful tool but may not be sufficiently sensitive or specific; combining it with monitoring of the provocative concentration of methacoline inducing a 20% fall in FEV_1 and possibly sputum induction may improve the accuracy of the diagnosis. Specific inhalation challenges in the laboratory or in the workplace are the reference standard for confirming the diagnosis of occupational asthma. They are safe when done under the close supervision of an expert physician by trained personnel. Any new case of occupational asthma should be considered as a sentinel event.

Definitions

Work-related asthma refers to asthma symptoms worsened at work. It includes asthma exacerbated at work, discussed in the next chapter, and occupational asthma (OA). Various definitions have been given to OA. The one proposed by Bernstein et al. [1] encompasses most of them: "Occupational asthma is a disease characterized by variable airflow limitation and/or hyperresponsiveness and/or inflammation due to causes and conditions attributable to a particular occupational environment and not to stimuli encountered outside the workplace". Two elements in this definition are important. The agent (identified or not) should be specific to the workplace and be causally related to the disease. Relevant agents are airborne dusts, gases, vapors

Occupational Asthma, edited by Torben Sigsgaard and Dick Heederik

or fumes [2]. This definition thus excludes asthma triggered by irritant mechanisms such as cold air or exercise. A previous history of asthma does not exclude the diagnosis of OA. Two types of OA are distinguished based on their appearance after a latency period or not. The most frequent type, which is usually quoted as OA, appears after a latency period leading to sensitization (either allergic as for most high- and certain low-molecular-weight agents or through unknown mechanisms). The other category does not require a latency period and includes irritant-induced asthma or reactive airways dysfunction syndrome (RADS), which may occur after single or multiple exposures to high concentrations of nonspecific irritants [3, 4] and is discussed in another chapter.

Investigation

As opposed to the traditional pneumoconiosis where the diagnosis is only based on exposure history and chest radiograph abnormalities, OA can be and should be confirmed by objective means. Indeed, the social consequences of making or refuting such a diagnosis are important for both the worker and its employer [5–7]. In order to prevent further deterioration of asthma, it is essential to withdraw the worker from exposure to the offending agent [8, 9]: this imposes a serious stress to the worker and his family and may mean loss of job or benefits or even moving to another town. On the other hand, removing a worker who does not have OA from exposure has the same consequences, whereas adequate environmental control (e.g., reduction of exposure to irritants) and better control of asthma may be sufficient to allow the worker to continue his job without loss of income.

The different steps involved in the investigation of OA are: history, pulmonary function tests, immunological tests, combined monitoring of peak expiratory flows (PEF), non-allergic bronchial responsiveness (NABR) and sputum induction, and specific bronchial challenges. Although specific inhalation challenges are considered the reference standard, all steps involved in the investigation have their own usefulness and they all add up to make the diagnosis, with combination of various elements strengthening its likelihood.

The purpose of this chapter is to review the different steps involved in the investigation of OA with a latency period.

History

The questionnaire is the basic, essential tool used in most epidemiological surveys and all individual assessments.

The classical history of OA is one of a worker whose asthma is worse at work, improving over weekends or holidays. However, this pattern is often absent as symptoms are also usually present outside the workplace, being triggered by exposure to irritants such as cold air, fumes or upon exercise. Furthermore, the process involved may be in use irregularly or the worker may be unaware that a specific process is involved as he is not involved directly with it. In many cases, symptoms are even more severe at home, awaking the subject at night, and weekends may not be long enough to allow recuperation. Finally, even workers without work-related asthma regularly report improvement of asthma during weekends and holidays, in 41% and 54% of cases, respectively [10]. A previous history of asthma may also postpone the diagnosis. Symptoms may develop after only a few weeks or after several years, duration of exposure tending to be shorter for low-molecular-weight chemicals [11].

The concomitant occurrence of rhino-conjunctivitis at work, especially in a worker exposed to high-molecular-weight chemicals who develops asthma is surely suggestive of OA [12]. Although rhinitis is as frequent with low- and high-molecular-weight agents, symptoms are usually more severe with the latter [12]. It often precedes or coincides with the development of OA, especially with high-molecular-weight chemicals [12]. Rash (urticaria or contact dermatitis) is sometimes associated with OA, usually on exposed surfaces (droplets) or by direct contact (e.g., latex gloves).

However, a history suggestive of OA, even in a worker exposed to a known sensitizer, is not sufficient to make the diagnosis: questionnaires are sensitive but not specific tools. Indeed, even in the hands of expert physicians, we showed in a prospective study of 162 workers referred for OA that the predictive value of a positive questionnaire was only 63%, while the predictive value of a negative questionnaire was 83% [13]. Therefore, in more than one third of cases, objective testing showed that the subjects did not have OA, although the initial questionnaire had been suggestive.

Pulmonary function tests and diagnosis of asthma

To make the diagnosis of OA, one must first confirm the diagnosis of asthma. Although the latter can be confirmed by the presence of reversible airflow obstruction, e.g., increase of FEV_1 greater than 12–15% after a beta-2 agonist, most workers investigated for OA have normal spirometry when seen in the clinic. Furthermore, pre- and post-shift monitoring of FEV_1 has not proven sensitive or specific enough to be a useful tool in the investigation of OA [14–16].

Increased non-allergic bronchial responsiveness (NABR) is the hallmark of asthma, but it is also present in other conditions such as rhinitis and chronic obstructive lung diseases. Therefore, alone, the presence of increased NABR does not make the diagnosis of OA. It may suggest that the subject has OA, common asthma, or one or other of the conditions listed above. There is a need for further confirmation of work-related asthma. However, the absence of increased NABR as assessed shortly (minutes, hours) after a work shift in a worker who complains of symptoms virtually excludes OA [17], although, in rare instances, specific inhalation challenges have been positive in workers without increased NABR [18, 19]. Even in the presence of OA, NABR may be normal in a worker who has left work for several days (a weekend may be enough [20]) or weeks/months. Return to work or even a specific inhalation test will then increase the bronchial responsiveness in the asthmatic range [21, 22].

Work visit

It is essential to obtain a list of the different agents used at work by the subject but also by colleagues, as the exposure may be indirect, and to find out if other workers have respiratory complaints. This can be done by asking the employer directly or the local health department for the material safety data sheets (MSDS) for the different products used in the plant. Unfortunately, these MSDS are often incomplete, lacking information on sensitizing chemicals found in small amounts that may be enough to trigger asthma [23].

Immunological testing

The presence of immediate skin reactivity or increased specific IgE or IgG antibodies may reflect sensitization and/or exposure to a suspected agent but it does not imply that the target organ (the bronchi in this instance) is involved. This has been shown for common allergens and occupational sensitizers such as snow crab [15, 24] and isocyanates [25]. These tests are, however, useful as they can support the diagnosis and may help to identify which agent mat be relevant. The problem is the lack of standardization for most allergens.

With most high-molecular-weight chemicals for which good extracts are available, such as cereals or psyllium, negative skin tests to these allergens cannot entirely exclude the diagnosis of OA but make it very unlikely. Indeed, the worker may still be sensitized to another agent found in the workplace or to another component of the offending agent. Conversely, a positive skin test does not confirm the diagnosis, as its predictive positive value is low. For example, in a study by Bardy et al. [15] the positive and negative predictive values of skin tests/radioallergosorbent test (RAST) to psyllium were 22/16% and 100/100%, respectively. In snow crab-workers' asthma, the odds for the presence of OA in a subject with positive skin tests to snow crab extract or RAST ratio >4.5 were respectively 69% and 79%, whereas the odds for the absence of OA in a subject with negative skin test or RAST ratio <4.5 were 76% and 73%, respectively [24]. With most low-molecular-weight chemicals, skin tests or specific IgE or IgG are either unavailable or not sufficiently sensitive or specific to refute or to make the diagnosis of OA. Other *in vitro* tests such as basophil histamine release or assay of monocyte chemoattractant protein-1 by peripheral blood mononuclear cells [26] may offer higher sensitivity or specificity but again they do not confirm the diagnosis of OA.

Even if specific inhalation challenges are considered the reference test, they are not always available, and combining various tests may increase the likelihood of a correct diagnosis. In the case of high-molecular-weight agents, combining a history highly suggestive of OA with a positive methacholine challenge and a positive skin test to a high-molecular-weight agent gives a post-test probability of >90% of disease and may be enough. On the other hand, negative combined tests results do not appear to provide clinicians with sufficient certainty to rule out OA [27].

Monitoring of PEF and NABR and sputum cell counts

The availability of portable, inexpensive devices has allowed physicians to monitor PEF at work and off-work. This approach was first used in the investigation of work-related asthma by S. Burge and colleagues [28, 29]. Coupling PEF monitoring and changes in NABR for periods at work and away from work has also been proposed [30–32] (Fig. 1). Recently, monitoring of eosinophils in sputum induction has also been proposed [33, 34] as a useful tool. The usefulness of PEF monitoring in diagnosing OA has been reviewed in various consensus reports [7, 35–37].

When compared to specific inhalation challenges as the reference, PEF monitoring has a sensitivity of around 64% and a specificity of 77%. Malo et al. [38] showed that sensitivity and specificity of PEF monitoring was optimal when PEF were measured every 2 hours at work and off-work. Observing the deterioration of asthma while at work is still the best way to evaluate changes in PEF [32, 39]. A computer-based system analysis of PEF has been developed by Gannon and colleagues and validated as a useful tool to assess work-related changes in PEF [40–42]. It is, however, sometimes difficult to distinguish between work-exacerbated asthma and OA, even by experts [43]. The poor sensitivity or specificity of PEF monitoring in certain subjects as compared to specific bronchial challenges can be explained by several means. Indeed, even if performed under close supervision of a technician, PEF may greatly underestimate or overestimate changes in airway caliber as assessed by FEV_1 [44–46]. Furthermore, PEF are effort dependent and thus require collaboration of the worker, which is not always obtained due to fear of loosing his job or malingering in order to get some compensation benefit. When PEF data are stored on a computer chip and subjects are unaware of this, two studies [47, 48] have shown that many workers will falsify their records as around 50% of values are inaccurately reported on diaries either in terms of the recorded value or of the timing of the measurement or as fabricated results.

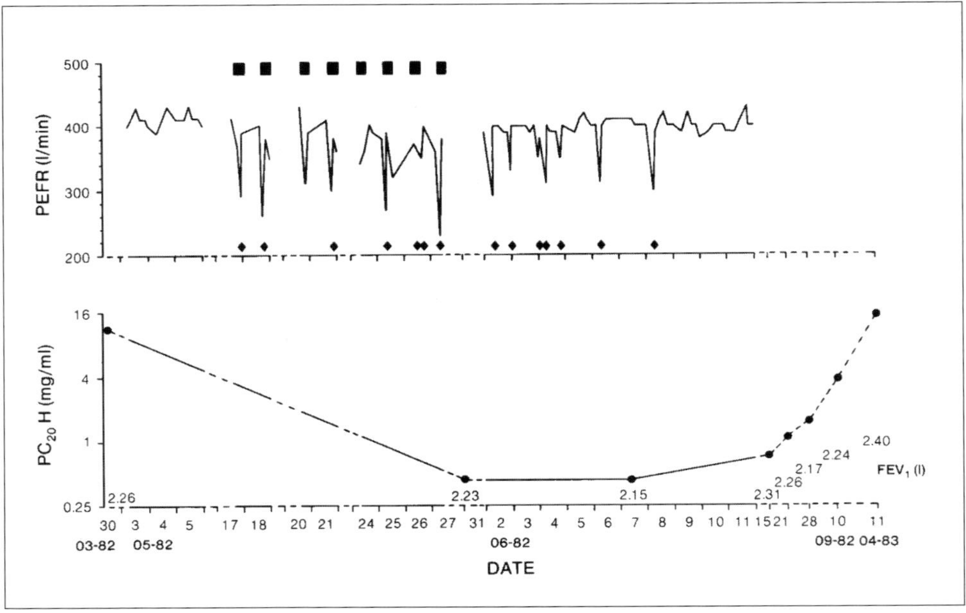

Figure 1.
Monitoring of PEF (PEFR; upper panel) and PC_{20}-histamine (lower panel) in a crab processing worker. Before returning to work, the subject was asymptomatic with borderline PC_{20}. Upon return to work, as illustrated by the black squares, the subject had a recurrence of asthma symptoms requiring rescue salbutamol (illustrated by the losanges) with significant changes in PEF and a significant fall in PC_{20}. Work withdrawal was associated with return to baseline of PEF and gradual, although very slow, recovery of PC_{20} over 1 year. This confirmed the diagnosis of occupational asthma. Reproduced with permission from [59].

The minimum period of monitoring should be at least 2 weeks at work and off-work to be able to draw some conclusions. In certain situations, particularly when asthma is severe or when the nature of the offending agent is unknown and intermittent, the interpretation of the monitoring may be difficult [32]. Subjects should be asked to take their beta-2 agonists on demand only, but should continue their inhaled steroids regularly. Indeed, reduction of inhaled steroids upon return to work may be associated with deterioration of asthma and reduction in PEF, which may be mistaken as diagnostic of OA. We usually avoid long-acting beta-2 agonists and leukotrienes antagonists, but allow the use of theophylline at the same dosage throughout the entire monitoring. In severe asthmatics, it may be necessary to withdraw the subject from work until his asthma is under control and on minimum treatment before returning him to work; deterioration of asthma may then suggest that asthma is caused by work.

The association of NABR monitoring to PEF monitoring at work and off-work is now frequently used in the investigation of OA [30–32]. NABR can be assessed by several means, but methacholine and histamine inhalation challenges with determination of the provocative concentration inducing a 20% fall in FEV_1 (PC_{20}) are the most reliable and are well standardized. Indeed, whereas exposure to irritants does not induce marked and prolonged changes in NABR, OA may be associated with significant and often long-lasting changes in NABR. However, Côté et al. [31] and Perrin et al. [32] showed that PC_{20} monitoring at and off-work did not improve the sensitivity or specificity of PEF monitoring in diagnosing OA. We recommend that monitoring of PEF is coupled to monitoring of NABR: indeed, when changes in PEF are associated with parallel changes in NABR, the diagnosis of OA is highly probable. If the monitoring of PEF and NABR are discordant, further investigations should be completed, such as specific bronchial challenges in the workplace or in the laboratory. When the monitoring of PEF and NABR shows no evidence of asthma in a symptomatic subject while at work, this is enough to exclude the diagnosis of OA.

As sputum eosinophils may increase following return to work in subjects with OA [33, 34, 49], we are regularly adding this parameter in our evaluation of workers. However, we tend to use a positive result as potentially indicating OA rather than confirming it; when there is a discrepancy between monitoring of PEF, NABR or sputum eosinophils, we tend to complete our investigation with specific inhalation challenges. In the absence of increased NABR and changes in airway caliber, an increased count of sputum eosinophils at work in a worker symptomatic of cough may suggest the diagnosis of eosinophilic occupational bronchitis [50, 51]. Unfortunately, monitoring of sputum induction is available in only a few centers and is of limited value. Finally, there is still no evidence that monitoring of exhaled NO is useful in the investigation of OA but this merits further investigation.

Although monitoring of PEF and NABR are useful tools, they are time consuming, require the subject's collaboration and may be hazardous in workers giving a history of severe asthma at work as exposure may not be titrated as easily as when the challenge is done in the laboratory. They are particularly useful as a screening procedure when the worker is exposed to several sensitizers or when the offending agent is unknown.

Specific inhalation challenges

Specific inhalation challenges (SIC) are still considered the reference test to confirm the diagnosis of OA [52–56]. Originally done in the laboratory and aiming at mimicking work exposure [57], they are now frequently done in the workplace [58, 59].

SIC are safe when performed under the close supervision of an expert physician and with trained personnel and are thus limited to specialized centers. Resuscitative measures should be available. When performed in the laboratory, the exposure chambers should be well ventilated and isolated to minimize exposure to the personnel. The tests can be carried out on an outpatient basis. Most challenges are done in an open fashion, the subject knowing the nature of the exposure. This is inevitable for workplace challenges but when challenges are done in the laboratory, we sometimes blind the exposure if we suspect that the subject is mimicking symptoms (particularly cough).

Although there is no standardized protocol, the methodology is well developed [52, 55, 56].

Drugs should be withheld before specific bronchial challenges according to standard recommendations [55] as with methacholine challenges [60]. Beta-2 agonist (oral and inhaled), inhaled ipratropium bromide and cromoglycate must be withheld for 8 hours. Inhaled long-acting beta-2 agonists, tiotropium and nedocromil, and leukotrienes antagonists should be discontinued for 48 hours. In most subjects, long-acting theophylline should be withheld for 48 hours (or 72 hours for once-a-day tablets), but may have to be continued in subjects who show too much variability in their spirometry throughout the day when they are withheld. If it is used, there should be daily serum monitoring to ensure a uniform effect. Inhaled (and occasionally oral) corticosteroids should be continued at their minimal dosage to keep asthma under control, but taken only in the evening of each challenge day at the same total dose. Although the dose of the agent required to induce a bronchial reaction may indeed be increased by theophylline or corticosteroids, these drugs would not abolish the response if the subject is sensitized.

While FEV_1 is the standard parameter used to assess changes in airway caliber, PEF are not reliable enough particularly in the late bronchial response as they may underestimate or overestimate changes [44]. While some investigators favor the use of airway resistance (R_{aw}), most consider that it is less reliable than FEV_1. In addition, we routinely measure lung volumes on the control day (total lung capacity, residual volume and functional residual capacity) to be able to confirm airways obstruction, as indicated by airway trapping and hyperinflation, during exposure to the offending agents in cases where simple spirometry is dubious (e.g., poor collaboration of the subject).

In all cases, spirometry should be monitored on a control day to ensure stability of airway caliber; in more severe asthmatics, the subject is first observed for at least 8 hours on a non-exposed day, whereas most subjects can be exposed on the first day to a control irritant, e.g., lactose powder, paint diluent, resin, etc., presented in the same way as the suspected agent [52, 55]. FEV_1 is monitored at baseline every 10 minutes for 1 hour, every 30 minutes for 1 hour, and then hourly for at least 8 hours after the end of exposure. If the subject show too much variability of his FEV_1 (>10%) during this control day or if the FEV_1 is too low (we usually require an FEV_1 >2.0 L or at least >1.5 L and >70% of predicted), the tests should be postponed and asthma controlled by adjusting the medication. At the end of the control day, a methacholine challenge test followed by sputum induction are done to determine the level of NABR as assessed by the PC_{20} dose and the profile of airway inflammation. The PC_{20} may help us determine the starting concentration to the offending agent on the next day, the lower the PC_{20}, the lower the exposure. In cases where allergic alveolitis is also suspected, monitoring of carbon monoxide lung diffusion capacity is measured on control and subsequent days in the morning and late afternoon, as well as monitoring of white blood cell counts.

Challenges preformed in the laboratory

When performed in the laboratory, specific bronchial challenges can be done in several ways, depending on the nature of the agent, i.e., powder, aerosol, liquid or gas. With powders, like flour, psyllium or red cedar, the subject may be exposed to a fine dust, mimicking work exposure by pouring the dust from one tray to another [57] or using a dust generator [61–63], which allows proper monitoring, regulation of exposure, establishment of dose-response curves, and reduces the risk of severe and/or irritant reactions. The agent may be diluted initially with an inert agent such as lactose to avoid severe reactions. Alternatively, the worker may be exposed to an aerosol of a crude extract. Exposure to non-powder agents is usually done by reproducing work environment, e.g., by nebulizing an aerosol of the isocyanates hardener or by having the worker breath over a bottle of methacrylate glue. Isocyanates and other gases can be generated in their gaseous form in a closed circuit generating chamber [64, 65] or a whole-body exposure chamber [66, 67]. Whenever possible, the level of exposure should be monitored to avoid high exposure and therefore irritant reactions.

Baseline spirometry on each exposure day should be reproducible, i.e., <10% of the control day. The exposure should be progressive (1 breath, 10–15 seconds, 1 minute, 2 minutes, 5 minutes, etc.). The total duration of exposure is a function of the type of agent and the history given by the subject. The dose may be conveniently increased sequentially by serial increases of the exposure period, and/or increasing the concentration of the agent. For high-molecular-weight chemicals for which positive skin tests can be elicited, exposure is increased progressively for up to 2 hours with in-between functional assessments, unless the subject gives a history suggestive of an isolated late asthmatic reaction. As on the control day, spirometry is assessed immediately and 10 minutes after each period of exposure. A significant reaction is defined as a 20% fall in FEV_1. At the end of exposure (whether it is after 2 hours or once the FEV_1 has dropped significantly by 20%), spirometry is performed as on the control day for up to 8 hours. With low-molecular-weight chemicals such as isocyanates, which are more often associated with isolated late responses [68], exposure should be more gradual and over a few days: one breath, 15 seconds, 45 seconds and 2 minutes on the first day, 30 minutes on the second day and 2 hours on a third day. However, this pattern of exposure may be modified by reducing the duration of subsequent exposures if there is a suggestion that the subject is starting to react. If there is no significant variation in FEV_1 on the last exposure day, NABR and sputum induction should be reassessed at the end of that day; if there is no significant change from baseline, there is no further exposure, whereas, if PC_{20} is significantly lower or if there is a significant increase in eosinophils, we repeat the exposure on the next day for up to 4 hours as the test may then be positive [69], sometimes even after a shorter exposure.

Tests in the workplace

Tests in the workplace are now done more frequently, especially when the relevant agent at work is unknown or when there are several potential sensitizing agents. They are also done in stepwise manner as the subject may experience a significant fall in FEV_1. Spirometry is performed in the same way throughout the day [58, 59]. Exposure to the offending agent is, however, less well controlled and monitored than in the laboratory, and it may be difficult to ensure that the subject is really exposed to the relevant agent at work. This may be, however, the only way to confirm the diagnosis of OA especially in cases where the nature of the offending agent is unknown.

Interpretation of the tests

A significant reaction is defined as a 20% fall in FEV_1. Typical patterns of bronchial reactions have been described [57, 68] (Fig. 2a). Immediate reactions are maximal between 10 and 30 minutes after exposure with complete recovery within 1–2 hours; although usually readily reversible by inhaled beta-2 agonists, they are actually the most dangerous as they can be severe and unpredictable, particularly in subjects for whom skin tests with the suspecting agent are not possible, stressing the importance of progressive exposure. Late reactions develop slowly and progressively either 1–2 hours (early late) or 4–8 hours (late) after exposure; they may occasionally be accompanied by fever and general malaise but extrinsic alveolitis should then be considered. Contrary to popular belief, they generally respond well to inhaled beta-2 agonist, although the response may be of shorter duration in some subjects [70]. Dual reactions are a combination of early and late. A recurrent nocturnal asthma pattern has also been described and is likely related to an increase in NABR following exposure [71].

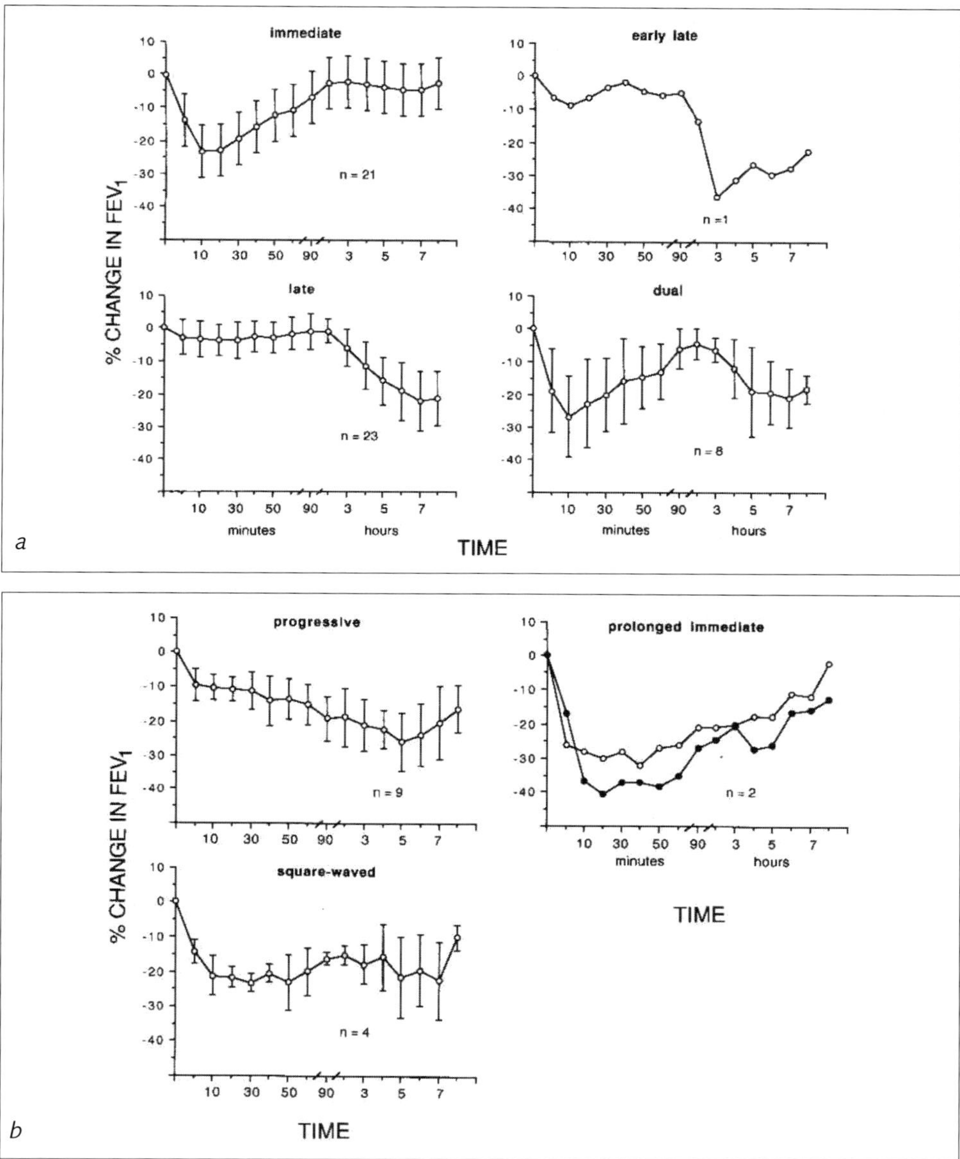

Figure 2.
Patterns of typical (a) and atypical (b) bronchial responses to specific inhalation challenges. Each point represents the mean % change in FEV_1 (n=number of subjects in each group) at several time points following the last inhalation of the responsible agent during a specific inhalation challenge. Reproduced with permission from [68].

Atypical patterns (Fig. 2b) have also been described with isocyanates and other low- or high-molecular-weight chemicals: they include the progressive type (starting within minutes after end of exposure and progressing over the next 7–8 hours), the square-waved reaction (with no recovery between the immediate and late components of the reaction) and finally the prolonged immediate type with slow recovery. Low-molecular-weight chemicals are more often associated with atypical patterns as compared to high-molecular-weight chemicals.

Irritant reactions are not well characterized but falls in FEV_1 that recover rapidly within 10 or 20 minutes are suggestive of an irritant pattern. It may be impossible to interpret results of specific bronchial challenges in subject with too much variability of FEV_1, stressing the importance of an adequate control day.

A positive test confirms the diagnosis of OA, whereas a negative test in the workplace, or in the laboratory, does not absolutely rule out the diagnosis of OA in a worker who has not been exposed to work for several months, as he may have become "desensitized" [22, 59, 69]; this is particularly true if there is a change in PC_{20} following the specific challenges [22, 69]. The worker should be returned to work with monitoring of PEF and bronchial responsiveness for at least a few weeks before excluding the diagnosis. False negative challenges in the laboratory may also be due to exposure to the wrong agent or administration of a forbidden drug (such as an inhaled beta-2 agonist) before the test. However, if the subject had his/her symptoms during the challenge procedure without any change in spirometry, these tests are conclusive and exclude the diagnosis of OA.

Conclusion

The diagnosis of OA should be based on objective means and cannot rely only on history or even on confirming the presence of asthma and positive skin tests. Monitoring of PEF, PC_{20} and sputum induction are useful tools but may not be sufficiently sensitive or specific. Specific inhalation challenges in the laboratory or in the workplace are the reference standard for confirming the diagnosis of OA, but should be done under the supervision of expert physicians.

Unanswered questions

- What is the role of exhaled NO in the investigation of OA?
- There is a need for a better characterization of the bronchial response to irritants by using indices such as NABR, sputum induction or exhaled NO.
- Duration of exposure to the agent in the laboratory needs to be better standardized. How long should the exposure be before we consider a challenge to be negative, 2, 4 hours?

- Monitoring the exposure is not always possible and this is clearly a limit of specific inhalation challenges as it may be sometimes difficult to exclude an irritant effect. There is thus a need to improve our capacity to do such monitoring.

References

1 Bernstein IL, Bernstein DI, Chan-Yeung M, Malo JL (2006): Defenition and classification of asthma in the workplace. In: IL Bernstein, M Chan-Yeung, JL Malo, DI Bernstein (eds): *Asthma in the Workplace and related conditions*. Taylor & Francis Group, New York, 1–8

2 Newman Taylor AJ (1980) Occupational asthma. *Thorax* 35: 241–245

3 Brooks SM, Weiss MA, Bernstein IL (1985) Reactive airways dysfunction syndrome (RADS). Persistent asthma syndrome after high level irritant exposures. *Chest* 88: 376–384

4 Brooks SM, Bernstein IL (1993): Reactive airways dysfunction syndrome or irritant-induced asthma. In: IL Bernstein, M Chan-Yeung, JL Malo, DI Bernstein (eds): *Asthma in the Workplace*. Marcel Dekker, New York, 533–549

5 Vandenplas O, Toren K, Blanc PD (2003) Health and socioeconomic impact of work-related asthma. *Eur Respir J* 22: 689–697

6 Larbanois A, Jamart J, Delwiche JP, Vandenplas O (2002) Socioeconomic outcome of subjects experiencing asthma symptoms at work. *Eur Respir J* 19: 1107–1113

7 Beach J, Rowe BH, Blitz S, Crumley E, Hooton N, Russell K, et al (eds) (2005) *Evidence Report/Technology Assessment No. 129. Diagnosis and management of work-related asthma.* Agency for Healthcare Research and Quality, Rockville, MD

8 Chan-Yeung M, Malo JL (1993): Natural history of occupational asthma. In: IL Bernstein, M Chan-Yeung, JL Malo, DI Bernstein (eds): *Asthma in the Workplace*. Marcel Dekker, New York, 299–322

9 Paggiaro PL, Vagaggini B, Bacci E, Bancalari L, Carrara M, Di Franco A, Giannini D, Dente FL, Giuntini C (1994) Prognosis of occupational asthma. *Eur Respir J* 7: 761–767

10 Tarlo SM, Liss G, Corey P, Broder I (1995) A workers compensation claim population for occupational asthma – Comparison of subgroups. *Chest* 107: 634–641

11 Malo JL, Ghezzo H, D'Aquino C, L'Archeveque J, Cartier A, Chan-Yeung M (1992) Natural history of occupational asthma: relevance of type of agent and other factors in the rate of development of symptoms in affected subjects. *J Allergy Clin Immunol* 90: 937–944

12 Malo JL, Lemiere C, Desjardins A, Cartier A (1997) Prevalence and intensity of rhinoconjunctivitis in subjects with occupational asthma. *Eur Respir J* 10: 1513–1515

13 Malo JL, Ghezzo H, L'Archeveque J, Lagier F, Perrin B, Cartier A (1991) Is the clinical history a satisfactory means of diagnosing occupational asthma? *Am Rev Respir Dis* 143: 528–532

14 Burge PS (1982) Single and serial measurements of lung function in the diagnosis of occupational asthma. *Eur J Respir Dis* 63 (Suppl 123): 47–59

15 Bardy JD, Malo JL, Séguin P, Ghezzo H, Desjardins J, Dolovich J, Cartier A (1987) Occupational asthma and IgE sensitization in a pharmaceutical company processing psyllium. *Am Rev Respir Dis* 135: 1033–1038

16 Malo JL, Cartier A (1988) Occupational asthma in workers of a pharmaceutical company processing spiramycin. *Thorax* 43: 371–377

17 Baur X, Huber H, Degens PO, Allmers H, Ammon J (1998) Relation between occupational asthma case history, bronchial methacholine challenge, and specific challenge test in patients with suspected occupational asthma. *Am J Ind Med* 33: 114–122

18 Smith AB, Brooks SM, Blanchard J, Bernstein IL, Gallagher J (1980) Absence of airway hyperreactivity to methacholine in a worker sensitized to toluene diisocyanate. *J Occup Med* 22: 327–331

19 Banks DE, Barkman WHJ, Butcher BT, Hammad YY, Rando RJ, Glindmeyer HWI, Jones RN, Weill H (1986) Absence of hyperresponsiveness to methacholine in a worker with methylene diphenyl diisocyanate (MDI)-induced asthma. *Chest* 89: 389–393

20 Cockcroft DW, Mink JT (1979) Isocyanate-induced asthma in an automobile spray painter. *Can Med Assoc J* 121: 602–604

21 Hargreave FE, Ramsdale EH, Pugsley SO (1984) Occupational asthma without bronchial hyperresponsiveness. *Am Rev Respir Dis* 130: 513–515

22 Lemiere C, Cartier A, Dolovich J, Chan-Yeung M, Grammer L, Ghezzo H, L'Archeveque J, Malo JL (1996) Outcome of specific bronchial responsiveness to occupational agents after removal from exposure. *Am J Respir Crit Care Med* 154: 329–333

23 Bernstein JA (2002) Material safety data sheets: Are they reliable in identifying human hazards? *J Allergy Clin Immunol* 110: 35–38

24 Cartier A, Malo JL, Ghezzo H, McCants M, Lehrer SB (1986) IgE sensitization in snow crab-processing workers. *J Allergy Clin Immunol* 78: 344–348

25 Cartier A, Grammer L, Malo JL, Lagier F, Ghezzo H, Harris K, Patterson R (1989) Specific serum antibodies against isocyanates: association with occupational asthma. *J Allergy Clin Immunol* 84: 507–514

26 Bernstein DI, Cartier A, Côté J, Malo JL, Boulet LP, Wanner M, Milot J, L'Archeveque J, Trudeau C, Lummus Z (2002) Diisocyanate antigen-stimulated monocyte chemoattractant protein-1 synthesis has greater test efficiency than specific antibodies for identification of diisocyanate asthma. *Am J Respir Crit Care Med* 166: 445–450

27 Beach J, Russell K, Blitz S, Hooton N, Spooner C, Lemiere C, Tarlo SM, Rowe BH (2007) A systematic review of the diagnosis of occupational asthma. *Chest* 131: 569–578

28 Burge PS, O'Brien I, Harries M (1979) Peak flow rate records in the diagnosis of occupational asthma due to isocyanates. *Thorax* 34: 317–323

29 Burge PS, O'Brien I, Harries M (1979) Peak flow rate records in the diagnosis of occupational asthma due to colophony. *Thorax* 34: 308–316

30 Cartier A, Pineau L, Malo JL (1984) Monitoring of maximum expiratory peak flow

rates and histamine inhalation tests in the investigation of occupational asthma. *Clin Allergy* 14: 193–196

31 Côté J, Kennedy S, Chan-Yeung M (1990) Sensitivity and specificity of PC20 and peak expiratory flow rate in cedar asthma. *J Allergy Clin Immunol* 85: 592–598

32 Perrin B, Lagier F, L'Archeveque J, Cartier A, Boulet LP, Côté J, Malo JL (1992) Occupational asthma: validity of monitoring of peak expiratory flow rates and non-allergic bronchial responsiveness as compared to specific inhalation challenge. *Eur Respir J* 5: 40–48

33 Girard F, Chaboillez S, Cartier A, Côté J, Hargreave FE, Labrecque M, Malo JL, Tarlo SM, Lemiere C (2004) An effective strategy for diagnosing occupational asthma: use of induced sputum. *Am J Respir Crit Care Med* 170: 845–850

34 Lemiere C (2004) The use of sputum eosinophils in the evaluation of occupational asthma. *Curr Opin Allergy Clin Immunol* 4: 81–85

35 Moscato G, Godnic-Cvar J, Maestrelli P, Malo JL, Burge PS, Coifman R (1995) Statement on self-monitoring of peak expiratory flows in the investigation of occupational asthma. Subcommittee on Occupational Allergy of the European Academy of Allergology and Clinical Immunology. American Academy of Allergy and Clinical Immunology. European Respiratory Society. American College of Allergy, Asthma and Immunology. *Eur Respir J* 8: 1605–1610

36 Bright P, Burge PS (1996) Occupational lung disease. 8. The diagnosis of occupational asthma from serial measurements of lung function at and away from work. *Thorax* 51: 857–863

37 Tarlo SM, Balmes J, Balkissoon R, Beach J, Beckett W, Bernstein D, Blanc PD, Brooks SM, Cowl CT, Daroowalla F, et al (2008) Diagnosis and management of work-related asthma: American College Of Chest Physicians Consensus Statement. *Chest* 134: 1S-41S

38 Malo JL, Côté J, Cartier A, Boulet LP, L'Archeveque J, Chan-Yeung M (1993) How many times per day should peak expiratory flow rates be assessed when investigating occupational asthma? *Thorax* 48: 1211–1217

39 Côté J, Kennedy S, Chan-Yeung M (1993) Quantitative *versus* qualitative analysis of peak expiratory flow in occupational asthma. *Thorax* 48: 48–51

40 Gannon PFG, Newton DT, Belcher J, Pantin CFA, Burge PS (1996) Development of OASYS-2 – A system for the analysis of serial measurement of peak expiratory flow in workers with suspected occupational asthma. *Thorax* 51: 484–489

41 Bright P, Newton DT, Gannon PF, Pantin CF, Burge PS (2001) OASYS-3: Improved analysis of serial peak expiratory flow in suspected occupational asthma. *Monaldi Arch Chest Dis* 56: 281–288

42 Baldwin DR, Gannon P, Bright P, Newton DT, Robertson A, Venables K, Graneek B, Barker RD, Cartier A, Malo JL, et al (2002) Interpretation of occupational peak flow records: Level of agreement between expert clinicians and Oasys-2. *Thorax* 57: 860–864

43 Chiry S, Cartier A, Malo JL, Tarlo SM, Lemiere C (2007) Comparison of peak expira-

tory flow variability between workers with work-exacerbated asthma and occupational asthma. *Chest* 132: 483–488

44 Bérubé D, Cartier A, L'Archeveque J, Ghezzo H, Malo JL (1991) Comparison of peak expiratory flow rate and FEV1 in assessing bronchomotor tone after challenges with occupational sensitizers. *Chest* 99: 831–836

45 Gautrin D, D'Aquino LC, Gagnon G, Malo JL, Cartier A (1994) Comparison between peak expiratory flow rates (PEFR) and FEV1 in the monitoring of asthmatic subjects at the outpatient clinic. *Chest* 106: 1419–1426

46 Moscato G, Dellabianca A, Paggiaro P, Bertoletti R, Corsico A, Perfetti L (1993) Peak expiratory flow monitoring and airway response to specific bronchial provocation tests in asthmatics. *Monaldi Arch Chest Dis* 48: 23–28

47 Malo JL, Trudeau C, Ghezzo H, L'Archeveque J, Cartier A (1995) Do subjects investigated for occupational asthma through serial peak expiratory flow measurements falsify their results. *J Allergy Clin Immunol* 96: 601–607

48 Quirce S, Contreras G, Dybuncio A, Chan-Yeung M (1995) Peak expiratory flow monitoring is not a reliable method for establishing the diagnosis of occupational asthma. *Am J Respir Crit Care Med* 152: 1100–1102

49 Lemiere C, Pizzichini MM, Balkissoon R, Clelland L, Efthimiadis A, O'Shaughnessy D, Dolovich J, Hargreave FE (1999) Diagnosing occupational asthma: Use of induced sputum. *Eur Respir J* 13: 482–488

50 Krakowiak AM, Dudek W, Ruta U, Palczynski C (2005) Occupational eosinophilic bronchitis without asthma due to chloramine exposure. *Occup Med (Lond)* 55: 396–398

51 Lemiere C, Efthimiadis A, Hargreave FE (1997) Occupational eosinophilic bronchitis without asthma: An unknown occupational airway disease. *J Allergy Clin Immunol* 100: 852–853

52 Cartier A, Malo JL (1993): Occupational challenge tests. In: IL Bernstein, M Chan-Yeung, JL Malo, DI Bernstein (eds): *Asthma in the Workplace*. Marcel Dekker, New York, 215–248

53 Chan-Yeung M, Malo JL (1987) Occupational asthma. *Chest* 91: 130S-136S

54 Canadian Thoracic Society (1989) Occupational asthma: Recommendations for diagnosis, management and assessment of impairment. *Can Med Assoc J* 140: 1029–1032

55 Cartier A, Bernstein IL, Burge PS, Cohn JR, Fabbri LM, Hargreave FE, Malo JL, McKay RT, Salvaggio JE (1989) Guidelines for bronchoprovocation on the investigation of occupational asthma. Report of the Subcommittee on Bronchoprovocation for Occupational Asthma. *J Allergy Clin Immunol* 84: 823–829

56 EAACI (1992) Guidelines for the diagnosis of occupational asthma. Subcommittee on 'Occupational Allergy' of the European Academy of Allergology and Clinical Immunology. *Clin Exp Allergy* 22: 103–108

57 Pepys J, Hutchcroft BJ (1975) Bronchial provocation tests in etiologic diagnosis and analysis of asthma. *Am Rev Respir Dis* 112: 829–859

58 Chan-Yeung M, McMurren T, Catonio-Begley F, Lam S (1993) Occupational asthma in a technologist exposed to glutaraldehyde. *J Allergy Clin Immunol* 91: 974–978

59 Cartier A, Malo JL, Forest F, Lafrance M, Pineau L, St-Aubin JJ, Dubois JY (1984) Occupational asthma in snow crab-processing workers. *J Allergy Clin Immunol* 74: 261–269

60 Crapo RO, Casaburi R, Coates AL, Enright PL, Hankinson JL, Irvin CG, MacIntyre NR, McKay RT, Wanger JS, Anderson SD, et al. (2000) Guidelines for methacholine and exercise challenge testing-1999. This official statement of the American Thoracic Society was adopted by the ATS Board of Directors, July 1999. *Am J Respir Crit Care Med* 161: 309–329

61 Cloutier Y, Lagier F, Lemieux R, Blais MC, St-Arnaud C, Cartier A, Malo JL (1989) New methodology for specific inhalation challenges with occupational agents in powder form. *Eur Respir J* 2: 769–777

62 Cloutier Y, Lagier F, Cartier A, Malo JL (1992) Validation of an exposure system to particles for the diagnosis of occupational asthma. *Chest* 102: 402–407

63 Cloutier Y, Malo JL (1992) Update on an exposure system for particles in the diagnosis of occupational asthma. *Eur Respir J* 5: 887–890

64 Vandenplas O, Malo JL, Cartier A, Perreault G, Cloutier Y (1992) Closed-circuit methodology for inhalation challenge tests with isocyanates. *Am Rev Respir Dis* 145: 582–587

65 Lemiere C, Cloutier Y, Perrault G, Drolet D, Cartier A, Malo JL (1996) Closed-circuit apparatus for specific inhalation challenges with an occupational agent, formaldehyde, in vapor form. *Chest* 109: 1631–1635

66 Banks DE, Tarlo SM, Masri F, Rando RJ, Weissman DN (1996) Bronchoprovocation tests in the diagnosis of isocyanate-induced asthma. *Chest* 109: 1370–1379

67 Sostrand P, Kongerud J, Eduard W, Nilsen T, Skogland M, Boe J (1997) A test chamber for experimental hydrogen fluoride exposure in humans. *Am Ind Hyg Assoc J* 58: 521–525

68 Perrin B, Cartier A, Ghezzo H, Grammer L, Harris K, Chan H, Chan-Yeung M, Malo JL (1991) Reassessment of the temporal patterns of bronchial obstruction after exposure to occupational sensitizing agents. *J Allergy Clin Immunol* 87: 630–639

69 Vandenplas O, Delwiche JP, Jamart J, Vandeweyer R (1996) Increase in non-specific bronchial hyperresponsiveness as an early marker of bronchial response to occupational agents during specific inhalation challenges. *Thorax* 51: 472–478

70 Malo JL, Ghezzo H, L'Archeveque J, Cartier A (1990) Late asthmatic reactions to occupational sensitizing agents: frequency of changes in nonspecific bronchial responsiveness and of response to inhaled beta 2-adrenergic agent. *J Allergy Clin Immunol* 85: 834–842

71 Cockcroft DW, Hoeppner VH, Werner GD (1984) Recurrent nocturnal asthma after bronchoprovocation with Western Red Cedar sawdust: association with acute increase in non- allergic bronchial responsiveness. *Clin Allergy* 14: 61–68

Work-exacerbated asthma

Paul K. Henneberger[1] *and Carrie A. Redlich*[2]

[1]National Institute for Occupational Safety and Health, Centers for Disease Control and Prevention, MS H2800, 1095 Willowdale Road, Morgantown, WV 26505, USA
[2]Occupational and Environmental Medicine and Pulmonary & Critical Care Medicine, Yale University School of Medicine, 135 College Street, New Haven, CT 06510, USA

Abstract

Exposures at work can contribute to both the onset and exacerbation of asthma. This chapter summarizes key information regarding work-exacerbated asthma (WEA), a common condition that has received little attention compared to new occupational asthma. WEA refers to pre-existing or concurrent asthma that is worsened by factors at work. WEA, as with asthma in general, is heterogeneous, with multiple phenotypes and triggers. The prevalence of WEA has ranged from about 15% to over 50% among working adults with asthma in published studies, but is rarely diagnosed by clinicians. WEA occurs in a wide range of industries and occupations, including education, services, manufacturing and construction, and can lead to job changes and unemployment. Multiple factors at work can exacerbate asthma, including various irritants, allergens, molds, cold and exertion. Cleaning products and building renovation in non-industrial workplaces such as schools and offices are commonly implicated. WEA can lead to substantial adverse outcomes, similar to OA. Management of WEA should focus on reducing work exposures and optimizing standard medical management.

Introduction and definitions

Asthma is a common disease, affecting up to approximately 15% of working-age adults [1]. Work-related asthma (WRA) comprises both occupational asthma (OA) in which exposures at work cause new onset asthma, and work-exacerbated asthma (WEA) in which existing asthma is aggravated by conditions at work. An estimated 15% of new adult onset asthma is attributable to exposure to sensitizers or irritants in the work environment [2, 3]. The literature on WRA has focused primarily on sensitizer-induced OA. Asthma exacerbations are common, and can be triggered by a number of factors, including workplace exposures. However, WEA has received less attention than OA. The purpose of this chapter is to summarize relevant

Occupational Asthma, edited by Torben Sigsgaard and Dick Heederik

information about WEA, including the definition and epidemiology of WEA, causative factors, natural history, and a suggested clinical approach for diagnosis and management of WEA.

WEA refers to pre-existing or concurrent asthma that is worsened by work-related factors [3]. A case of 'concurrent asthma' has onset while the individual is employed, but the onset is not attributable to work. As with asthma in general, definitions of WEA have varied depending on the clinical, research, or public health setting, but all depend on defining "asthma" and "asthma exacerbation". This can be challenging, given that asthma is a heterogeneous syndrome that involves multiple phenotypes, multiple factors can exacerbate asthma, and that exacerbations can vary from brief worsening of symptoms to severe episodes requiring hospitalization or resulting in death. Key features of asthma include airway inflammation, airway hyperresponsiveness (reversible airflow obstruction), and recurrent symptoms of wheezing, chest tightness or cough [4, 5]. Clinical studies are more likely to use objective tests such as reversible airflow obstruction on spirometry and medication usage to define asthma. Epidemiological studies are more likely to use self-reports of doctor-diagnosed asthma and asthma symptoms. Work-relatedness is primarily assessed by self-reports of symptoms or medication use relative to work, or occasionally by physiologic indicators such as work-related changes in peak flow rates.

Prevalence of WEA

The prevalence of WEA has been investigated using several approaches. A relatively small but growing number of studies have evaluated the frequency of WEA in general populations of asthmatics and provide estimates of the prevalence of WEA among adult asthmatics (Tab. 1) [6–14]. The prevalence of WEA estimated from these studies was quite variable, as shown in Table 1, ranging from 14% to 38% among all adults with asthma, and from 14% to over 50% among working adults with asthma, a more appropriate at risk group (denominator). The populations studied, age ranges, asthma definitions, geographic locales, and criteria for work exacerbation vary in these studies, as noted in Table 1. Asthma was defined as doctor-diagnosed asthma in most studies, with access to medical records to identify cases, except for studies that selected participants from the general population. Work exacerbation was generally based on self-reported asthma symptoms that had worsened in relation to work, typically within the past year; however, these reports rarely included the frequency or severity of exacerbation.

The frequency of WEA has also been expressed as a percentage of all WRA cases, with a denominator that includes both OA and WEA cases (Tab. 2) [15–26]. Most of these studies were conducted in clinical referral settings or relied on surveillance or worker compensation systems for identifying cases of WRA. Estimates

Table 1. Prevalence of WEA among adults with asthma (selected studies)

Reference	Setting*	No. of asthma cases	Age (years)	Criteria for WEA (self-reported on questionnaire unless indicated otherwise)	Prevalence of WEA among	
					All adults with asthma	Working adults with asthma
Abramson 1995 [6]	G Pop	159	43 mean	Respiratory symptoms at work	20%	NA[§]
Blanc 1999 [7]	G Pop	160	20–44	Report chest tightness at work	38%	NA
Bolen 2007 [8]	HMO	95 all employed	18–44, 34 mean	Pattern of serial peak expiratory flow rate consistent with WEA	NA	14%
Goh 1994 [9]	Clinics	802	20–54	Work environment is asthma trigger	27%	NA
Henneberger 2002 [12]	HMO	1,461	18–44	Current work environment makes asthma worse	25%	NA
Henneberger 2003 [10]	G Pop	42 28 employed	18–65, 42 mean	Coughing or wheezing is worse at work than when not at work	14%	21%
Henneberger 2006 [11]	HMO	598 OA excluded	18–44	Relevant exposure and work-related pattern of symptoms or medication use	23%	24%
Mancuso 2003 [13]	Primary care	102 all employed	39 mean	At least one of several job conditions makes asthma worse	NA	58%
Saarinen 2003 [14]	NHI system	969 OA excluded	20–65, 43 mean	Asthma symptoms caused or worsened by work at least weekly in past month	NA	20%

* Abbreviations for setting: G Pop, general population; HMO, health maintenance organization; NHI, national health insurance
§ NA, not applicable

Table 2. Prevalence of WEA among all work-related asthma (WRA) cases (selected studies)

Reference	Clinical setting*	Age (years)	Criteria for WEA†	No. with WRA	% with WEA
Caldeira 2006 [15]	1922 subjects selected from birth cohort	23–25	Pre-existing asthma worsened by exposure at work	81	36%
Curwick 2006 [16]	Workers compensation (WA)	43 median	SENSOR Criteria	301	45%
de Fatima 2007 [17]	Cleaners	37 mean F, 34 mean M	Pre-existing asthma, and cleaning-related sx	26	58%
Fletcher 2006 [18]	OHC (NY)	20–60, 43 mean	SENSOR Criteria	454	14%
Goe 2004§ [19]	SENSOR surveillance	18–70+	SENSOR Criteria	1101	19%,
Larbanois 2002 [20]	Referral clinic	32–54	Asthma sx temporally related to work exposure and negative SIC	157	45%
Lemiere 2007 [21]	Referral clinic	Adults	Aggravation of asthma sx at work, negative SIC	351	41%
Pechter 2005§ [22]	SENSOR cases in health care	41 median	SENSOR Criteria	305	23%
Reinisch 2001§ [23]	Survey of physician first reports (CA)	18–65+	SENSOR Criteria	444	35%
Rosenman 2003§ [24]	SENSOR cases cleaning products	18–70+	SENSOR Criteria	236	20%
Tarlo 1995 [26]	Worker compensation	Mean ~40	Asthma worse at work, with or without prior asthma, no sensitizer exposure. Objective testing common	469	50%
Tarlo 2000 [25]	Asthma clinic	Mean 46	Work-related sx, irritants or other aggravating factors, no sensitizer exposure. Objective testing common	51	49%

* Abbreviations Clinical Setting: OHC system, occupational health clinic; Referral clinic, clinic for suspected work-related asthma; Worker compensation, data from worker compensation system.

† Abbreviations for Criteria WEA: rx, medications; sx, symptoms; SIC, specific inhalation challenge

§ A subset of subjects reported in [9]. SENSOR, Sentinel Event Notification Systems for Occupational Risks. Data from CA, MA, MI, NJ, unless otherwise specified.

SENSOR criteria WEA, asthma in 2 years before new occupational setting, asthma symptoms work-related, more asthma symptoms or medications in new setting of prevalence of WEA as a percentage of all WRA cases ranged from 14% to over 50%, as shown in Table 2. These estimates were highly dependent on factors such as physician recognition, referral patterns, reporting system, and local workers compensation laws. WEA typically is not diagnosed by clinicians in settings where it is not clearly recognized as a condition under worker's compensation rules, such as in New York State and many other states in the United States [18]. Where WEA is recognized, as in the Canadian province of Ontario, or more recently in the province of Quebec, the number of cases of WEA compared to OA tends to rise [21, 25, 26].

The prevalence of WEA has also been described in selected groups of asthmatic workers, such as office workers, cleaners, or construction workers (Tab. 3), with up to 70% of asthmatics reporting exacerbation of their asthmatic symptoms related to their work [17, 27–32]. As with the other clinical and epidemiological studies, the worker populations and diagnostic criteria were variable.

Exposures and WEA

As with non-work-related asthma, a number of diverse exposures and factors have been associated with WEA (Tab. 4). Overall, most commonly reported are various irritant mixed exposures, such as dusts, second-hand smoke, solvents, cleaning products, and fumes at work [9, 18, 25–27]. Common allergens and molds, frequently in settings with inadequate indoor air quality such as office buildings and schools, have also been reported as triggers for asthma symptoms [3, 18, 28]. In addition, non-chemical conditions can also exacerbate asthma at work, including extremes of temperature, physical exertion, emotional stress, and viral infections [3, 11, 14, 25–27, 33].

There are few quantitative data regarding the levels of work exposures that trigger asthma, and comparisons between studies and with different definitions or criteria for WRA can be difficult. However, together these studies indicate that exposures associated with WEA, as compared to new onset OA, were less likely to be specific sensitizing agents, and more likely to be irritant exposures [3, 9, 25]. The irritants associated with WEA typically occur at lower levels than those reported to cause new onset irritant-induced OA [3].

WEA has been reported in a wide range of industries and occupations, including public administration, wholesale and retail trade, cleaning, manufacturing, education, and construction [7, 9, 12, 14, 27]. Several studies have suggested a healthy worker effect, where asthmatic workers leave workplaces with more asthma triggers [10, 12, 34]. Although the specific asthma triggers can be difficult to identify, it is clear that WEA can occur in numerous different work settings, including non-industrial workplaces such as office buildings, schools, and laboratories.

Table 3. Prevalence of WEA among selected asthmatics in certain jobs or work settings (selected studies)

Reference	Type of workers/ work setting	Age (years)	Criteria for WEA (self-reported on questionnaire unless indicated otherwise)	Number asthmatics	Prevalence WEA among asthmatics
Berger 2006 [27]	Low income inner city patients	18–55	Asthma worse at current or most recent job (janitors, security guards, clerks, restaurant workers, textile workers)	301	51%
Cox-Ganser 2005 [28]	Office workers	46 mean	Work-related asthma symptoms in water-damaged building	67	34%
De Fatima 2007 [17]	Cleaners	37 mean F 34 mean M	Cleaning-related asthma symptoms	39	38% (46% females/ 18% males)
Gouge 1994 [29]	Soldiers in Iraq	21–44	Exacerbation of asthma symptoms	10	70%
Jacobs 2007 [30]	Swimming pool workers	16–65 40.5 mean	In last 1 year more asthma attacks and asthma medications, compared to Dutch population	624 working at pools (number with asthma unclear)	OR = 2.6 asthma attack $p < 0.05$
Kreiss 2006 [31]	Cosmetic workers	42 mean	Report asthma worse with workplace exposure or activities	175 108 pre/67 post hire	28% pre-hire asthmatics 58% post-hire asthmatics
Sauni 2001 [32]	Construction workers	18–64	Symptoms worse at work or occupational dust cause symptoms	76	68% worse at work, 66% dust causes symptoms

Table 4. Selected industries, jobs and exposures associated with WEA

Selected industries / Jobs associated with WEA
Technical, sales and administrative support
Public administration, teaching
Laboratory and medical technicians
Cleaners, janitors
Manufacturing (textile workers, operators, laborers)
Selected exposures associated with WEA
Second-hand smoke
Dusts
Smoke, welding fumes
Chemicals (cleaning products, paints, solvents, acids, ammonia)
Common allergens / molds
Abnormal temperatures
Physically strenuous work
Viral respiratory infections

WEA should also be considered in the context of non-work-related asthma exacerbations, which are common, and quite variable in severity, time course and etiology. A number of factors and/or triggers can exacerbate asthma, including viral infections, allergens, irritants, non-compliance with medications, exercise, stress, or other medical conditions (e.g., gastroesophageal reflux or sinusitis) [35]. In both settings many of these exposures are preventable, but in the work setting the patient typically has less control over the environment.

Clinical characteristics and natural history of WEA

The clinical characteristics and natural history of WEA have received much less attention than those related to OA. Several studies have now compared clinical characteristics of patients with WEA to those with OA or to other asthmatics. The study populations, selection and diagnostic criteria, and other methodological features have been quite variable, making findings within and between studies difficult to interpret and compare. A limited number of studies comparing WEA and OA have found predominantly similarities between these groups, including similar levels of asthma severity, airway hyperresponsiveness, medication usage, and needs for healthcare [9, 20, 21, 26, 36].

Similarly, the few studies that have evaluated removal from exposure or more long-term outcomes in WEA have generally found outcomes similar to those for OA, with persistent asthma but improved symptoms and reduced airway inflammation away from exposure [36, 37], although some differences have also been noted, such as higher doses of inhaled corticosteroids in WEA [36]. These findings may reflect selection criteria for the two groups of patients.

A relatively small number of studies have also compared WEA to other asthma cases. Overall, these studies have tended to find more asthmatic symptoms and/or more frequent or more severe asthma exacerbations in asthmatics with WEA compared to other asthmatics [11, 14, 21, 38]. However, some of these same studies have found less severe asthma in WEA using different criteria for asthma severity, and other studies have found less frequent asthma exacerbations in subjects with WEA [11, 25].

Socioeconomic impact

Recent studies have begun to evaluate the social and financial consequences of WEA, comparing WEA to asthma unrelated to work or to occupational asthma [9, 20, 39]. Again, comparisons within and between studies is difficult, as the studies were based on different patient populations, asthma severities, age ranges, and diagnostic criteria. Despite these limitations, studies have generally found that WEA is associated with similar outcomes to those of OA in terms of prolonged unemployment, loss of income, and frequent job changes [9, 20, 39]. However, other studies have reported less frequent job changes for WEA subjects [9, 20, 26].

Diagnosis, management and prevention of WEA

Clinical studies addressing optimal strategies for diagnosing and managing WEA are limited, with the great majority of prior studies addressing sensitizer OA. An expert panel assembled by the American College of Chest Physicians recently published a consensus document on the diagnosis and management of work-related asthma, including WEA [3]. Relevant conclusions are summarized briefly. WEA should be considered in any patient with worsening asthma and/or work-related asthma symptoms. The diagnosis of asthma should be clarified, based on the clinical history, typical symptoms and exam findings, and documentation of reversible airflow obstruction or airway hyperresponsiveness (e.g., bronchodilator response or methacholine challenge test), although this can be difficult to demonstrate in some asthmatics. A careful occupational and medical history is essential. Information on job exposures, type of industry, ventilation, the onset and timing of symptoms in relationship to work, medication use, symptoms in co-workers, and use of protective equipment should be obtained. History of asthma, childhood asthma, atopy, rhinitis and sinusitis should also be clarified, with particular focus on the first onset of asthmatic symptoms, clinical course and triggers.

The relationship between work and asthma exacerbations should be assessed, most commonly by careful documentation of changes in symptoms and medication use temporally related to work, including specific tasks or jobs at work. More severe exacerbations may be documented by health care visits or physiological changes (e.g., in peak expiratory flow rate or forced expiratory volume in one second). Additional sources of exposure information include Material Safety Data Sheet (often abbreviated as MSDS), a union, the employer (with patient's permission), and government agencies. WEA frequently is due to a mixture of substances rather than a single substance, such as encountered in work settings with several irritant gases, construction dust from multiple materials, or many types of cleaning products in use.

WEA should be distinguished from OA, especially if a specific sensitizing agent is identified at work. This can be challenging if the asthma is longstanding and the worker is no longer at the suspect job, since chronic asthma tends to respond non-specifically to multiple triggers. Factors at work and outside work that trigger the asthma should be identified. Thus allergy testing may be useful in atopic asthmatics.

Data on management and prevention of WEA is also very limited. The goal is to improve asthmatic symptoms by reducing work triggers and optimizing asthma treatment. If unsuccessful, a change to a job with fewer triggers may be necessary. Prevention also focuses on reducing work exposures and factors that can trigger asthma, and potentially modifying a worker's job to avoid triggers such as cold weather.

Summary

WEA refers to pre-existing or concurrent asthma that is worsened by work factors. WEA is common in both industrial and non-industrial settings, but has received less attention than OA that is caused by work. A review of the current literature on WEA demonstrates that the prevalence of WEA among working adults is variable, ranging from approximately 15% to 50%. Numerous different exposures or conditions at work can exacerbate asthma. WEA clinically shares many features with OA, including persistent asthma and adverse socioeconomic outcomes (prolonged unemployment, reduction in income). Management of WEA should focus on reducing work exposures and optimizing standard medical management, with a change in jobs only if necessary.

References

1 Moorman JE, Rudd RA, Johnson CA, King M, Minor P, Bailey C, Scalia MR, Akinbami LJ (2007) National surveillance for asthma – United States, 1980–2004. *MMWR Surveill Summ* 56: 1–54

2 Balmes J, Becklake M, Blanc P, Henneberger P, Kreiss K, Mapp C, Milton D, Schwartz D, Toren K, Viegi G (2003) American Thoracic Society Statement: Occupational contribution to the burden of airway disease. *Am J Respir Crit Care Med* 167: 787–797

3 Tarlo SM, Balmes J, Balkissoon R, Beach J, Beckett W, Bernstein D, Blanc PD, Brooks SM, Cowl CT, Daroowalla F et al (2008) Diagnosis and management of work-related asthma: American College of Chest Physicians Consensus Statement. *Chest* 134: 1S-41S

4 Kavura MS, Wiedemann HP (2005) Asthma. In: RB George, RW Light, MA Matthay, RA Matthay (eds): *Chest Medicine*. Lippincott Williams& Wilkins, Philadelphia, 131–162

5 Bateman ED, Hurd SS, Barnes PJ, Bousquet J, Drazen JM, FitzGerald M, Gibson P, Ohta K, O'Byrne P, Pedersen SE et al (2008) Global strategy for asthma management and prevention: GINA executive summary. *Eur Respir J* 31: 143–178

6 Abramson MJ, Kutin JJ, Rosier MJ, Bowes G (1995) Morbidity, medication and trigger factors in a community sample of adults with asthma. *Med J Aust* 162: 78–81

7 Blanc PD, Ellbjar S, Janson C, Norback D, Norrman E, Plaschke P, Toren K (1999) Asthma-related work disability in Sweden. The impact of workplace exposures. *Am J Respir Crit Care Med* 160: 2028–2033

8 Bolen AR, Henneberger PK, Liang X, Sama SR, Preusse PA, Rosiello RA, Milton DK (2007) The validation of work-related self-reported asthma exacerbation. *Occup Environ Med* 64: 343–348

9 Goh LG, Ng TP, Hong CY, Wong ML, Koh K, Ling SL (1994) Outpatient adult bronchial asthma in Singapore. *Singapore Med J* 35: 190–194

10 Henneberger PK, Deprez RD, Asdigian N, Oliver LC, Derk S, Goe SK (2003) Workplace exacerbation of asthma symptoms: Findings from a population-based study in Maine. *Arch Environ Health* 58: 781–788

11 Henneberger PK, Derk SJ, Sama SR, Boylstein RJ, Hoffman CD, Preusse PA, Rosiello RA, Milton DK (2006) The frequency of workplace exacerbation among health maintenance organisation members with asthma. *Occup Environ Med* 63: 551–557

12 Henneberger PK, Hoffman CD, Magid DJ, Lyons EE (2002) Work-related exacerbation of asthma. *Int J Occup Environ Health* 8: 291–296

13 Mancuso CA, Rincon M, Charlson ME (2003) Adverse work outcomes and events attributed to asthma. *Am J Ind Med* 44: 236–245

14 Saarinen K, Karjalainen A, Martikainen R, Uitti J, Tammilehto L, Klaukka T, Kurppa K (2003) Prevalence of work-aggravated symptoms in clinically established asthma. *Eur Respir J* 22: 305–309

15 Caldeira RD, Bettiol H, Barbieri MA, Terra-Filho J, Garcia CA, Vianna EO (2006)

Prevalence and risk factors for work related asthma in young adults. *Occup Environ Med* 63: 694–699
16 Curwick CC, Bonauto DK, Adams DA (2006) Use of objective testing in the diagnosis of work-related asthma by physician specialty. *Ann Allergy Asthma Immunol* 97: 546–550
17 de Fatima Macaira E, Algranti E, Medina Coeli Mendonca E, Antonio Bussacos M (2007) Rhinitis and asthma symptoms in non-domestic cleaners from the Sao Paulo metropolitan area, Brazil. *Occup Environ Med* 64: 446–453
18 Fletcher AM, London MA, Gelberg KH, Grey AJ (2006) Characteristics of patients with work-related asthma seen in the New York State Occupational Health Clinics. *J Occup Environ Med* 48: 1203–1211
19 Goe SK, Henneberger PK, Reilly MJ, Rosenman KD, Schill DP, Valiante D, Flattery J, Harrison R, Reinisch F, Tumpowsky C et al (2004) A descriptive study of work aggravated asthma. *Occup Environ Med* 61: 512–517
20 Larbanois A, Jamart J, Delwiche JP, Vandenplas O (2002) Socioeconomic outcome of subjects experiencing asthma symptoms at work. *Eur Respir J* 19: 1107–1113
21 Lemiere C, Forget A, Dufour MH, Boulet LP, Blais L (2007) Characteristics and medical resource use of asthmatic subjects with and without work-related asthma. *J Allergy Clin Immunol* 120: 1354–1359
22 Pechter E, Davis LK, Tumpowsky C, Flattery J, Harrison R, Reinisch F, Reilly MJ, Rosenman KD, Schill DP, Valiante D et al (2005) Work-related asthma among health care workers: Surveillance data from California, Massachusetts, Michigan, and New Jersey, 1993–1997. *Am J Ind Med* 47: 265–275
23 Reinisch F, Harrison RJ, Cussler S, Athanasoulis M, Balmes J, Blanc P, Cone J (2001) Physician reports of work-related asthma in California, 1993–1996. *Am J Ind Med* 39: 72–83
24 Rosenman KD, Reilly MJ, Schill DP, Valiante D, Flattery J, Harrison R, Reinisch F, Pechter E, Davis L, Tumpowsky CM et al (2003) Cleaning products and work-related asthma. *J Occup Environ Med* 45: 556–563
25 Tarlo SM, Leung K, Broder I, Silverman F, Holness DL (2000) Asthmatic subjects symptomatically worse at work: Prevalence and characterization among a general asthma clinic population. *Chest* 118: 1309–1314
26 Tarlo SM, Liss G, Corey P, Broder I (1995) A workers' compensation claim population for occupational asthma. Comparison of subgroups. *Chest* 107: 634–641
27 Berger Z, Rom WN, Reibman J, Kim M, Zhang S, Luo L, Friedman-Jimenez G (2006) Prevalence of workplace exacerbation of asthma symptoms in an urban working population of asthmatics. *J Occup Environ Med* 48: 833–839
28 Cox-Ganser JM, White SK, Jones R, Hilsbos K, Storey E, Enright PL, Rao CY, Kreiss K (2005) Respiratory morbidity in office workers in a water-damaged building. *Environ Health Perspect* 113: 485–490
29 Gouge SF, Daniels DJ, Smith CE (1994) Exacerbation of asthma after pyridostigmine during Operation Desert Storm. *Mil Med* 159: 108–111

30 Jacobs JH, Spaan S, van Rooy GB, Meliefste C, Zaat VA, Rooyackers JM, Heederik D (2007) Exposure to trichloramine and respiratory symptoms in indoor swimming pool workers. *Eur Respir J* 29: 690–698

31 Kreiss K, Esfahani RS, Antao VC, Odencrantz J, Lezotte DC, Hoffman RE (2006) Risk factors for asthma among cosmetology professionals in Colorado. *J Occup Environ Med* 48: 1062–1069

32 Sauni R, Oksa P, Vattulainen K, Uitti J, Palmroos P, Roto P (2001) The effects of asthma on the quality of life and employment of construction workers. *Occup Med (Lond)* 51: 163–167

33 Jajosky RA, Harrison R, Reinisch F, Flattery J, Chan J, Tumpowsky C, Davis L, Reilly MJ, Rosenman KD, Kalinowski D et al (1999) Surveillance of work-related asthma in selected U.S. states using surveillance guidelines for state health departments – California, Massachusetts, Michigan, and New Jersey, 1993–1995. *MMWR CDC Surveill Summ* 48: 1–20

34 Petsonk EL, Daniloff EM, Mannino DM, Wang ML, Short SR, Wagner GR (1995) Airway responsiveness and job selection: A study in coal miners and non-mining controls. *Occup Environ Med* 52: 745–749

35 Lemanske RF, Jr., Busse WW (2006) 6. Asthma: Factors underlying inception, exacerbation, and disease progression. *J Allergy Clin Immunol* 117: S456–461

36 Pelissier S, Chaboillez S, Teolis L, Lemiere C (2006) Outcome of subjects diagnosed with occupational asthma and work-aggravated asthma after removal from exposure. *J Occup Environ Med* 48: 656–659

37 Girard F, Chaboillez S, Cartier A, Cote J, Hargreave FE, Labrecque M, Malo JL, Tarlo SM, Lemiere C (2004) An effective strategy for diagnosing occupational asthma: Use of induced sputum. *Am J Respir Crit Care Med* 170: 845–850

38 Breton CV, Zhang Z, Hunt PR, Pechter E, Davis L (2006) Characteristics of work related asthma: Results from a population based survey. *Occup Environ Med* 63: 411–415

39 Cannon J, Cullinan P, Newman Taylor A (1995) Consequences of occupational asthma. *BMJ* 311: 602–603

Natural history and prognosis

Dennis Nowak

Institute and Outpatient Clinic for Occupational, Social and Environmental Medicine, Clinical Centre, Ludwig Maximilian University, Munich, Germany

Abstract

In patients with occupational asthma, the rate of symptomatic recovery after avoidance of exposure to the respective agents is only about one third, worsening with increasing age. Likewise, persistent nonspecific bronchial hyperresponsiveness at long-term follow-up is found in about three quarters of these patients. The situation is even worse if patients with occupational asthma are left in the same workplace. These clinical and functional data are supported by investigations demonstrating inflammation and airway remodeling in the course of occupational asthma despite inhaled steroid medication. Given the frequently adverse outcome of occupational asthma, much more effort should be taken to avoid the disease.

Introduction

The present chapter focuses on factors modifying the onset and the course of occupational asthma (OA) under various conditions. Scientific data in this field are limited due to various selection processes in a setting in which medical as well as social, legal and compensational aspects may affect outcomes. Furthermore, small study sizes, different disease mechanisms, various agents, heterogeneous observation times, and varying treatment schemes contribute to limited consistency and generalizability. Nevertheless, some practical conclusions can be drawn based on published evidence.

Onset of disease

In a follow-up of the International Study on Asthma and Allergies in Childhood (ISAAC) II cohort study in Germany, we demonstrated that, surprisingly, pre-existing asthma, allergic rhinitis or atopic dermatitis did not influence job choices of teenagers [1]. Therefore, reasonable prevention by avoiding specific high-risk jobs does not seem to occur at least in this population.

Occupational Asthma, edited by Torben Sigsgaard and Dick Heederik

Individual factors and predisposing conditions contributing to an increased risk for OA due to high- and low-molecular-weight agents are discussed in the respective chapters.

Mainly, the nature of the agent and the intensity of exposure are predictors regarding the onset of disease. In their frequently cited but – unfortunately – not renewed review on the natural history of OA, Chan-Yeung and Malo [2] concluded from the literature on the onset of OA that the majority of patients develop asthma within the first 1–2 years of exposure, but that new cases can still occur after more than 10 years of exposure. On average, sensitization to low-molecular-weight agents seems to require a shorter interval than sensitization to high-molecular-weight compounds. Amongst the latter group, workers exposed to laboratory animal proteins most frequently develop sensitization during the first 2 years of exposure, but bakers exposed to flour do not, indicating that animal allergens are much more potent sensitizers than flour [3]. In workers exposed to high-molecular-weight agents such as laboratory animal dust, symptoms of rhinitis frequently precede the onset of asthma symptoms, without this being a general condition, as shown in a recent follow-up study of bakers' apprentices [4]. This is less frequent with exposure to low-molecular weight agents [5–7]. Riu and coworkers [8] demonstrated that the onset of rhinitis was highest among those currently employed in a high risk job for less than 10 months. Thus, even short exposures, e.g., in holiday jobs, may predispose to occupational rhinitis and indicate an increased risk of developing OA.

Outcome of patients after cessation of exposure

Recently, Rachiotis and co-workers [9] conducted a systematic review of the published literature on the symptomatic and functional outcomes of OA after avoidance of exposure to the causative agents. They identified 39 original studies documenting complete recovery from asthma ($n = 1681$ patients) and 28 with improvement in nonspecific bronchial hyperresponsiveness ($n = 695$ patients). The mean duration of follow-up was 31 (range 6–240) months in studies of symptomatic recovery and 37 (range 6–240) months amongst studies of nonspecific bronchial hyperresponsiveness. However, there is not much information on quantification of exposure prior to and after what is called cessation. Hence, data should be interpreted with caution.

According to this review, rates of symptomatic recovery varied broadly, with a pooled estimate of 32% (95% CI 26–38%). These rates were lower with increasing age and among clinic-based populations. Symptomatic outcomes worsened with increasing age and – not significantly – with the duration of symptomatic exposure: Patients with the shortest durations of exposure (≤76 months) had a slightly higher rate of recovery, but still it was on average only 36% (95% CI 25–50%). The fact that on average only one third of patients with OA will recover fully from their disease, despite avoidance of the causative agent, seems not to be related to the duration of avoidance (Fig. 1).

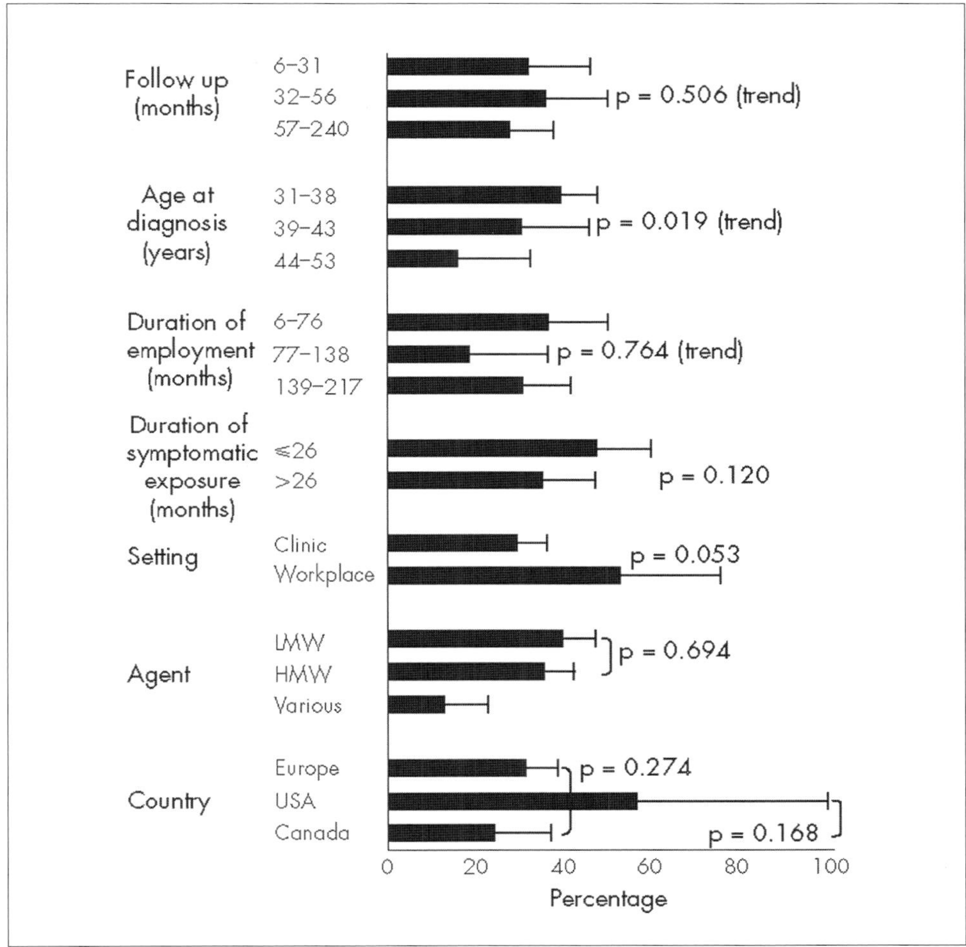

Figure 1.
Determinants of complete symptomatic recovery from occupational asthma after cessation of exposure and a mean follow-up time of 31 (range 6–240) months. Data were collected in a systematic review of the literature, based on 39 studies with 1681 patients. The mean proportion of subjects with complete symptomatic recovery from asthma at follow-up was 32% (HMW, high-molecular-weight, LMW, low-molecular-weight). Reproduced from [9] with permission from BMJ Publishing Group Ltd.

Persistent nonspecific bronchial hyperresponsiveness at follow-up was present in 73% of patients (95% CI 66–79%). This figure was higher in patients whose disease was due to high-molecular-weight agents (approximately 90%) as compared to those with disease due to low-molecular-weight agents (approximately 65%) (Fig. 2).

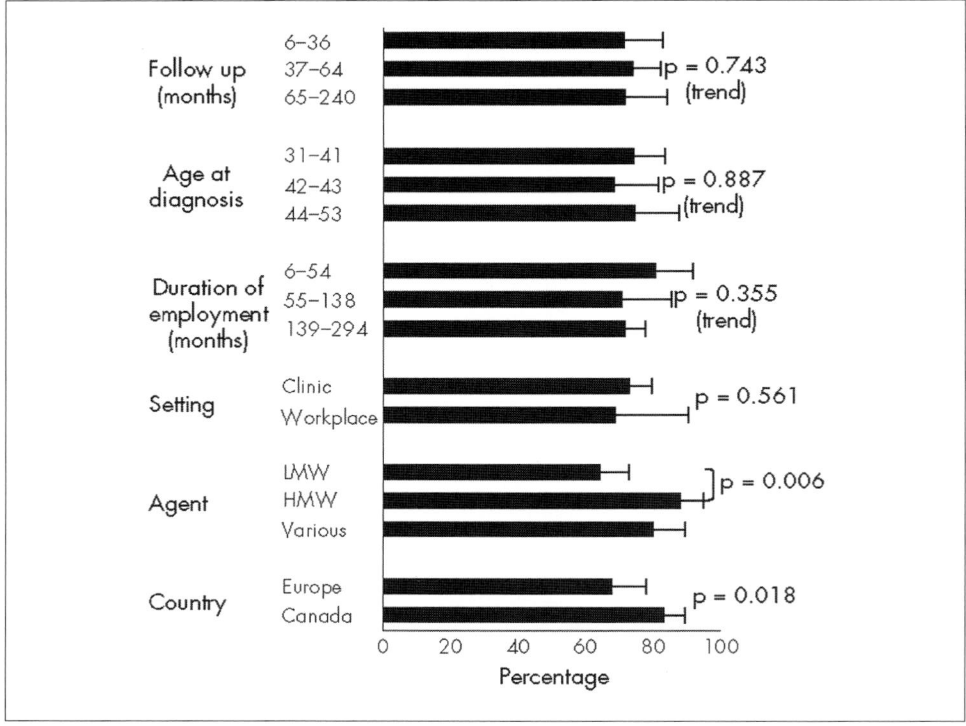

Figure 2.
Determinants of persistent nonspecific bronchial hyperresponsiveness in patients with occupational asthma after cessation of exposure and a mean follow-up time of 37 (range 6–240) months. The mean proportion of subjects with persistent nonspecific bronchial hyperresponsiveness was 73%. (HMW, high-molecular-weight, LMW, low-molecular-weight.) Reproduced from [9] with permission from BMJ Publishing Group Ltd.

Descatha and coworkers performed a pooled analysis of factors associated with severity of OA with a latency period at diagnosis [10]. Their study population consisted of 229 consecutive subjects with OA recruited by four occupational health departments and divided into two groups according to the severity of disease at the time of diagnosis. On multivariate analysis, only a longer duration of symptoms before diagnosis was slightly but significantly associated with a higher asthma severity (OR 1.12, 95% CI 1.05–1.18).

In the specific setting of routine surveillance programs in high-risk populations, OA due, for example, to isocyanates can be diagnosed earlier and is often associated with better outcome compared to the absence of such a program [11].

In the majority of patients sensitized to occupational agents, nonspecific bronchial hyperresponsiveness persists even several years after the end of exposure. In these patients it is of particular practical importance to know whether or not they may nevertheless respond to their specific agent. They may! Lemière and coworkers demonstrated that, despite treatment [12, 13], the absence of asthmatic symptoms and normal nonspecific airway responsiveness, subjects with a history of OA to high-molecular-weight agents, e.g., flour, guar gum and psyllium, and high levels of specific IgE to these agents responded within a few minutes after specific bronchial challenges. Thus, patients with OA due to high-molecular-weight agents should persistently avoid specific exposure even when they have become asymptomatic and nonspecific airway responsiveness has returned to the normal range. Probably, persistent immunological sensitization is a unique factor in causing persistence of disease in these subjects [14].

Outcome of patients with continuous exposure

Patients with OA generally deteriorate if they are left in the same workplace. This was demonstrated, for example, in patients with cedar asthma after an average follow-up of 6.5 years; one third of these patients showed marked deterioration [15]. Anees and coworkers [16] investigated the course of spirometric changes in patients with OA predominantly due to low-molecular-weight agents. In 90 subjects in whom FEV_1 measurements had been performed at least 1 year before removal from exposure (median 2.9 years), the mean rate of decline in FEV_1 was 101 ml/year. One year after removal from exposure, FEV_1 had improved by a mean of 12.3 ml. The mean decline in FEV_1 was 26.6 ml/year in 86 subjects in whom measurements were made for at least 1 year following removal from exposure, similar to the rate of decline in healthy adults. Remarkably, the decline in FEV_1 was not significantly worse in current smokers than in those who had never smoked, and was not affected by the use of inhaled corticosteroids.

These data seem to contrast findings of Marabini et al. [17] who reported that regular treatment with inhaled corticosteroids and long-acting bronchodilators seemed to prevent respiratory deterioration over a 3-year period in workers with mild-to-moderate persistent OA who were still exposed at work to the occupational cause of their disease. However, this was a small-scale study with only ten subjects available for follow-up, with ten others retiring or changing jobs. Thus, a selection process may have contributed to the somewhat surprisingly favorable outcome. Additionally, as the authors state, some of the patients reported a reduction of exposure to the offending agent. Therefore, conclusions from these data should be drawn with great caution.

Inflammation and airway remodeling in the course of occupational asthma

Maghni and coworkers found that patients with OA who retain their bronchial hyperresponsiveness for several years after removal from exposure to the causing agent exhibit persistent airway inflammation with eosinophilia and neutrophilia in induced sputum [18]. Thus, inflammation seemed to be self-sustained even in the absence of exposure to the asthmagenic agent. Maestrelli commented on these data that low-molecular-weight chemicals responsible for occupational sensitization once inhaled may attach to proteins, although these compounds are unlikely to remain in the body for years [19]. The same was considered even more valid when the sensitizing agent is a protein. Therefore, if the mechanism of airway inflammation in these patients with persistent asthma is independent of exogenous stimulation, allergen avoidance alone will not be sufficient to produce a favorable outcome.

Saetta and co-workers [20] studied airway wall remodeling in sensitized subjects with OA caused by diisocyanates both at the time of diagnosis, and 6–21 months after cessation of exposure to toluene diisocyanate. The cessation of exposure to the sensitizing agent was associated with a reduced, but still – compared to normal – pathologically increased thickness of the basement membrane and with a reduced number of subepithelial fibroblasts, mast cells, and lymphocytes in the bronchial mucosa, suggesting a remodeling of the airway wall with the avoidance of the specific stimulus.

In a comparable setting, Piirilä and coworkers investigated inflammatory changes in patients with diisocyanate-induced asthma after initiation of inhaled steroid treatment at a mean period of 7 months (range 3–60 months) after cessation of exposure [21]. The count of mast cells in bronchial mucosa decreased and that of macrophages increased. During the first year, interleukin (IL)-4 level in mucosa was significantly higher than in controls, but its level decreased during follow-up. IL-6, IL-15, and tumor necrosis factor-α mRNA levels were significantly higher in patients with bronchial hyperresponsiveness as compared to those without. Therefore, inflammation may persist in diisocyanate-induced asthma despite inhaled steroid medication.

Fatal outcomes

Besides anaphylaxis to occupational sensitizers, OA may be a fatal condition: Exposure to diisocyanates [22, 23], baking flour [24] and shark cartilage dust [25] has been reported to cause death in sensitized workers. Whether or not the patient reported by Chester et al. [26] was sensitized to diisocyanates or an irritative mechanism caused his fatality is not known. Stanbury and coworkers recently reported an acute death of a young asthmatic waitress associated with work-related environmental tobacco smoke in a bar [27].

Outcome of reactive airways dysfunction syndrome

Malo and coworkers studied the long-term outcomes of acute irritant-induced asthma [28]. In this cohort study of 35 subjects, the causal agent was chlorine in the majority ($n=20$). At reassessment after a mean interval of 14 ± 5 years, all subjects reported respiratory symptoms, and 24 (two thirds) were on inhaled steroids. There were no significant improvements in FEV_1 and FEV_1/FVC values. Among 23 subjects with methacholine tests at follow-up, only 6 had normal levels of responsiveness. Greven et al. [29] investigated respiratory effects among 138 emergency services first responders and residents with exposure to combustion products in the aftermath of a chemical waste depot fire. Identified by telephone interview 6 years later, subjects with persistent respiratory symptoms were suspected as having reactive airways dysfunction syndrome (RADS). Persistent respiratory symptoms and bronchial responsiveness were associated with exposure to combustion products of that fire. Thus, the long-term adverse outcome of RADS should generally be taken more into consideration when managing incidents to limit exposure to airway irritants.

Conclusion

Available data on the prognosis of OA suggest that on average, only one third of patients will lose their symptoms, and nonspecific bronchial hyperresponsiveness may persist in the majority. Although data are insufficiently consistent to allow individually tailored advice with a high positive predictive value, there is evidence that continued exposure, once the disease has developed, leads to a worse prognosis, and that early removal from exposure is associated with a better prognosis. Recently published evidence-based guidelines for the prevention, identification, and management of OA [30] therefore summarize that:

- symptoms and functional impairment of OA caused by various agents may persist for many years after avoidance of further exposure to the causative agent (evidence 2+),
- the likelihood of improvement or resolution of symptoms or of preventing deterioration is greater in workers who have

- no further exposure to the causative agent (evidence 2++),
- relatively normal lung function at the time of diagnosis (evidence 2+),
- shorter duration of symptoms prior to diagnosis (evidence 2+).

References

1 Radon K, Huemmer S, Dressel H, Windstetter D, Weinmayr G, Weiland S, Riu E, Vogelberg C, Leupold W, von Mutius E, Goldberg M, Nowak D (2006) Do respiratory symptoms predict job choices in teenagers? *Eur Respir J* 27: 774–778

2 Chan-Yeung M, Malo JL (1999) Natural history of occupational asthma. In: IL Bernstein, M Chan-Yeung, JL Malo, DI Bernstein (eds): *Asthma in the Workplace*. Marcel Dekker, New York, 299–322

3 Gautrin D, Ghezzo H, Infante-Rivard C, Malo JL (2000) Incidence and determinants of IgE-mediated sensitization in apprentices: a prospective study. *Am J Respir Crit Care Med* 162: 1222–1228

4 Skjold T, Dahl R, Juhl B, Sigsgaard T (2008) The incidence of respiratory symptoms and sensitisation in baker apprentices. *Eur Respir J* 32: 452–459

5 Gautrin D, Ghezzo H, Infant-Rivard C, Malo JL (2001) Natural history of sensitization, symptoms and diseases in apprentices exposed to laboratory animals. *Eur Respir J* 17: 904–908

6 Rodier F, Gautrin D, Ghezzo H, Malo HL (2003) Incidence of occupational rhinoconjunctivitis and risk factors in animal-health apprentices. *J Allergy Clin Immunol* 112: 1105–1111

7 Malo JL, Lemière C, Desjardins A, Cartier A (1997) Prevalence and intensity of rhinoconjunctivitis in subjects with occupational asthma. *Eur Respir J* 10: 1513–1515

8 Riu E, Dressel H, Windstetter D, Weinmayr G, Weiland S, Vogelberg C, Leupold W, von Mutius E, Nowak D, Radon K (2007) First months of employment and new onset of rhinitis in adolescents. *Eur Respir J* 30: 549–555

9 Rachiotis G, Savani R, Brant A, MacNeill SJ, Newman Taylor A, Cullinan P (2007) Outcome of occupational asthma after cessation of exposure: a systematic review. *Thorax* 62: 147–152

10 Descatha A, Leproust H, Choudat D, Garnier R, Pairon JC, Ameille J (2007) Factors associated with severity of occupational asthma with a latency period at diagnosis. *Allergy* 62: 795–801

11 Tarlo SM, Liss GM (2002) Diisocyanate-induced asthma: Diagnosis, prognosis, and effects of medical surveillance measures. *Appl Occup Environ Hyg* 17: 902–908

12 Lemière C, Cartier A, Malo JL, Lehrer SB (2000) Persistent specific bronchial reactivity to occupational agents in workers with normal nonspecific bronchial reactivity. *Am J Respir Crit Care Med* 162: 976–980

13 Lemière C (2003) Persistence of bronchial reactivity to occupational agents after remov-

al from exposure and identification of associated factors. *Ann Allergy Asthma Immunol* 90: 52–55

14 Mapp CE, Boschetto P, Maestrelli P, Fabbri LM (2005) Occupational asthma. State of the art. *Am J Respir Crit Care Med* 172: 280–305

15 Coté J, Kennedy S, Chan-Yeung M (1990) Outcome of patients with red cedar asthma with continuous exposure. *Am Rev Respir Dis* 141: 373–376

16 Anees W, Moore VC, Burge PC (2006) FEV_1 decline in occupational asthma. *Thorax* 61: 751–755

17 Marabini A, Siracusa A, Stopponi R, Tacconi C, Abbritti G (2003) Outcome of occupational asthma in patients with continuous exposure. A 3-year longitudinal study during pharmacologic treatment. *Chest* 124: 2372–2376

18 Maghni K, Lemière C, Ghezzo H, Yuquan W, Malo JL (2004) Airway inflammation after cessation of exposure to agents causing occupational asthma. *Am J Respir Crit Care Med* 169: 367–372

19 Maestrelli P (2004) Natural history of adult-onset asthma. Insights from model of occupational asthma. *Am J Respir Crit Care Med* 169: 331–332

20 Saetta M, Maestrelli P, Turato G, Mapp CE, Milani GF, Pivirotto F, Fabbri LM, di Stefano A (1995) Airway wall remodeling after cessation of exposure to isocyanates in sensitized asthmatic subjects. *Am J Respir Crit Care Med* 151: 489–494

21 Piirilä PL, Meuronen A, Majuri ML, Luukkonen R, Mäntylä T, Wolff HJ, Nordman H, Alenius H, Laitinen A (2008) Inflammation and functional outcome in diisocyanate-induced asthma after cessation of exposure. *Allergy* 63: 583–591

22 Fabbri LM, Danieli D, Crescioli S, Bevilaqua P, Meli S, Saetta M, Mapp CE (1988) Fatal asthma in a subject sensitized to toluene diisocyanate. *Am Rev Respir Dis* 137: 1494–1498

23 Carino M, Aliani M, Licitra C, Sarno N, Ioli F (1997) Death due to asthma at workplace in a diphenylmethane diisocyanate-sensitized subject. *Respiration* 64: 111–113

24 Ehrlich RI (1994) Fatal asthma in a baker: A case report. *Am J Ind Med* 26: 799–802

25 Ortega HG, Kreiss K, Schill DP, Weissman DN (2002) Fatal asthma from powdering shark cartilage and review of occupational asthma literature. *Am J Ind Med* 42: 50–54

26 Chester DA, Hanna EA, Pickelman BG, Rosenman KD (2005) Asthma death after spraying polyurethane truck bedliner. *Am J Ind Med* 48: 78–84

27 Stanbury M, Chester D, Hanna EA, Rosenman KD (2008) How many deaths will it take? A death from asthma associated with work-related environmental tobacco smoke. *Am J Ind Med* 51: 111–116

28 Malo JL, L'Archeveque J, Castellanos L, Lavoie K, Ghezzo H, Maghni K (2009) Long-term outcomes of acute irritant-induced asthma. *Am J Respir Crit Care Med* 179: 923–928

29 Greven F, Kerstjens HA, Duijm F, Eppinga P, de Meer G, Heederik D (2009) Respiratory effects in the aftermath of a major fire in a chemical waste depot. *Scand J Work Environ Health* 35: 368–375

30 Nicholson PJ, Cullinan P, Newman Taylor AJ, Burge PS, Boyle C (2005) Evidence based

guidelines for the prevention, identification, and management of occupational asthma. *Occup Environ Med* 62: 290–299

Mechanisms of allergic occupational asthma

Xaver Baur

Ordinariat und Zentralinstitut für Arbeitsmedizin und Maritime Medizin, Universität Hamburg, Hamburg, Germany

Abstract

High-molecular-weight agents are a major cause of allergic occupational asthma in the workplace. High-molecular-weight agents comprise proteins from plant, microorganism or animal origin in the 10–60 kDa range. A few occupational asthma allergens are man-made chemicals such as isocyanates or acid anhydrides. Allergens with a major public health relevance are derived from flour, latex, enzymes and laboratory animals. The structures of antigenic determinants and mechanisms of many occupational allergens have been elucidated, whereas those of others, e.g. of platinum, recognized by immunocompetent cells are still obscure.

The underlying immune mechanisms of allergic occupational asthma correspond to type I allergy, i.e., antigen recognition and processing by antigen-presenting cells, induction of the Th2 immune response resulting in the production of antigen-specific IgE antibodies, and finally release and generation of bronchospastic and inflammatory mediators by mast and other cells.

The pathological mechanisms of allergic and non-allergic occupational asthma are relevant to diagnostics, management, and prevention, and are also briefly covered in this chapter. Related to this chapter is a useful listing of know occupational allergens, of high and low molecular weight, included in an Appendix.

Introduction

Asthma characterized by variable airflow obstruction due to immunological mechanisms against agents occurring in the workplace is called 'allergic occupational asthma' (allergic OA) (Fig. 1). Immunological mechanisms associated with allergen-specific IgE antibodies have been identified for most causative high-molecular weight (HMW) and for some causative low-molecular weight (LMW) occupational agents. The importance of other immunological mechanisms initiating airway inflammation without detectable IgE antibodies needs further investigations (see below).

Typically, allergic OA has a latency period, which differs from 'non-allergic OA' that is caused by exposure to irritant (non-allergenic) gases, fumes or particles (Tab. 1). Non-allergic OA or irritant OA encompasses the reactive airways dysfunction syndrome (RADS), sometimes even occurring after a single exposure but also after multiple exposure events to high concentrations of nonspecific irritants.

Occupational Asthma, edited by Torben Sigsgaard and Dick Heederik

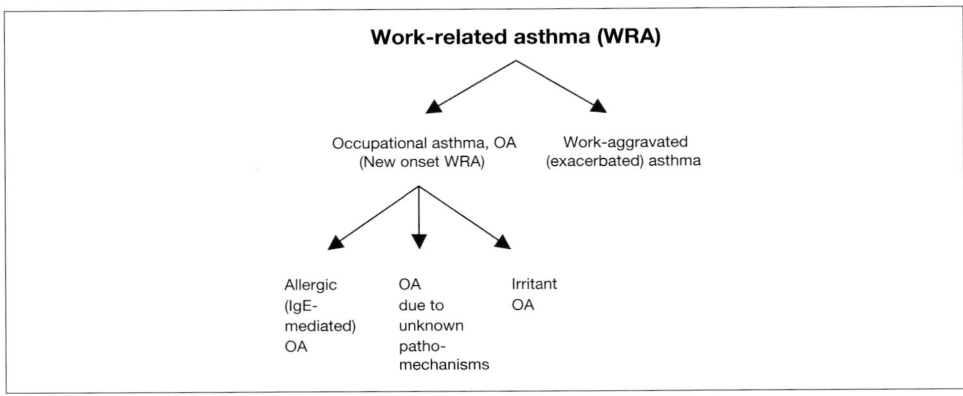

Figure 1.
Schematic representation of occupational asthma (OA) as part of work-related asthma.

Table 1. Specific aspects of allergic occupational asthma (OA) and differences in comparison with non-allergic (irritant) OA

	Allergic OA	**Non-allergic (irritant-induced) OA**
Causes	Mainly HMW and some LMW agents	Airway irritants
Mechanisms	Specific IgE antibodies	Acute or chronic irritant injury to bronchial mucosa
Essential features	Latency period of exposure and sensitization prior to onset of symptoms	Mostly sudden onset without latency period; evidence for chronic low-dose pathogenesis (rare)
Evidence of causal relationship	Specific IgE antibodies, positive skin prick test results	Temporal relationship between exposure to irritant agents and the (mostly rapid) onset of asthma symptoms
Diagnostics	Assessment of obstructive ventilation pattern, bronchial hyperresponsiveness, and eosinophilic inflammation associated with exposure Serial PEFR plus symptom diary Specific inhalation challenge	Assessment of obstructive ventilation pattern, and bronchial hyperresponsiveness associated with exposure (Serial PEFR, if possible during relevant exposure) (Specific inhalation challenge rarely of diagnostic value)
Outcome	Improvement or normalisation after removal from exposure source; airway hyperresponsiveness may persist	Improvement after removal from exposure source; frequently persistent airway hyperresponsiveness

HMW, High-molecular weight; LMW, low-molecular-weight; PEFR, peak expiratory flow recordings

Pathophysiology and immunology of allergic OA

Initial pathophysiological mechanisms of allergic OA differ fundamentally from irritant OA (Tab. 1), although similar inflammatory changes have been described for the chronic course of both disorders. Furthermore, there is no difference between asthma caused by allergens from the general environment and asthma caused by occupational allergens, as shown by various investigations including sputum cytology, bronchoalveolar lavage (BAL) analyses, bronchial biopsies and postmortem lung tissue studies.

The most relevant involved mechanisms, cells and cytokines, are shown in Figure 2.

Inhaled occupational allergens gain access to the viable airway epithelium where they engage and activate local dendritic cells, which keep mucosal surfaces under surveillance. Allergens are processed by these cells, bind to major histocompatibility complex class II (MHC-II) molecules, and their fragments (highly polymorphic

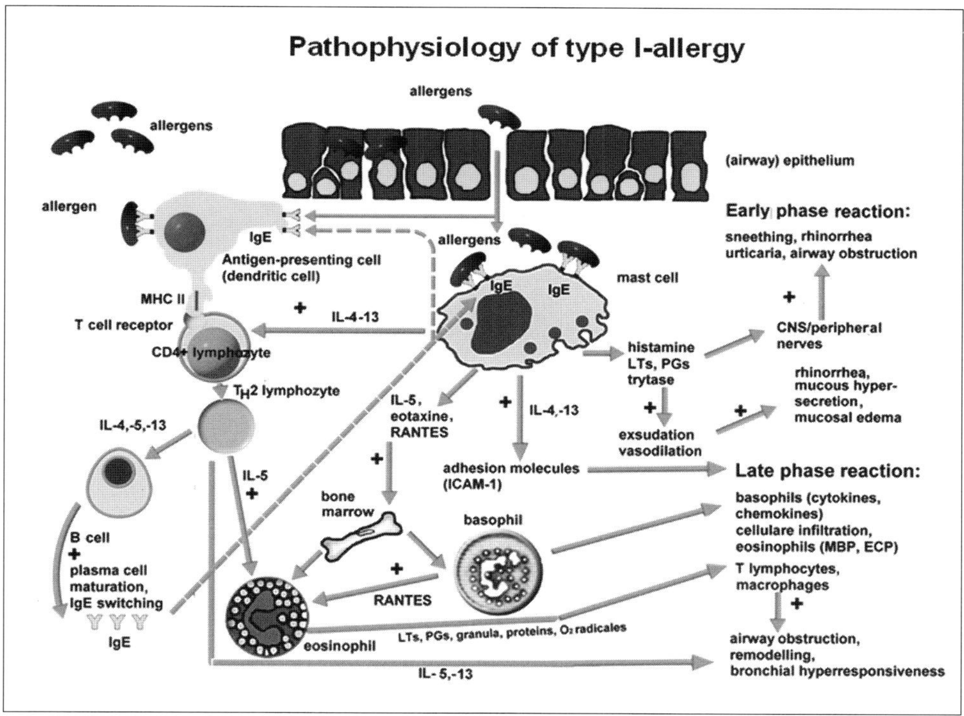

Figure 2.
Scheme on immune mechanisms, mediators and pathophysiology of type I allergy.

short peptides) are then transported by these cells to regional lymph nodes and presented to T lymphocytes, which recognize them by their T cell receptors (TCR). The cytokine milieu is critical to T cell differentiation in Th1 or Th2 responses. IL-12 production leads to Th1 phenotypes, and increased IL-4/IL-13 production leads to Th2 phenotypes. The Th2-dominant cytokine response drives the synthesis and secretion of allergen-specific IgE antibodies by B cells (plasma cells). IgE regulates the expression of its own high-affinity IgE receptors (FcεRI) and low-affinity IgE receptor (CD23) on the surface of mast cells, basophils and possibly of macrophages, dendritic cells, eosinophils and platelets. IgE-dependent up-regulation of FcεRI and CD23 receptors subsequently amplifies immunological reactions. It leads to a greater release of mast cell and basophil mediators at lower concentrations of a specific allergen. Upon new exposure, the allergen cross-links between these specific IgE antibodies on cell surfaces, gives rise to a cascade of events, and leads to an inflammatory cell activation with subsequent synthesis and/or release of a variety of preformed mediators (e.g., histamine) and newly formed inflammatory ones (e.g., prostaglandins, leukotrienes). These mediators orchestrate the inflammatory reaction in bronchial mucosa and submucosa (Fig. 2).

An interesting finding is the cleavage of the tight junction protein occludin by allergenic proteases, e.g., from house dust mites or moulds, which damage the airway epithelium barrier and subsequently increase epithelial permeability and stimulation of the release of mediators. This also orchestrates local immune responses and the inflammatory process [1, 2].

Airway remodeling, as typically found in bronchial asthma [3, 4], also takes place in OA. It can be interpreted as an exaggerated and uncontrolled injury repair process influenced by type and intensity of airway injury and modulated by host as well as genetic factors. It involves epithelial changes, increases in smooth muscle mass and subepithelial collagen deposition, proteoglycans and elastin content, angiogenesis, cartilage changes, goblet cell and glandular hyperplasia. Airway modeling may lead to persistently increased airway responsiveness and mucous production, airflow limitation, and probably to a decline in lung function [5]. Besides its detrimental effect it may protect against excessive bronchoconstriction and inflammation.

Typical morphological findings in airways of allergic OA patients include:

- epithelial desquamation or hyperplasia;
- an increased number of inflammatory cells, especially of eosinophils, in mucosal and submucosal layers (demonstrated by bronchial biopsies); they are also found in sputum and BAL;
- evidence for the activation of eosinophils and lymphocytes;
- increased airway wall thickening;
- increased thickness of the basement membrane, especially of the reticular layer due to interstitial cross-linked collagens produced by myofibroblasts;

- airway smooth muscle hyperplasia, hypertrophia, an increased secretion of cytokines as well as growth factors recruiting inflammatory cells and stimulating the production of extracellular matrix proteins; submucosal and peribronchial vessels are dilated, congested and exhibit thickening of arterial media [4];
- increased NO concentrations in exhaled air (FeNO) after exposure to causative allergens, isocyanates, ozone, swine confinements [6].

It should be noted, however, that there is no consistency with regard to the parallel changes in inflammatory cell counts and/or their activation status on the one hand and asthma severity on the other hand.

Exposure cessation does not always lead to an improvement of abnormal morphological and cellular changes and clinical findings [7]. Subepithelial collagen thickening may reverse after exposure termination and treatment with inhaled steroids.

Determinants of allergic OA

Atopy affecting approximately one third of the population, and defined as the tendency to produce specific IgE antibodies to environmental allergens like those from house dust mites, pollen, and cat or dog fur, modifies the risk of allergic OA resulting from HMW sensitizers as found in bakers (especially in those with hay fever) [8–12], laboratory animal workers (in those sensitized to pets) [13–16], subjects exposed to detergent enzymes, certain reactive dyes, latex [17], and other HMW allergens [18]. In contrast, atopy does not modify the risk for developing asthma caused by isocyanates, acid anhydrides, platinum salts or plicatic acid of red cedar wood. An increasing number of studies show convincing evidence for exposure-response relationships in allergic OA, with higher exposure levels associated with specific sensitization, symptoms, and obstructive ventilation patterns [19–30]. The exposure-response relationships show mostly a linear shape, but bell-shaped relations have also been described for some OA allergens [12]. There is a need for prospective studies with more detailed investigations on dose and timing of occupational exposures.

Recently there has been increased interest in the role of specific genes and gene-environment interactions, which are often complex and non-linear. Generally, most studies on allergic asthma are small and replication studies have seldom been published. Mostly candidate gene studies have been performed focusing on polymorphisms in genes responsible for metabolism of chemicals (like for isocyanates) or genes coding for certain steps in immunological pathways such as antigen presentation [human leukocyte antigen (HLA) genes]. Very few gene environment studies have been conducted. One of the more interesting ones refers to a promoter single nucleotide polymorphism in the CD14 gene (–159 T to C). This polymorphism and exposure to endotoxin were found to be associated with a decreased frequency of allergic asthma in children living on farms [31–33]. One early study showed that α-1-antitrypsin alleles were associated increased hyperresponsiveness in farming students only, indicating a gene-environment interaction [34]. Recent studies provide strong evidence for a genetic basis of increased skin and mucosa permeability in atopics. This involves defects of filaggrin, facilitating terminal differentiation of the epidermis and formation of a skin barrier [35, 36]. Its mutations are linked with eczema-associated asthma and asthma severity [37]. Furthermore, overexpression of Th2 cytokines down-regulates filaggrin expression [38].

Other polymorphisms that code for genes of HLA class II or transmembrane proteins or respiratory anti-oxidant mechanisms may also explain susceptibility to a number of causative occupational agents; however, respective definitive risk factors cannot be provided yet [39–44]. Genetic studies and gene-environment studies are, at the moment, mainly of mechanistic interest. Applications for risk profiling, diagnosis or personalized treatment or prevention over the short term are not expected.

Cigarette smoking increases the risk of specific sensitization and OA due to several LMW agents [45–49]. This was shown in workers of platinum refineries [50, 51], snow-crab processing plants [52], and subjects exposed to tetrachlorophthalic anhydride [53] or *Ispaghula* dust [54].

Allergic occupational rhinitis frequently occurs as a co-morbid condition in allergic OA. Typically, allergic occupational rhinitis or rhinoconjunctivitis develop before the onset of allergic OA, indicating an increased OA risk in affected subjects [22, 26, 55–60].

Occupational allergens

List of known occupational allergens

There are about 350 OA-inducing allergens, mainly HMW compounds representing airborne (glyco)proteins from plants, microorganisms, and animals (see Tab. 2), and eliciting IgE-mediated hypersensitivity. Several LMW agents may also elicit IgE responses; some of them thus seem to be complete allergens. Other LMW agents such as acid anhydrides and isocyanates form allergenic conjugates upon reaction with autologous human proteins. Specific IgE antibody responses may be directed against the newly formed structures (especially against the binding regions of such conjugates behaving as new antigenic determinants) or against the haptenic ligand (the latter was shown for phthalic acid anhydride and himic anhydride). There is evidence that ring structures, positions of double bonds and methyl group substitutions are critical determinants of IgE-mediated sensitization [61, 62]. Many of the allergenic LMW agents also behave as irritants, i.e., OA may be due to the IgE-mediated pathway or, especially at high concentrations, due to irritative effects. This

Table 2. Allergenic agents reported to cause OA: Groups and important examples (Complete list available at: http://www.uke.uni-hamburg.de/institute/arbeitsmedizin/ →Publikationen "Allergenic agents reported to cause occupational asthma") (accessed 6 November 2009)

Group	Important examples
Microorganisms and their products	Aspergillus enzymes, e.g., fungal α-amylase, detergent enzymes
Plants	Flour, grain Latex Wood dust Flowers
Animals	Rats, mice Cows Birds Storage mites Insects Seafood
Chemicals	Isocyanates Acid anhydrides Metal dust, e.g., platinum salts Synthetic drugs Hairdressing chemicals

means that the detection of respective IgE antibodies is a specific but not necessarily a sensitive diagnostic marker of OA caused by such LMW agents.

For some occupational agents such as plicatic acid and morphine, respective IgE antibodies seem not correlated with clinical findings. This unexpected finding raises the question of the specificity of IgE tests used or the absence of IgE.

For details on OA-inducing occupations and confinements comprising some specific, heterogeneous or unidentified allergens, see the Appendix.

Clinical aspects

Exposure of a sensitized and hyperresponsive subject to a causative allergen elicits an early asthmatic reaction, which is characterized by smooth muscle contraction, mucosal edema and an inflammatory response. A late asthmatic reaction may take place several hours afterwards, which is associated with a prolific influx of inflammatory cells and followed by remarkable and long-term inflammatory reactions and an increase in bronchial hyperresponsiveness.

Diagnosis of allergic occupational asthma

The initial suspicion of OA is mostly expressed by the general practitioner, pneumologist, allergologist or occupational or factory physician due to work-related asthma symptoms. Diagnostic measures should be performed before the worker leaves her/his workplace since prolonged avoidance of contact with the causative substance(s) can reduce susceptibility and lead to false-negative diagnostic results. A basic clinical examination and environmental evaluation should be performed in any suspicious case. If there is evidence for an occupational cause of asthmatic symptoms and/or disorders a more detailed assessment should follow to establish a working hypothesis of the disorder. Evaluation tests will confirm or definitely negate the provisional diagnosis. These measures usually require considerable effort and expertise. For details, see Figure 3 and 4. One should realize that specific mechanisms involved in the different phenotypes of OA related to different causes determine to some extent the sequence and choice for specific diagnostic procedures. This makes the diagnosis a complicated process and the likelihood of making wrong

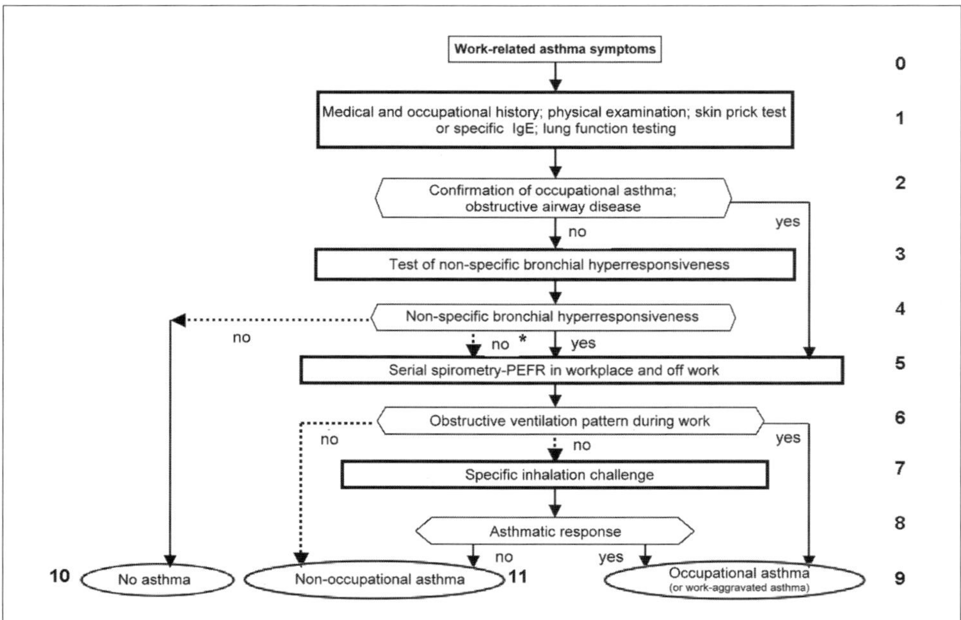

Figure 3.
*Stepwise scheme for the diagnostic procedure to confirm or exclude OA. * Consider possibility of false-negative testing of nonspecific bronchial hyperresponsiveness. In case of positive allergological test results, the diagnosis is allergic OA.*

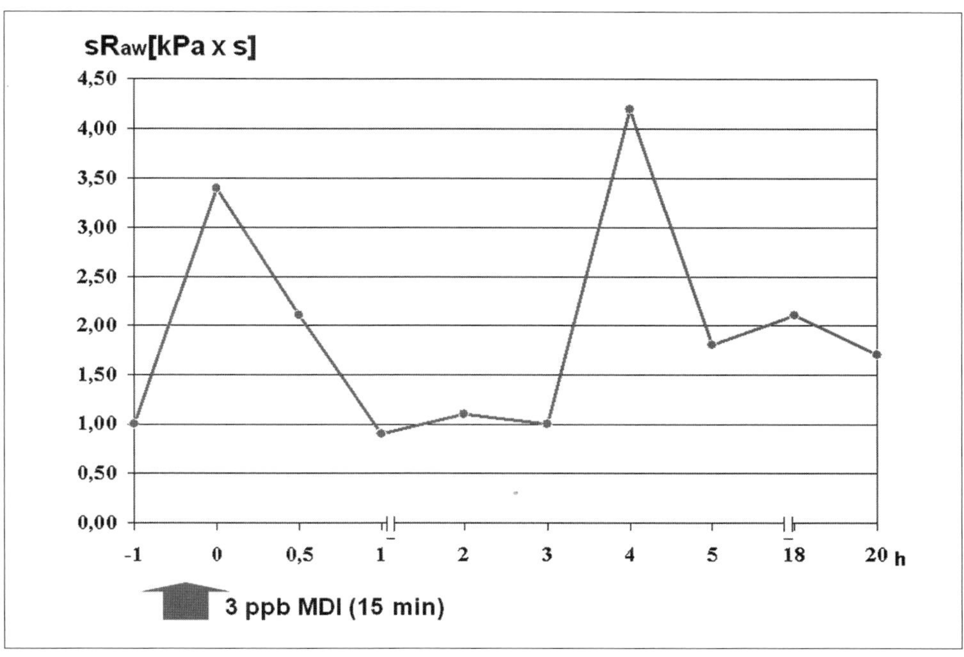

Figure 4.
Specific inhalation challenge test by the isocyanate MDI eliciting a dual asthmatic response. The 51-year-old foam worker has suffered from work-related asthma attacks for 15 months as well as from nocturnal asthmatic symptoms that could not clearly be related to a causative agent so far.

decisions is always present. In brief, the diagnostic workup consists of the following steps with some relevant details for each step related to mechanisms:

- The detailed occupational history and the detailed medical history (Tab. 1 and 3) are the central parts of the diagnostic algorithm;
- Allergic OA has to be differentiated from irritant OA (see basic toxicological information for an agent, check medical literature, interpret results of allergological tests);
- Commercially available well-standardized allergen extracts should be used for allergological testing and specific inhalative challenge tests; mostly they have to be supplemented by self-made extracts of HMW agents occurring in the workplace;
- The use of standardized and sensitive methods for the measurement of specific IgE antibodies in serum is highly recommended if the routine skin prick testing is not possible or its results are not reliable;

Table 3. Components of the medical, occupational, and environmental history

Components of the medical, occupational, and environmental history
A. History of the present illness 1. Detailed record of the circumstances resulting in the onset and worsening of disease 2. Temporal relationships between recurrent exposures and disease exacerbations 3. Course and rate of airway diseases in the particular workplace/branch 4. Asthma severity at the time of initial evaluation
B. Medical history 1. Premorbid medical history, e.g., childhood asthma, hay fever, pet allergy 2. Associated symptoms and concomitant diseases
C. Occupational and environmental history 1. Type (quality) of noxious substances in the workplace (e.g., allergens, irritants, carcinogens, etc.) 2. Intensity (concentrations) of exposure by inhalation, and skin contact 3. Cumulative dose during working life 4. Use of protective equipment

- The course of lung function parameters and symptoms before, during and after occupational exposure has to be evaluated in detail. Further, exact analyses of all medical reports before, during and after employment including medical surveillance data should be performed; Table 4 gives an overview on indications and further details of specific inhalative challenge tests.
- If the occupational exposure generated a new onset of asthma or a significant aggravation of preexisting asthma, the disorder and its deteriorating proportion have to be reported to the responsible insurance institution for occupational diseases, be recognized and compensated as an occupational disease (respective national legal definitions and regulations have to be observed).

New diagnostic tools

New additional diagnostic tools include measurements of the fraction of exhaled nitrous oxide (FeNO), and analyses of induced sputum and exhaled breath condensate during occupational exposure. These methods have been shown to provide valuable information on occupationally induced allergic airway diseases and differential diagnoses [63, 64].

Table 4. Overview of specific inhalative challenge tests: indications, methodology, advantages and limitations

Indications	- uncertain diagnosis and unclear etiology - the respective information is necessary for preventive and/or therapeutic measures or compensation.
Methodology	- generate constant, well-defined non-irritative air concentrations - start with a concentration that is expected not to cause a response and increase it in several ~15-min intervals, each with an ~3-fold increase in concentration up to the workplace atmosphere level or OEL (TLV) - monitor air concentration continuously with validated equipment, e.g., isocyanates by an MDA 7700 device.
Advantages	- Identification/exclusion of an individual occupational agent as OA cause.
Limitations	- High concentrations of an irritative agent may lead to unspecific effects, i.e., to a false-positive result - A false-negative result may occur due to: • anti-asthmatic treatment • a long latency period • use of an inappropriate substance or too low concentration of the causative agent • cumulative effects of an occupational agent over days or of several agents with additive effects present in the workplace (the latter two cannot be reproduced in the laboratory).

OEL, occupational exposure limit; TLV, threshold limit value

Appendix: Occupational asthma-inducing occupations and work environments comprising some specific, heterogeneous or unidentified allergens

Animal confinements and farm working

The prevalence of rat allergy among laboratory animal workers ranges from 12% to 31% [65]. Cross-sectional and cohort studies revealed that the exposure levels to rat urinary aeroallergens correlated positively with the frequency of positive skin test results as well as with work-related upper and lower airway responses [8, 66–68]. Atopic workers had a more than threefold increased sensitization risk at low allergen levels than non-atopics. Major allergens in rat excreta and epithelium involve $\alpha 2\mu$-globulin (17 kDa), prealbumin (21 kDa) and a 23-kDa protein. Similar results were reported for mouse allergens/urinary proteins [65, 69]. An increase in asthma prevalence also occurs in farm animal confinements [70–73]. Cow allergens were reported to be a major cause of respiratory allergies of farmers [74–76]. Concentrations as low as 1–20 μg (atopics), and 25–50 μg (non-atopics) of the major cow allergen Bos d 2 per gram dust were found to be significantly associated with specific IgE antibodies [77]. Furthermore, Rautiainen et al. [78] reported that the level of antibodies to bovine epithelial allergens among exposed subjects reflects the level of clinical allergies.

Working in swine confinements [79–83], poultry confinements [84, 85], poultry slaughter houses [86, 87] or contact with raw poultry [88] causes lung function declines and OA. Further, a dose-response relationship between daily working hours inside animal houses and symptoms was established for pig farmers [82]. However, recent publications indicate that endotoxins represent the predominant cause of obstructive airway diseases in poultry and swine confinement workers [81, 89]. Irritating gases such as ammonia and NO_x may also elicit OA in these environments. Thus, animal and farm working is associated with an increased prevalence of OA and also of chronic obstructive pulmonary disease [82]. In addition to specific animal allergens, causative exposures in animal confinements comprise hay and grain dusts and other animal feed as well as storage mites [90]. Allergic reactions and irritant OA have to be differentiated in these workers [91].

For flour mill workers, Peretz et al. [12] also described a positive association between exposure to up to ~10 μg EQ/m^3 and sensitization, but a decline in sensitization at higher concentrations The healthy worker effect may have contributed to these findings [92, 93]. Recently, Cullinan et al. [23] reported an annual incidence of work-related chest symptoms of 4.1%, and their association with a positive skin prick test to flour or α-amylase of 1% (sensitization to α-amylase was a little more frequent than that to flour). Interestingly, predominantly atopics became symptomatic and sensitized to α-amylase; and exclusively atopics were sensitized to flour.

Industrial enzyme production

A variety of natural and an increasing number of genetically modified recombinant enzymes produced on a large-scale behave as potent inhalative allergens [94]. These include many mould enzymes, detergent enzymes derived from *Bacillus subtilis* and other bacteria as well as plant proteins such as bromelain (a pineapple protease) or papain (derived from the papaya fruit). The latter enzyme is used as meat tenderizer and capable of sensitizing workers in industrial kitchens. Obviously all enzymes have to be regarded as inhalative allergens affecting mainly pharmaceutical factory and laboratory workers [95].

Fungal α-amylase, derived from *Aspergillus oryzae* is widely used as a baking additive; sensitizing air concentrations in bakeries are in the ng/m^3 range. In the late 1960s, the introduction of alkaline heat-stable enzymes (proteases, amylases, cellulases) in the detergent industry was associated with estimated enzyme air concentrations in the workplace of ~300 ng/m^3 and higher; 40–50% of the workers were sensitized and developed asthma and/or rhinitis. Follow-up studies showed high exposures (estimates were based on the dustiness of workplace atmospheres) and atopy to be related with an increased sensitization incidence. The highest sensitization occurred within the first 2 years of observation, although follow-up was short [96]. Nevertheless, Cullinan et al. [24] found 19% of detergent workers exposed to enzymes (the geometric mean concentration was 4.25 ng/m^3) to be sensitized; 16% had work-related respiratory symptoms. In 2007, ACGIH [97] published a threshold limit value (TLV)-short-term exposure limit (STEL)-C (ceiling) of 0.06 µg/m^3 for the bacterial protease subtilisin.

More recently, it has been established that aeroallergens containing proteases may have a critical role in overcoming airway tolerogenic mechanisms that ordinarily exclude allergic responses to inhaled allergens. Proteases, e.g., from mites and moulds, probably do not only behave as typical allergens. They permit allergic responses by enhancing antigen presentation *via* the degradation of tight junction structures. Moreover, protease activation of epithelial cell protease-activated receptors (PARs) may facilitate allergic responses to aeroallergens by directly inducing the expression of chemokines required for maximal leukocytic activation and infiltration. The latter may induce a non-allergic, innate inflammatory response *via* the release of pro-inflammatory cytokines.

Floricultures, florists; greenhouses

Floriculture and greenhouse workers have an increased risk of sensitization and OA [82, 98–101]. Many fresh or dry flowers and non-flowering green plants were found to cause OA, frequently also rhinitis, and/or dermatitis including: amaryllis (*Amaryllis hippeastrum*) [102], asparagus (*Asparagus officinalis*) [103], aster (*Asteraceae*) [98, 104, 105], baby's breath (*Gypsophila paniculata*) [106–108], bells of Ireland (pollen, *Molucella laevis*) [109], canari palm pollen (*Phoenix canariensis*) [110], carnation (*Dianthus caryophillus*) [111–113], *Carthamus tinctorius* and yarrow (*Achillea millefolium*) [114], Christmas cactus (*Schlumbergia*) [115], *Chrysanthemum leucanthemum*, *Chrysanthemum* spp. and other flowers [105, 116–118], compositae such as chamomile (*Matricaria chamomilla*) [104], Easter lily (*Lilium longiflorum*) [119, 120], eggplant (*Solanum melongena*) [121], freesia (*Freesia hybrida*) [117, 122, 123], *G. paniculata* [108], German statice (*Limonium tataricum*) [124], hyacinth (*Hyacinthus orientalis*) [125], Liliaceae [102], Madagascar jasmine (*Stephanotis floribunda*) [126], mimosa pollen (*Acacia floribunda*) [104, 127], narcissus (*Narcissus pseudonarcissus*) [128], paprika (*Fructus capsici*) [122], pea, sweetpea (*Lathyrus odoratus*) [129], peach (*Prunus persica*) [130], poppy (*Papaver somniferum*) [131], rose (*Rosa* sp.) [132, 133], safflower (*Carthamus tinctorius*) [114], saffron pollen (*Crocus sativus*) [134], spathe flowers (*Spathiphyllum wallisii*) [135], statice (*Limonium tataricum*) [124], sunflower (*Helianthus annus*) [136–138], *Tetranychus urticae* [139], tulip (*Tulipa*) [117, 140, 141], umbrella tree (*Schefflera*) [142], various decorative flowers [98, 104, 117], weeping fig (*Ficus benjamina*) [142–144].

The predatory mites *Amblyseius cucumeris* [145], *Phytoseiulus persimilis* and *Hypoaspis* [146, 147] were also reported to cause OA among horticulturists working in greenhouses.

Further causative allergen sources are the red spider mite (*Tetranychus urticae*) [139, 148] and biopesticides containing *Bacillus thuringiensis* or *Verticillium lecanii* [149]. Furthermore, high indoor temperatures und humidity in greenhouse facilities may result in intensive mould growth, particularly of *Cladosporium herbarum*, penicillium, aspergillus and alternaria spp., which have been shown to be associated with an increased asthma prevalence [150]. For more details, see chapter "Exposure to moulds".

Exposure to other important plant allergens

A variety of plant components and plant products represent important occupational respiratory allergens, e.g., baking flour, grain and soy bean dust, natural latex. They also comprise aniseed powder [151], asparagus [103], banha [152], carrot [153], chicory [154], fenugreek [155], garlic dust [156, 157], ginseng [158], aromatic herbs [159], hobs [160], ipecacuanha [161], kapok [162], licorice roots [163], lycopodium powder [164], 'Maiko' (derived from the tuberous root of devil's tongue) [165], mushroom powder [166, 167], onion [168], peach leaves [130], pectin powder [169], potato [170], freeze-dried raspberry [171], rose hips [133], sanyak [172], sarsaparilla root [173], various spices such as coriander, mace [174], fermented tea [175–177], green tea [178, 179], herbal teas (sage, chamomile, dog, rose, mint and others). Vegetable gums derived from plant materials and containing carbohydrates produce mucilage upon reaction with water. They are frequently used in the industry and in pharmacies. Exposed workers may develop respiratory allergies inducing OA. Mostly printers exposed to acacia gum [180–183], hairdressers having contact to karaya [184], pharmaceutical workers and nurses handling psyllium seeds [185–196] and carpet manufacturers in contact with guar gum [197] are affected.

Hairdressing salons

OA-inducing hairdressing chemicals comprise persulfate salts, p-phenylenediamine, reactive dyes, henna, other dyes and natural latex and hairdressers are thus exposed to a complex mixture of HMW and LMW sensitizers and irritants [198–206].

Drug-manufacturing plants

Drug manufacturing and application may be associated with the generation of airborne dust containing particles of raw materials, intermediate or end products capable of causing OA. These materials and products include amoxicillin, amprolium (the latter also causes asthma in poultry feed mixers), ceftazidine, cephalosporins, cimetidine, hydralazine, ipecacuanha, isonicotinic acid hydrazide, methyl dopa, mitoxantrone, opiate compounds, penicillamine, penicillin and ampicillin, phenylglycine acid chloride, piperacillin, psyllium, salbutamol intermediate, spiramycin, tetracycline and tylosin tartrate. An IgE-mediated mechanism has not been proven for all of these compounds.

Isocyanate application

Isocyanates are increasingly used for the production of polyurethane foam, elastomers, adhesives, varnishes, coatings, insecticides and many other products. These highly reactive chemicals have become the number 1 of occupational airway sensitizers in several western countries. The study by Petsonk et al. [207] should be mentioned, which evaluated respiratory health in a new wood products-manufacturing plant using diphenylmethane-4,4'-diisocyanate (MDI) and its prepolymer. In the follow-up survey 15 out of 56 workers (27%) in areas with the highest potential exposures to liquid isocyanates had an onset of asthma-like symptoms. In addition, 47% of workers with MDI skin staining and 19% without skin staining developed such symptoms, which were associated with variable airflow limitation and specific IgE to MDI-HSA, while controls did not develop any OA cases. Our cross-sectional studies performed in two factories showed in comparison to the group exposed to 5–10 ppb MDI significantly fewer symptomatic subjects, lung function impairments and specific IgE antibodies in the group exposed to less than 5 ppb toluene diisocyanate (TDI) [208]. Tarlo et al. [209] found evidence for higher isocyanate exposures in facilities with OA claims. In another study [210], specific sensitization did not occur at TDI concentrations $\leq$0.02 ppm over 3 years, whereas elevated antibody levels were found in subjects who experienced accidental exposures without a clear exposure-response relationship. There is evidence that dermal exposure to isocyanates can induce OA [211, 212]. Only a minority of symptomatic isocyanate workers show IgE antibodies to diisocyanate-HSA conjugates [213–218]. Several authors observed isocyanate exposure-dependent lung function declines in the occupational exposure limit (OEL) range [219–223]. It is worth mentioning that in most western countries OELs for monomer diisocyanate exposure have been set at 10 ppb. From the clinical point of view, this value seems to be too high. According to literature, 5–2.5 ppb considering all isocyanates in a particular workplace would be health-based levels [224, 225]. OELs for isocyanates should consider gaseous as well as aerosol forms and also the increasingly used polyisocyanates or oligomers causing similar disorders as monomeric diisocyanates. Moreover, the prevention of isocyanate skin contact is obviously also an effective measure to reduce the risk of respiratory disorders. The TLV-time weighted averages (TWAs) currently proposed by ACGIH (2007) [97] are for TDI 0.005 ppm (TLV-STEL 0.02 ppm), for MDI 0.005 ppm and for HDI 0.005 ppm based on monomer exposure.

References

1 Tai HY, Tam MF, Chou H, Peng HJ, Su SN, Perng DW, Shen HD (2006) Pen ch 13 allergen induces secretion of mediators and degradation of occludin protein of human lung epithelial cells. *Allergy* 61: 382–388

2 Wan H, Winton HL, Soeller C, Tovey ER, Gruenert DC, Thompson PJ, Stewart GA, Taylor GW, Garrod DR, Cannell MB et al (1999) Der p 1 facilitates transepithelial allergen delivery by disruption of tight junctions. *J Clin Invest* 104: 123–133

3 Bergeron C, Boulet LP (2006) Structural changes in airway diseases: Characteristics, mechanisms, consequences, and pharmacologic modulation. *Chest* 129: 1068–1087

4 James AL, Wenzel S (2007) Clinical relevance of airway remodelling in airway diseases. *Eur Respir J* 30: 134–155

5 Portengen L, Hollander A, Doekes G, de Meer G, Heederik D (2003) Lung function decline in laboratory animal workers: The role of sensitisation and exposure. *Occup Environ Med* 60: 870–875

6 Baur X, Barbinova L (2006) Isocyanate-induced increase of exhaled NO (FeNO). P3631. ERS Annual congress. *Eur Respir J* 28: 619s-620s

7 Suni Y, Foley S, Daigle S, L'Archevêque J, Olivenstein R, Letuvé S, Malo J, Hamid Q (2007) Structural changes and airway remodelling in occupational asthma at a mean interval of 14 years after cessation of exposure. *Clin Exp Allergy* 37: 1781–1787

8 Cullinan P, Lowson D, Nieuwenhuijsen MJ, Gordon S, Tee RD, Venables KM, McDonald JC, Newman Taylor AJ (1994) Work related symptoms, sensitisation, and estimated exposure in workers not previously exposed to laboratory rats. *Occup Environ Med* 51: 589–592

9 Droste J, Vermeire P, Van Sprundel M, Bulat P, Braeckman L, Myny K, Vanhoorne M (2005) Occupational exposure among bakery workers: Impact on the occurrence of work-related symptoms as compared with allergic characteristics. *J Occup Environ Med* 47: 458–465

10 Houba R, Heederik DJ, Doekes G, van Run PE (1996) Exposure-sensitization relationship for alpha-amylase allergens in the baking industry. *Am J Respir Crit Care Med* 154: 130–136

11 Nieuwenhuijsen MJ, Heederik D, Doekes G, Venables KM, Newman Taylor AJ (1999) Exposure-response relations of alpha-amylase sensitisation in British bakeries and flour mills. *Occup Environ Med* 56: 197–201

12 Peretz C, de Pater N, de Monchy J, Oostenbrink J, Heederik D (2005) Assessment of exposure to wheat flour and the shape of its relationship with specific sensitization. *Scand J Work Environ Health* 31: 65–74

13 Cullinan P, Lowson D, Nieuwenhuijsen MJ, Sandiford C, Tee RD, Venables KM, McDonald JC, Newman Taylor AJ (1994) Work related symptoms, sensitisation, and estimated exposure in workers not previously exposed to flour. *Occup Environ Med* 51: 579–583

14 Gautrin D, Ghezzo H, Infante-Rivard C, Malo JL (2002) Host determinants for the development of allergy in apprentices exposed to laboratory animals. *Eur Respir J* 19: 96–103

15 Heederik D, Venables KM, Malmberg P, Hollander A, Karlsson AS, Renstrom A, Doekes G, Nieuwenhijsen M, Gordon S (1999) Exposure-response relationships for work-related sensitization in workers exposed to rat urinary allergens: Results from a pooled study. *J Allergy Clin Immunol* 103: 678–684

16 Snippe RJ, Gijsbers JHJ, van Drooge H, Preller E (2001) *Chemische allergenen in Nederland. Een onderzoek naar de blootstelling aan diisocyanaten en zuuranhydriden in Nederland.* Ministerie van Sociale Zaken en Werkgelegenheid, Directie Voorlichting, Bibliotheek en Documentatie, Den Haag

17 Archambault S, Malo JL, Infante-Rivard C, Ghezzo H, Gautrin D (2001) Incidence of sensitization, symptoms, and probable occupational rhinoconjunctivitis and asthma in apprentices starting exposure to latex. *J Allergy Clin Immunol* 107: 921–923

18 Newman Taylor AJ, Nicholson PJ (2004) *Guidelines for the prevention, identification & management of occupational asthma: Evidence review & recommendations.* British Occupational Health Research Foundation, London

19 Barbinova L, Baur X (2007) Possible influence of occupational exposure to high and low molecular-weight asthmagens on the atopic status. *Eur Respir J* 30: 4s

20 Brisman J, Jarvholm B, Lillienberg L (2000) Exposure-response relations for self reported asthma and rhinitis in bakers. *Occup Environ Med* 57: 335–340

21 Cathcart M, Nicholson P, Roberts D, Bazley M, Juniper C, Murray P, Randell M (1997) Enzyme exposure, smoking and lung function in employees in the detergent industry over 20 years. Medical Subcommittee of the UK Soap and Detergent Industry Association. *Occup Med (Lond)* 47: 473–478

22 Cullinan P, Cook A, Gordon S, Nieuwenhuijsen MJ, Tee RD, Venables KM, McDonald JC, Newman Taylor AJ (1999) Allergen exposure, atopy and smoking as determinants of allergy to rats in a cohort of laboratory employees. *Eur Respir J* 13: 1139–1143

23 Cullinan P, Cook A, Nieuwenhuijsen MJ, Sandiford C, Tee RD, Venables KM, McDonald JC, Newman Taylor AJ (2001) Allergen and dust exposure as determinants of work-related symptoms and sensitization in a cohort of flour-exposed workers; a case-control analysis. *Ann Occup Hyg* 45: 97–103

24 Cullinan P, Harris JM, Newman Taylor AJ, Hole AM, Jones M, Barnes F, Jolliffe G (2000) An outbreak of asthma in a modern detergent factory. *Lancet* 356: 1899–1900

25 Heederik D, Houba R (2001) An exploratory quantitative risk assessment for high molecular weight sensitizers: Wheat flour. *Ann Occup Hyg* 45: 175–185

26 Houba R, Heederik D, Doekes G (1998) Wheat sensitization and work-related symptoms in the baking industry are preventable. An epidemiologic study. *Am J Respir Crit Care Med* 158: 1499–1503

27 Nieuwenhuijsen M, Baur X, Heederik D (2006) Environmental monitoring: General considerations, exposure-response relationships, and risk assessment. In: IL Bernstein, M Chan-Yeung, JL Malo, DI Bernstein (eds): *Asthma in the Workplace*. Taylor & Francis, New York, 253–274

28 Ortega HG, Daroowalla F, Petsonk EL, Lewis D, Berardinelli S Jr, Jones W, Kreiss K, Weissman DN (2001) Respiratory symptoms among crab processing workers in Alaska: Epidemiological and environmental assessment. *Am J Ind Med* 39: 598–607

29 Osterman K, Zetterstrom O, Johansson SG (1982) Coffee worker's allergy. *Allergy* 37: 313–322

30 Vanhanen M, Tuomi T, Nordman H, Tupasela O, Holmberg PC, Miettinen M, Mutanen P, Leisola M (1997) Sensitization to industrial enzymes in enzyme research and production. *Scand J Work Environ Health* 23: 385–391

31 Martinez FD (2007) CD14, endotoxin, and asthma risk: Actions and interactions. *Proc Am Thorac Soc* 4: 221–225

32 Moore WC, Peters SP (2007) Update in asthma 2006. *Am J Respir Crit Care Med* 175: 649–654

33 Schaub B, Lauener R, von Mutius E (2006) The many faces of the hygiene hypothesis. *J Allergy Clin Immunol* 117: 969–977; quiz 978

34 Sigsgaard T, Brandslund I, Omland O, Hjort C, Lund ED, Pedersen OF, Miller MR (2000) S and Z alpha1–antitrypsin alleles are risk factors for bronchial hyperresponsiveness in young farmers: An example of gene/environment interaction. *Eur Respir J* 16: 50–55

35 Candi E, Schmidt R, Melino G (2005) The cornified envelope: A model of cell death in the skin. *Nat Rev Mol Cell Biol* 6: 328–340

36 Irvine AD (2007) Fleshing out filaggrin phenotypes. *J Invest Dermatol* 127: 504–507

37 Palmer CN, Ismail T, Lee SP, Terron-Kwiatkowski A, Zhao Y, Liao H, Smith FJ, McLean WH, Mukhopadhyay S (2007) Filaggrin null mutations are associated with increased asthma severity in children and young adults. *J Allergy Clin Immunol* 120: 64–68

38 Howell MD, Kim BE, Gao P, Grant AV, Boguniewicz M, Debenedetto A, Schneider L, Beck LA, Barnes KC, Leung DY (2007) Cytokine modulation of atopic dermatitis filaggrin skin expression. *J Allergy Clin Immunol* 120: 150–155

39 Balboni A, Baricordi OR, Fabbri LM, Gandini E, Ciaccia A, Mapp CE (1996) Association between toluene diisocyanate-induced asthma and DQB1 markers: A possible role for aspartic acid at position 57. *Eur Respir J* 9: 207–210

40 Bignon JS, Aron Y, Ju LY, Kopferschmitt MC, Garnier R, Mapp C, Fabbri LM, Pauli G, Lockhart A, Charron D et al (1994) HLA class II alleles in isocyanate-induced asthma. *Am J Respir Crit Care Med* 149: 71–75

41 Horne C, Quintana PJ, Keown PA, Dimich-Ward H, Chan-Yeung M (2000) Distribution of DRB1 and DQB1 HLA class II alleles in occupational asthma due to western red cedar. *Eur Respir J* 15: 911–914

42 Jeal H, Draper A, Jones M, Harris J, Welsh K, Taylor AN, Cullinan P (2003) HLA associations with occupational sensitization to rat lipocalin allergens: A model for other animal allergies? *J Allergy Clin Immunol* 111: 795–799

43 Mapp CE, Beghe B, Balboni A, Zamorani G, Padoan M, Jovine L, Baricordi OR, Fabbri LM (2000) Association between HLA genes and susceptibility to toluene diisocyanate-induced asthma. *Clin Exp Allergy* 30: 651–656

44 Mapp CE, Fryer AA, De Marzo N, Pozzato V, Padoan M, Boschetto P, Strange RC, Hemmingsen A, Spiteri MA (2002) Glutathione S-transferase GSTP1 is a susceptibility gene for occupational asthma induced by isocyanates. *J Allergy Clin Immunol* 109: 867–872

45 Bernstein DI (1997) Allergic reactions to workplace allergens. *JAMA* 278: 1907–1913

46 Heederik K, Portegen L, Meijer E, Doekes G, De Meer G (1999) *Beroepsgebonden allergische luchtwegaandoeningen. Literaturstudie in opdracht van het Ministerie van Sociale Zaken en Werkgelegenheid.* Ministerie van Sociale Zaken in Werkgelegenheid, Wageningen

47 Nielsen GD, Olsen O, Larsen ST, Lovik M, Poulsen LK, Glue C, Brandorff NP, Nielsen PJ (2005) IgE-mediated sensitisation, rhinitis and asthma from occupational exposures. Smoking as a model for airborne adjuvants? *Toxicology* 216: 87–105

48 Portengen L (2004) *Risk modification and combined exposures in occupational respiratory allergy (Proefschrift).* University of Utrecht, Institute for Risk Assessment Sciences, Utrecht

49 Siracusa A, Desrosiers M, Marabini A (2000) Epidemiology of occupational rhinitis: Prevalence, aetiology and determinants. *Clin Exp Allergy* 30: 1519–1534

50 Merget R, Kulzer R, Dierkes-Globisch A, Breitstadt R, Gebler A, Kniffka A, Artelt S, Koenig HP, Alt F, Vormberg R et al (2000) Exposure-effect relationship of platinum salt allergy in a catalyst production plant: Conclusions from a 5-year prospective cohort study. *J Allergy Clin Immunol* 105: 364–370

51 Venables KM, Dally MB, Nunn AJ, Stevens JF, Stephens R, Farrer N, Hunter JV, Stewart M, Hughes EG, Newman Taylor AJ (1989) Smoking and occupational allergy in workers in a platinum refinery. *BMJ* 299: 939–942

52 Cartier A, Malo JL, Forest F, Lafrance M, Pineau L, St-Aubin JJ, Dubois JY (1984) Occupational asthma in snow crab-processing workers. *J Allergy Clin Immunol* 74: 261–269

53 Venables KM, Topping MD, Howe W, Luczynska CM, Hawkins R, Taylor AJ (1985) Interaction of smoking and atopy in producing specific IgE antibody against a hapten protein conjugate. *Br Med J (Clin Res Ed)* 290: 201–204

54 Zetterstrom O, Osterman K, Machado L, Johansson SG (1981) Another smoking hazard: Raised serum IgE concentration and increased risk of occupational allergy. *Br Med J (Clin Res Ed)* 283: 1215–1217

55 Cortona G, Pisati G, Dellabianca A, Moscato G (2001) [Respiratory occupational allergies: The experience of the Hospital Operative Unit of Occupational Medicine in Lombardy from 1990 to 1998]. *G Ital Med Lav Ergon* 23: 64–70

56 Gautrin D, Ghezzo H, Infante-Rivard C, Malo JL (2001) Natural history of sensitization, symptoms and occupational diseases in apprentices exposed to laboratory animals. *Eur Respir J* 17: 904–908

57 Gautrin D, Infante-Rivard C, Ghezzo H, Malo JL (2001) Incidence and host determinants of probable occupational asthma in apprentices exposed to laboratory animals. *Am J Respir Crit Care Med* 163: 899–904

58 Grammer LC, Ditto AM, Tripathi A, Harris KE (2002) Prevalence and onset of rhinitis and conjunctivitis in subjects with occupational asthma caused by trimellitic anhydride (TMA). *J Occup Environ Med* 44: 1179–1181

59 Karjalainen A, Martikainen R, Klaukka T, Saarinen K, Uitti J (2003) Risk of asthma among Finnish patients with occupational rhinitis. *Chest* 123: 283–288

60 Malo JL, Lemiere C, Desjardins A, Cartier A (1997) Prevalence and intensity of rhinoconjunctivitis in subjects with occupational asthma. *Eur Respir J* 10: 1513–1515

61 Zhang XD, Lotvall J, Skerfving S, Welinder H (1997) Antibody specificity to the chemical structures of organic acid anhydrides studied by *in-vitro* and *in-vivo* methods. *Toxicology* 118: 223–232

62 Zhang XD, Welinder H, Jonsson BA, Skerfving S (1998) Antibody responses of rats after immunization with organic acid anhydrides as a model of predictive testing. *Scand J Work Environ Health* 24: 220–227

63 Barbinova L, Baur X (2006) Increase in exhaled nitric oxide (eNO) after work-related isocyanate exposure. *Int Arch Occup Environ Health* 79: 387–395

64 Lemiere C, Pelissier S, Tremblay C, Chaboillez S, Thivierge M, Stankova J, Rola-Pleszczynski M (2004) Leukotrienes and isocyanate-induced asthma: A pilot study. *Clin Exp Allergy* 34: 1684–1689

65 Bush RK, Wood RA, Eggleston PA (1998) Laboratory animal allergy. *J Allergy Clin Immunol* 102: 99–112

66 Nieuwenhijsen MJ, Putcha V, Gordon S, Heederik D, Cullinan P, Venables KM, Newman Taylor AJ (2001) Exposure-response relationships in laboratory animal workers. In: G-NRCfEa Health (ed): *Thirteenth conference of the International Society for Environmental Epidemiology.* Neuherberg, Garmisch-Partenkirchen, A18

67 Nieuwenhuijsen MJ, Putcha V, Gordon S, Heederik D, Venables KM, Cullinan P, Newman-Taylor AJ (2003) Exposure-response relations among laboratory animal workers exposed to rats. *Occup Environ Med* 60: 104–108

68 Hollander A, Heederik D, Doekes G (1997) Respiratory allergy to rats: Exposure-response relationships in laboratory animal workers. *Am J Respir Crit Care Med* 155: 562–567

69 Thulin H, Bjorkdahl M, Karlsson AS, Renstrom A (2002) Reduction of exposure to laboratory animal allergens in a research laboratory. *Ann Occup Hyg* 46: 61–68

70 Hoppin JA, Umbach DM, London SJ, Alavanja MC, Sandler DP (2003) Animal production and wheeze in the Agricultural Health Study: Interactions with atopy, asthma, and smoking. *Occup Environ Med* 60: e3

71 Hoppin JA, Umbach DM, London SJ, Alavanja MC, Sandler DP (2004) Diesel exhaust, solvents, and other occupational exposures as risk factors for wheeze among farmers. *Am J Respir Crit Care Med* 169: 1308–1313

72 Monso E, Riu E, Radon K, Magarolas R, Danuser B, Iversen M, Morera J, Nowak D (2004) Chronic obstructive pulmonary disease in never-smoking animal farmers working inside confinement buildings. *Am J Ind Med* 46: 357–362

73 Portengen L, Preller L, Tielen M, Doekes G, Heederik D (2005) Endotoxin exposure and atopic sensitization in adult pig farmers. *J Allergy Clin Immunol* 115: 797–802

74 Terho EO, Husman K, Vohlonen I, Rautalahti M, Tukiainen H (1985) Allergy to storage mites or cow dander as a cause of rhinitis among Finnish dairy farmers. *Allergy* 40: 23–26

75 Terho EO, Vohlonen I, Husman K, Rautalahti M, Tukiainen H, Viander M (1987) Sensitization to storage mites and other work-related and common allergens among Finnish dairy farmers. *Eur J Respir Dis* 152: 165–174

76 Virtanen T, Vilhunen P, Husman K, Mantyjarvi R (1988) Sensitization of dairy farmers to bovine antigens and effects of exposure on specific IgG and IgE titers. *Int Arch Allergy Appl Immunol* 87: 171–177

77 Hinze S, Bergmann KC, Lowenstein H, Hansen GN (1996) [Different threshold concentrations for sensitization by cattle hair allergen Bos d 2 in atopic and non-atopic farmers]. *Pneumologie* 50: 177–181

78 Rautiainen M, Virtanen T, Ruoppi P, Nuutinen J, Mantyjarvi R (1997) Humoral responses to bovine dust in dairy farmers with allergic rhinitis. *Acta Otolaryngol* (Suppl) 529: 169–172

79 Schwartz DA, Donham KJ, Olenchock SA, Popendorf WJ, Van Fossen DS, Burmeister LF, Merchant JA (1995) Determinants of longitudinal changes in spirometric function among swine confinement operators and farmers. *Am J Respir Crit Care Med* 151: 47–53

80 Cormier Y, Coll B, Laviolette M, Boulet LP (1996) Reactive airways dysfunction syndrome (RADS) following exposure to toxic gases of a swine confinement building. *Eur Respir J* 9: 1090–1091

81 Vogelzang PF, van der Gulden JW, Folgering H, Kolk JJ, Heederik D, Preller L, Tielen MJ, van Schayck CP (1998) Endotoxin exposure as a major determinant of lung function decline in pig farmers. *Am J Respir Crit Care Med* 157: 15–18

82 Radon K, Monso E, Weber C, Danuser B, Iversen M, Opravil U, Donham K, Hartung J, Pedersen S, Garz S et al (2002) Prevalence and risk factors for airway diseases in farmers – Summary of results of the European Farmers' Project. *Ann Agric Environ Med* 9: 207–213

83 Dosman JA, Lawson JA, Kirychuk SP, Cormier Y, Biem J, Koehncke N (2004) Occupa-

tional asthma in newly employed workers in intensive swine confinement facilities. *Eur Respir J* 24: 698–702

84 Danuser B, Wyss C, Hauser R, von Planta U, Folsch D (1988) [Lung function and symptoms in employees of poultry farms]. *Soz Praventivmed* 33: 286–291

85 Danuser B, Weber C, Kunzli N, Schindler C, Nowak D (2001) Respiratory symptoms in Swiss farmers: An epidemiological study of risk factors. *Am J Ind Med* 39: 410–418

86 Perfetti L, Cartier A, Malo JL (1997) Occupational asthma in poultry-slaughterhouse workers. *Allergy* 52: 594–595

87 Borghetti C, Magarolas R, Badorrey I, Radon K, Morera J, Monso E (2002) [Sensitization and occupational asthma in poultry workers]. *Med Clin (Barc)* 118: 251–255

88 Schwartz HJ (1994) Raw poultry as a cause of occupational dermatitis, rhinitis, and asthma. *J Asthma* 31: 485–486

89 Hagmar L, Schutz A, Hallberg T, Sjoholm A (1990) Health effects of exposure to endotoxins and organic dust in poultry slaughter-house workers. *Int Arch Occup Environ Health* 62: 159–164

90 Cuthbert OD, Jeffrey IG, McNeill HB, Wood J, Topping MD (1984) Barn allergy among Scottish farmers. *Clin Allergy* 14: 197–206

91 Baur X (2008) Airborne allergens and irritants in the workplace. In: AB Kay, AP Kaplan, J Bousquet, PG Holt (eds): *Allergy and allergic diseases*. Blackwell Publishing, 1017–1122

92 Heederik D, Doekes G, Nieuwenhuijsen MJ (1999) Exposure assessment of high molecular weight sensitisers: Contribution to occupational epidemiology and disease prevention. *Occup Environ Med* 56: 735–741

93 Heederik D, Thorne PS, Doekes G (2002) Health-based occupational exposure limits for high molecular weight sensitizers: How long is the road we must travel? *Ann Occup Hyg* 46: 439–446

94 Baur X (2005) Enzymes as occupational and environmental respiratory sensitisers. *Int Arch Occup Environ Health* 78: 279–286

95 Vanhanen M (2001) *Exposure, sensitization and allergy to industrial enzymes: Department of Pulmonology*. Helsinki University Central Hospital, Helsinki

96 Juniper CP, How MJ, Goodwin BF, Kinshott AK (1977) *Bacillus subtilis* enzymes: A 7–year clinical, epidemiological and immunological study of an industrial allergen. *J Soc Occup Med* 27: 3–12

97 American Conference of Governmental and Industrial Hygienists (2007) *TLVs and BEIs*. ACGIH, Cincinnati

98 Goldberg A, Confino-Cohen R, Waisel Y (1998) Allergic responses to pollen of ornamental plants: High incidence in the general atopic population and especially among flower growers. *J Allergy Clin Immunol* 102: 210–214

99 Monso E, Magarolas R, Radon K, Danuser B, Iversen M, Weber C, Opravil U, Donham KJ, Nowak D (2000) Respiratory symptoms of obstructive lung disease in European crop farmers. *Am J Respir Crit Care Med* 162: 1246–1250

100 Groenewoud GC, de Jong NW, van Oorschot-van Nes AJ, Vermeulen AM, van

Toorenenbergen AW, Mulder PG, Burdorf A, de Groot H, van Wijk RG (2002) Prevalence of occupational allergy to bell pepper pollen in greenhouses in the Netherlands. *Clin Exp Allergy* 32: 434–440

101 Monso E, Schenker M, Radon K, Riu E, Magarolas R, McCurdy S, Danuser B, Iversen M, Saiki C, Nowak D (2003) Region-related risk factors for respiratory symptoms in European and Californian farmers. *Eur Respir J* 21: 323–331

102 Jansen AP, Visser FJ, Nierop G, de Jong NW, Waanders-de Lijster de Raadt J, Vermeulen A, van Toorenenbergen AW (1996) Occupational asthma to amaryllis. *Allergy* 51: 847–849

103 Tabar AI, Alvarez-Puebla MJ, Gomez B, Sanchez-Monge R, Garcia BE, Echechipia S, Olaguibel JM, Salcedo G (2004) Diversity of asparagus allergy: Clinical and immunological features. *Clin Exp Allergy* 34: 131–136

104 de Jong NW, Vermeulen AM, Gerth van Wijk R, de Groot H (1998) Occupational allergy caused by flowers. *Allergy* 53: 204–209

105 Akpinar-Elci M, Elci OC, Odabasi A (2004) Work-related asthma-like symptoms among florists. *Chest* 125: 2336–2339

106 Antepara I, Jauregui I, Urrutia I, Gamboa PM, Gonzalez G, Barber D (1994) Occupational asthma related to fresh *Gypsophila paniculata. Allergy* 49: 478–480

107 Schroeckenstein DC, Meier-Davis S, Yunginger JW, Bush RK (1990) Allergens involved in occupational asthma caused by baby's breath (*Gypsophila paniculata*). *J Allergy Clin Immunol* 86: 189–193

108 Twiggs JT, Yunginger JW, Agarwal MK, Reed CE (1982) Occupational asthma in a florist caused by the dried plant, baby's breath. *J Allergy Clin Immunol* 69: 474–477

109 Miesen WM, van der Heide S, Kerstjens HA, Dubois AE, de Monchy JG (2003) Occupational asthma due to IgE mediated allergy to the flower *Molucella laevis* (Bells of Ireland). *Occup Environ Med* 60: 701–703

110 Blanco C, Carrillo T, Quiralte J, Pascual C, Martin Esteban M, Castillo R (1995) Occupational rhinoconjunctivitis and bronchial asthma due to *Phoenix canariensis* pollen allergy. Allergy 50: 277–280

111 Sanchez-Guerrero IM, Escudero AI, Bartolom B, Palacios R (1999) Occupational allergy caused by carnation (*Dianthus caryophyllus*). *J Allergy Clin Immunol* 104: 181–185

112 Cistero-Bahima A, Enrique E, Alonso R, del Mar San Miguel M, Bartolome B (2000) Simultaneous occupational allergy to a carnation and its parasite in a greenhouse worker. *J Allergy Clin Immunol* 106: 780

113 Sanchez-Fernandez C, Gonzalez-Gutierrez ML, Esteban-Lopez MI, Martinez A, Lombardero M (2004) Occupational asthma caused by carnation (*Dianthus caryophyllus*) with simultaneous IgE-mediated sensitization to *Tetranychus urticae. Allergy* 59: 114–115

114 Compes E, Bartolome B, Fernandez-Nieto M, Sastre J, Cuesta J (2006) Occupational asthma from dried flowers of *Carthamus tinctorious* (safflower) and *Achillea millefolium* (yarrow). *Allergy* 61: 1239–1240

115 Paulsen E, Skov PS, Bindslev-Jensen C, Voitenko V, Poulsen LK (1997) Occupational type I allergy to Christmas cactus (*Schlumbergera*). *Allergy* 52: 656–660
116 Groenewoud GC, de Jong NW, Burdorf A, de Groot H, van Wyk RG (2002) Prevalence of occupational allergy to Chrysanthemum pollen in greenhouses in the Netherlands. *Allergy* 57: 835–840
117 Piirila P, Keskinen H, Leino T, Tupasela O, Tuppurainen M (1994) Occupational asthma caused by decorative flowers: Review and case reports. *Int Arch Occup Environ Health* 66: 131–136
118 Ueda A, Tochigi T, Ueda T, Aoyama K, Manda F (1992) Immediate type of allergy in statis growers. *J Allergy Clin Immunol* 90: 742–748
119 Vidal C, Polo F (1998) Occupational allergy caused by *Dianthus caryophillus*, *Gypsophila paniculata*, and *Lilium longiflorum*. *Allergy* 53: 995–998
120 Piirila P, Kanerva L, Alanko K, Estlander T, Keskinen H, Pajari-Backas M, Tuppurainen M (1999) Occupational IgE-mediated asthma, rhinoconjunctivitis, and contact urticaria caused by Easter lily (*Lilium longiflorum*) and tulip. *Allergy* 54: 273–277
121 Gil M, Hogendijk S, Hauser C (2002) Allergy to eggplant flower pollen. *Allergy* 57: 652
122 van Toorenenbergen AW, Dieges PH (1984) Occupational allergy in horticulture: Demonstration of immediate-type allergic reactivity to freesia and paprika plants. *Int Arch Allergy Appl Immunol* 75: 44–47
123 van Toorenenbergen AW, Dieges PH (1985) Immunoglobulin E antibodies against coriander and other spices. *J Allergy Clin Immunol* 76: 477–481
124 Quirce S, Garcia-Figueroa B, Olaguibel JM, Muro MD, Tabar AI (1993) Occupational asthma and contact urticaria from dried flowers of *Limonium tataricum*. *Allergy* 48: 285–290
125 Piirila P, Hannu T, Keskinen H, Tuppurainen M (1998) Occupational asthma to hyacinth. *Allergy* 53: 328–329
126 van der Zee JS, de Jager KS, Kuipers BF, Stapel SO (1999) Outbreak of occupational allergic asthma in a *Stephanotis floribunda* nursery. *J Allergy Clin Immunol* 103: 950–952
127 Ariano R, Panzani RC, Amedeo J (1991) Pollen allergy to mimosa (*Acacia floribunda*) in a Mediterranean area: An occupational disease. *Ann Allergy* 66: 253–256
128 Goncalo S, Freitas JD, Sousa I (1987) Contact dermatitis and respiratory symptoms from *Narcissus pseudonarcissus*. *Contact Dermatitis* 16: 115–116
129 Jansen A, Vermeulen A, van Toorenenbergen AW, Dieges PH (1995) Occupational asthma in horticulture caused by *Lathyrus odoratus*. *Allergy Proc* 16: 135–139
130 Garcia BE, Lombardero M, Echechipia S, Olaguibel JM, Diaz-Perales A, Sanchez-Monge R, Barber D, Salcedo G, Tabar AI (2004) Respiratory allergy to peach leaves and lipid-transfer proteins. *Clin Exp Allergy* 34: 291–295
131 Moneo I, Alday E, Ramos C, Curiel G (1993) Occupational asthma caused by *Papaver somniferum*. *Allergol Immunopathol (Madr)* 21: 145–148

132 Demir AU, Karakaya G, Kalyoncu AF (2002) Allergy symptoms and IgE immune response to rose: An occupational and an environmental disease. *Allergy* 57: 936–939
133 Kwaselow A, Rowe M, Sears-Ewald D, Ownby D (1990) Rose hips: A new occupational allergen. *J Allergy Clin Immunol* 85: 704–708
134 Feo F, Martinez J, Martinez A, Galindo PA, Cruz A, Garcia R, Guerra F, Palacios R (1997) Occupational allergy in saffron workers. *Allergy* 52: 633–641
135 Kanerva L, Makinen-Kiljunen S, Kiistala R, Granlund H (1995) Occupational allergy caused by spathe flower (*Spathiphyllum wallisii*). *Allergy* 50: 174–178
136 Bousquet J, Dhivert H, Clauzel AM, Hewitt B, Michel FB (1985) Occupational allergy to sunflower pollen. *J Allergy Clin Immunol* 75: 70–74
137 Atis S, Tutluoglu B, Sahin K, Yaman M, Kucukusta AR, Oktay I (2002) Sensitization to sunflower pollen and lung functions in sunflower processing workers. *Allergy* 57: 35–39
138 Jimenez A, Moreno C, Martinez J, Martinez A, Bartolome B, Guerra F, Palacios R (1994) Sensitization to sunflower pollen: Only an occupational allergy? *Int Arch Allergy Immunol* 105: 297–307
139 Navarro AM, Delgado J, Sanchez MC, Orta JC, Martinez A, Palacios R, Martinez J, Conde J (2000) Prevalence of sensitization to *Tetranychus urticae* in greenhouse workers. *Clin Exp Allergy* 30: 863–866
140 Krüsmann W, Hausen BM (1987) Tulpenallergy vom Soforttyp mit Asthma bronchiale und Rhinokonjunktivitis. *Allergologie* 10: 549–551
141 Lahti A (1986) Contact urticaria and respiratory symptoms from tulips and lilies. *Contact Dermatitis* 14: 317–319
142 Grob M, Wuthrich B (1998) Occupational allergy to the umbrella tree (*Schefflera*). *Allergy* 53: 1008–1009
143 Axelsson G, Skedinger M, Zetterstrom O (1985) Allergy to weeping fig – A new occupational disease. *Allergy* 40: 461–464
144 Axelsson IG, Johansson SG, Zetterstrom O (1987) Occupational allergy to weeping fig in plant keepers. *Allergy* 42: 161–167
145 Groenewoud GC, de Graaf in 't Veld C, vVan Oorschot-van Nes AJ, de Jong NW, Vermeulen AM, van Toorenenbergen AW, Burdorf A, de Groot H, Gerth van Wijk R (2002) Prevalence of sensitization to the predatory mite *Amblyseius cucumeris* as a new occupational allergen in horticulture. *Allergy* 57: 614–619
146 Johansson E, Kolmodin-Hedman B, Kallstrom E, Kaiser L, van Hage-Hamsten M (2003) IgE-mediated sensitization to predatory mites in Swedish greenhouse workers. *Allergy* 58: 337–341
147 Kronqvist M, Johansson E, Kolmodin-Hedman B, Oman H, Svartengren M, van Hage-Hamsten M (2005) IgE-sensitization to predatory mites and respiratory symptoms in Swedish greenhouse workers. *Allergy* 60: 521–526
148 Delgado J, Orta JC, Navarro AM, Conde J, Martinez A, Martinez J, Palacios R (1997) Occupational allergy in greenhouse workers: Sensitization to *Tetranychus urticae*. *Clin Exp Allergy* 27: 640–645

149 Doekes G, Larsen P, Sigsgaard T, Baelum J (2004) IgE sensitization to bacterial and fungal biopesticides in a cohort of Danish greenhouse workers: The BIOGART study. *Am J Ind Med* 46: 404–407
150 Monso E (2004) Occupational asthma in greenhouse workers. *Curr Opin Pulm Med* 10: 147–150
151 Fraj J, Lezaun A, Colas C, Duce F, Dominguez MA, Alonso MD (1996) Occupational asthma induced by aniseed. *Allergy* 51: 337–339
152 Kim SH, Jeong H, Kim YK, Cho SH, Min KU, Kim YY (2001) IgE-mediated occupational asthma induced by herbal medicine, Banha (*Pinellia ternata*). *Clin Exp Allergy* 31: 779–781
153 Quirce S, Blanco R, Diez-Gomez ML, Cuevas M, Eiras P, Losada E (1997) Carrot-induced asthma: Immunodetection of allergens. *J Allergy Clin Immunol* 99: 718–719
154 Cadot P, Kochuyt AM, Deman R, Stevens EA (1996) Inhalative occupational and ingestive immediate-type allergy caused by chicory (*Cichorium intybus*). *Clin Exp Allergy* 26: 940–944
155 Dugué J, Bel J, Figueredo M (1993) Le fenugrec responsable d'un nouvel asthme professionnel. *La Presse Médicale* 22: 922
156 Lybarger JA, Gallagher JS, Pulver DW, Litwin A, Brooks S, Bernstein IL (1982) Occupational asthma induced by inhalation and ingestion of garlic. *J Allergy Clin Immunol* 69: 448–454
157 Anibarro B, Fontela JL, De La Hoz F (1997) Occupational asthma induced by garlic dust. *J Allergy Clin Immunol* 100: 734–738
158 Subiza J, Subiza JL, Escribano PM, Hinojosa M, Garcia R, Jerez M, Subiza E (1991) Occupational asthma caused by Brazil ginseng dust. *J Allergy Clin Immunol* 88: 731–736
159 Lemiere C, Cartier A, Lehrer SB, Malo JL (1996) Occupational asthma caused by aromatic herbs. *Allergy* 51: 647–649
160 Newmark FM (1978) Hops allergy and terpene sensitivity: An occupational disease. *Ann Allergy* 41: 311–312
161 Luczynska CM, Marshall PE, Scarisbrick DA, Topping MD (1984) Occupational allergy due to inhalation of ipecacuanha dust. *Clin Allergy* 14: 169–175
162 Kern DG, Kohn R (1994) Occupational asthma following kapok exposure. *J Asthma* 31: 243–250
163 Cartier A, Malo JL, Labrecque M (2002) Occupational asthma due to liquorice roots. *Allergy* 57: 863
164 Catilina P, Chamoux A, Gabrillargues D, Catilina MJ, Royfe MH, Wahl D (1988) Contribution à l'étude des asthmas d'origine professionnelle: L'asthme à la poudre de lycopode. *Arch Mal Prof* 49: 143–148
165 Kobayashi S (1980) Different aspects of occupational asthma in Japan. In: CA Frazier (ed): *Occupational asthma*. van Nostrand-Reinhold, New York, 229–244
166 Symington IS, Kerr JW, McLean DA (1981) Type I allergy in mushroom soup processors. *Clin Allergy* 11: 43–47

167 Michils A, De Vuyst P, Nolard N, Servais G, Duchateau J, Yernault JC (1991) Occupational asthma to spores of Pleurotus cornucopiae. *Eur Respir J* 4: 1143–1147
168 Valdivieso R, Subiza J, Varela-Losada S, Subiza JL, Narganes MJ, Martinez-Cocera C, Cabrera M (1994) Bronchial asthma, rhinoconjunctivitis, and contact dermatitis caused by onion. *J Allergy Clin Immunol* 94: 928–930
169 Cohen AJ, Forse MS, Tarlo SM (1993) Occupational asthma caused by pectin inhalation during the manufacture of jam. *Chest* 103: 309–311
170 Quirce S, Diez Gomez ML, Hinojosa M, Cuevas M, Urena V, Rivas MF, Puyana J, Cuesta J, Losada E (1989) Housewives with raw potato-induced bronchial asthma. *Allergy* 44: 532–536
171 Sherson D, Andersen B, Hansen I, Kjoller H (2003) Occupational asthma due to freeze-dried raspberry. *Ann Allergy Asthma Immunol* 90: 660–663
172 Park HS, Kim MJ, Moon HB (1994) Occupational asthma caused by two herb materials, *Dioscorea batatas* and *Pinellia ternata*. *Clin Exp Allergy* 24: 575–581
173 Vandenplas O, Depelchin S, Toussaint G, Delwiche JP, Weyer RV, Saint-Remy JM (1996) Occupational asthma caused by sarsaparilla root dust. *J Allergy Clin Immunol* 97: 1416–1418
174 Sastre J, Olmo M, Novalvos A, Ibanez D, Lahoz C (1996) Occupational asthma due to different spices. *Allergy* 51: 117–120
175 Uragoda CG (1970) Tea maker's asthma. *Br J Ind Med* 27: 181–182
176 Roberts JA, Thomson NC (1988) Tea-dust induced asthma. *Eur Respir J* 1: 769–770
177 Cartier A, Malo JL (1990) Occupational asthma due to tea dust. *Thorax* 45: 203–206
178 Shirai T, Reshad K, Yoshitomi A, Chida K, Nakamura H, Taniguchi M (2003) Green tea-induced asthma: Relationship between immunological reactivity, specific and non-specific bronchial responsiveness. *Clin Exp Allergy* 33: 1252–1255
179 Shirai T, Sato A, Hara Y (1994) Epigallocatechin gallate. The major causative agent of green tea-induced asthma. *Chest* 106: 1801–1805
180 Bohner CB, Sheldon JM, Trenis JW (1941) Sensitivity to gum acazia, with a report of ten cases of asthma in printers. *Allergy* 12: 290–294
181 Hinault G, Blacque-Bélair A, Buffe D (1961) L'asthme à la gomme arabique dans un grand atelier de typographie. *J Franc Méd Chir Thor* 15: 51–61
182 Gaultier M, Fournier E, Gervais P, Vignolet (1960) Un cas d'asthme à la gomme arabique. Histoire clinique, tests cutanés, épreuves fonctionnelles respiratoires. *Arch Mal Prof* 21: 55–56
183 Fowlers PBS (1952) Printer's asthma. *Lancet* 2: 755–757
184 Bullen SS (1934) Perennial hay fever from indian gum (Karaya gum). *J Allergy* 5: 484–487
185 Bardy JD, Malo JL, Seguin P, Ghezzo H, Desjardins J, Dolovich J, Cartier A (1987) Occupational asthma and IgE sensitization in a pharmaceutical company processing psyllium. *Am Rev Respir Dis* 135: 1033–1038
186 Malo JL, Cartier A, L'Archeveque J, Ghezzo H, Lagier F, Trudeau C, Dolovich J (1990)

Prevalence of occupational asthma and immunologic sensitization to psyllium among health personnel in chronic care hospitals. *Am Rev Respir Dis* 142: 1359–1366

187 Gauss WF, Alarie JP, Karol MH (1985) Workplace allergenicity of a psyllium-containing bulk laxative. *Allergy* 40: 73–76

188 Scott D (1987) Psyllium-induced asthma. Occupational exposure in a nurse. *Postgrad Med* 82: 160–161

189 Terho EO, Torkko M (1980) Occupational asthma from psyllium laxatives. *Duodecim* 96: 1213–1216

190 Schwartz HJ (1989) Effect of chronic chromolyn sodium therapy in a beautician with occupational asthma. *J Occup Med* 31: 112–114

191 Bernton HS (1970) The allergenicity of psyllium seed. Report of a case. *Med Ann Dist Columbia* 39: 313–317

192 Nelson WL (1987) Allergic events among health care workers exposed to psyllium laxatives in the workplace. *J Occup Med* 29: 497–499

193 Breton JL, Leneutre F, Esculpavit G, Abourjaili M (1989) [A new cause of occupational asthma in a pharmacist]. *Presse Med* 18: 433

194 Busse WW, Schoenwetter WF (1975) Asthma from psyllium in laxative manufacture. *Ann Intern Med* 83: 361–362

195 Freeman GL (1994) Psyllium hypersensitivity. *Ann Allergy* 73: 490–492

196 Morgan MS, Arlian LG, Vyszenski-Moher DL, Deyo J, Kawabata T, Fernandez-Caldas E (1995) English plantain and psyllium: Lack of cross-allergenicity by crossed immunoelectrophoresis. *Ann Allergy Asthma Immunol* 75: 351–359

197 Malo JL, Cartier A, L'Archeveque J, Ghezzo H, Soucy F, Somers J, Dolovich J (1990) Prevalence of occupational asthma and immunologic sensitization to guar gum among employees at a carpet-manufacturing plant. *J Allergy Clin Immunol* 86: 562–569

198 Gelfand HH (1963) Respiratory allergy due to chemical compounds encountered in the rubber, lacquer, shellac, and beauty culture industries. *J Allergy Clin Immunol* 34: 374–381

199 Pepys J, Hutchcroft BJ, Breslin AB (1976) Asthma due to inhaled chemical agents – Persulphate salts and henna in hairdressers. *Clin Allergy* 6: 399–404

200 Starr JC, Yunginger J, Brahser GW (1982) Immediate type I asthmatic response to henna following occupational exposure in hairdressers. *Ann Allergy* 48: 98–99

201 Blainey AD, Ollier S, Cundell D, Smith RE, Davies RJ (1986) Occupational asthma in a hairdressing salon. *Thorax* 41: 42–50

202 Parra FM, Igea JM, Quirce S, Ferrando MC, Martin JA, Losada E (1992) Occupational asthma in a hairdresser caused by persulphate salts. *Allergy* 47: 656–660

203 Bolhaar ST, Mulder M, van Ginkel CJ (2001) IgE-mediated allergy to henna. *Allergy* 56: 248

204 Hollund BE, Moen BE, Lygre SH, Florvaag E, Omenaas E (2001) Prevalence of airway symptoms among hairdressers in Bergen, Norway. *Occup Environ Med* 58: 780–785

205 Munoz X, Cruz MJ, Orriols R, Bravo C, Espuga M, Morell F (2003) Occupational asthma due to persulfate salts: Diagnosis and follow-up. *Chest* 123: 2124–2129

206 Moscato G, Galdi E (2006) Asthma and hairdressers. *Curr Opin Allergy Clin Immunol* 6: 91–95

207 Petsonk EL, Wang ML, Lewis DM, Siegel PD, Husberg BJ (2000) Asthma-like symptoms in wood product plant workers exposed to methylene diphenyl diisocyanate. *Chest* 118: 1183–1193

208 Latza U, Baur X, Malo JL (2002) Isocyanate-induced health effects In: JV Bakke, JO Norén, S Thorud, TB Aasen (eds): *International consensus report on: Isocyanates – Risk assessment and management.* Norwegian Labour Inspection Authority Gjovik, 237–251

209 Tarlo SM, Liss GM, Dias C, Banks DE (1997) Assessment of the relationship between isocyanate exposure levels and occupational asthma. *Am J Ind Med* 32: 517–521

210 Karol MH (1981) Survey of industrial workers for antibodies to toluene diisocyanate. *J Occup Med* 23: 741–747

211 Rattray NJ, Botham PA, Hext PM, Woodcock DR, Fielding I, Dearman RJ, Kimber I (1994) Induction of respiratory hypersensitivity to diphenylmethane-4,4'-diisocyanate (MDI) in guinea pigs. Influence of route of exposure. *Toxicology* 88: 15–30

212 Vanoirbeek JA, Tarkowski M, Ceuppens JL, Verbeken EK, Nemery B, Hoet PH (2004) Respiratory response to toluene diisocyanate depends on prior frequency and concentration of dermal sensitization in mice. *Toxicol Sci* 80: 310–321

213 Zammit-Tabona M, Sherkin M, Kijek K, Chan H, Chan-Yeung M (1983) Asthma caused by diphenylmethane diisocyanate in foundry workers. Clinical, bronchial provocation, and immunologic studies. *Am Rev Respir Dis* 128: 226–230

214 Baur X, Marek W, Ammon J, Czuppon AB, Marczynski B, Raulf-Heimsoth M, Roemmelt H, Fruhmann G (1994) Respiratory and other hazards of isocyanates. *Int Arch Occup Environ Health* 66: 141–152

215 Cartier A, Grammer L, Malo JL, Lagier F, Ghezzo H, Harris K, Patterson R (1989) Specific serum antibodies against isocyanates: Association with occupational asthma. *J Allergy Clin Immunol* 84: 507–514

216 Grammer LC, Eggum P, Silverstein M, Shaughnessy MA, Liotta JL, Patterson R (1988) Prospective immunologic and clinical study of a population exposed to hexamethylene diisocyanate. *J Allergy Clin Immunol* 82: 627–633

217 Karol MH (1983) Concentration-dependent immunologic response to toluene diisocyanate (TDI) following inhalation exposure. *Toxicol Appl Pharmacol* 68: 229–241

218 Keskinen H, Tupasela O, Tiikkainen U, Nordman H (1988) Experiences of specific IgE in asthma due to diisocyanates. *Clin Allergy* 18: 597–604

219 Peters JM (1970) Studies of isocyanate toxicity. *Proc R Soc Med* 63: 372–375

220 Wegman DH, Peters JM, Pagnotto L, Fine LJ (1977) Chronic pulmonary function loss from exposure to toluene diisocyanate. *Br J Ind Med* 34: 196–200

221 Wegman DH, Musk AW, Main DM, Pagnotto LD (1982) Accelerated loss of FEV-1 in polyurethane production workers: A four-year prospective study. *Am J Ind Med* 3: 209–215

222 Diem JE, Jones RN, Hendrick DJ, Glindmeyer HW, Dharmarajan V, Butcher BT, Sal-

vaggio JE, Weill H (1982) Five-year longitudinal study of workers employed in a new toluene diisocyanate manufacturing plant. *Am Rev Respir Dis* 126: 420–428

223 Omae K, Higashi T, Nakadate T, Tsugane S, Nakaza M, Sakurai H (1992) Four-year follow-up of effects of toluene diisocyanate exposure on the respiratory system in polyurethane foam manufacturing workers. II. Four-year changes in the effects on the respiratory system. *Int Arch Occup Environ Health* 63: 565–569

224 Baur X (1996) Occupational asthma due to isocyanates. *Lung* 174: 23–30

225 Bernstein DI, Korbee L, Stauder T, Bernstein JA, Scinto J, Herd ZL, Bernstein IL (1993) The low prevalence of occupational asthma and antibody-dependent sensitization to diphenylmethane diisocyanate in a plant engineered for minimal exposure to diisocyanates. *J Allergy Clin Immunol* 92: 387–396

Mechanisms of occupational asthma caused by low-molecular-weight chemicals

Vanessa De Vooght, Valérie Hox, Benoit Nemery and Jeroen A. J. Vanoirbeek

K. U. Leuven, Faculty of Medicine, School of Public Health, Occupational, Environmental and Insurance Medicine, Research Unit for Lung Toxicology, Leuven, Belgium

Abstract

Understanding the pathogenesis and working mechanisms of occupational asthma (OA) is crucial towards optimizing prevention and management of the disease. The study of the sensitizing and asthma-inducing properties of low-molecular-weight (LMW) agents is evolving quickly. So far, experimental research has shown that OA caused by sensitization to LMW agents does not completely fit the pathways of the traditional allergic model, in which there is a central role for immunoglobulin E. Furthermore, recent evidence indicates that chemical respiratory allergens may induce respiratory tract sensitization by routes other than inhalation, such as dermal exposure. Knowledge on OA induced by LMW is increasing, but the pathogenesis remains largely vague. Dendritic cells, T cells, eosinophils, and several cytokines and chemokines are likely involved as in atopic asthma. However, through subtle differences in T cell subpopulations, cytokine balances and effector cells involved chemical-induced OA may well depend on processes that might differ substantially from those of atopic asthma. Furthermore, the involvement of the transient receptor potential channels in chemical-induced OA and irritant-induced asthma is intriguing. Further research in both humans and animals remains necessary to clarify the process of sensitization by LMW allergens and the mode of action inducing the OA phenotype.

Introduction

The lungs are the primary target for a diverse spectrum or work-related dusts, gases, fumes and vapors. Depending on the amount inhaled and on their physical-chemical properties, these agents have the capacity to cause annoyance, irritation, corrosive changes and/or sensitization in the respiratory tract. Occupational asthma (OA) is a type of asthma due to causes and conditions attributable to a particular work environment, rather than stimuli encountered outside the workplace [1]. It is characterized by a reversible airway obstruction of the airways associated with bronchial hyperresponsiveness upon inhalation of workplace-related agents [2]. OA has been implicated (directly or indirectly) in 9–15% of the cases of adult asthma, making OA one of the most common presentations of occupational lung diseases

Occupational Asthma, edited by Torben Sigsgaard and Dick Heederik

in many industrialized countries [3]. More than 350 agents have been reported to cause OA [4].

Traditionally, OA is divided into two types. The first type is immunologically mediated (or allergic) OA, in which sensitization against a workplace agent occurs after a "latency period". Immunologically mediated OA can be further divided into the well-known classical IgE-mediated form, and the more elusive "poly-immunological" cellular form (non-IgE-mediated). The second type, non-allergic OA or "irritant-induced" OA, is caused by exposure to irritant chemicals to which the host does not become sensitized. In its most typical presentation, irritant-induced asthma (IIA) is characterized by the absence of a latency period, because it is initiated by a sudden, acute exposure to high concentrations of an irritant. This form of IIA is often called reactive airways dysfunction syndrome (RADS). Other forms of IIA, caused by repeated exposures to irritants, are more controversial. Besides these forms of OA, some exposures at work may also lead to pharmacological bronchoconstriction and reflex bronchospasms [1, 5], but these reactions will not be discussed further.

The prevalence of OA depends mainly on the causative agent and the intensity of exposure [6, 7], and to some extent also on the distribution of individual-dependent factors, such as atopy and smoking status [8]. The highest prevalence of immunologically mediated OA has been reported in the detergent industry (up to 50%), in which workers are exposed to proteolytic enzymes. In cohorts of laboratory animal workers, prevalences of 30% of OA have been described. However, the prevalence of OA is generally much lower. In most occupational cohorts, prevalence varies between 9 and 15% [1]. Non-immunological OA is generally considered to occur less frequently than immunologically mediated asthma. The proportion of IIA among patients referred to an occupational lung disease clinic has been reported to be 2–3% [9, 10]. When criteria were expanded to one or more exposures to high levels of irritant, the prevalence of IIA doubled to 6%, accounting for 17% of all OA patients participating in a study of Tarlo and Broder [10]. One of the largest epidemiological studies published on IIA, concerns workers of the New York City Fire Department who were exposed to a variety of airway irritants during the rescue mission after the collapse of the World Trade Center on 11 September 2001: 16% of a sample of these workers met the criteria for IIA [11].

Depending on their molecular mass, agents causing OA can be divided into two categories: (a) biological agents of high molecular mass (HMW) (>5 kDa), such as proteins, glycoproteins and polysaccharides, and (b) chemicals of low molecular mass (LMW) (<5 kDa), such as synthetic chemicals, natural compounds, drugs and metals. HMW compounds generally induce OA *via* IgE-dependent mechanisms comparable with asthma induced by pollen or house dust mite allergens [12, 13], whereas many (although not all) LMW compounds appear to induce OA *via* pathways that do not involve IgE-dependent mechanisms.

Pathophysiology

Immunologically mediated OA

LMW chemicals comprise an important subset of etiological agents of OA, including approximately 100 chemical entities [4]. Isocyanates, acid anhydrides, plicatic acid from western red cedar, colophony fume, metals, complex platinum salts, persulfate salts, and some acrylates are just a few examples of important chemicals causing OA.

Since LMW agents are non-immunogenic in their native state, it is assumed that they must form a stable association with proteins to initiate an immune response. These protein-hapten conjugates can be recognized and internalized by professional antigen-presenting cells (APC) such as dendritic (DC) or Langerhans cells. Like most HMW agents, these conjugates are presented to T cells, which initiate an immune response and, possibly, asthma *via* an IgE-mediated mechanism or another mechanism. Complex platinum salts and trimellitic anhydride (TMA) are LMW asthmagens that are generally considered to induce asthma *via* specific IgE antibodies. These agents most likely possess a unique inherent ability to react directly (or indirectly, after metabolic activation) with functional groups present on human proteins [14, 15]. Not only albumin, but also other proteins such as keratine and tubuline can serve as carriers to render LMW agents immunogenic [15, 16].

Wisnewski et al. [17, 18] showed that LMW asthmagens can conjugate with proteins present on the surface of epithelial cells, thereby permitting presentation of LMW asthmagens to the immune system in a hapten-like manner. This may facilitate the uptake of the protein-hapten conjugates by professional APC to initiate the T cell response. If this is true for these LMW agents, then overall, the mechanism by which LMW antigens are presented to T cells and the following cascade of B cell activation plus IgE class switching, cross-linking of antigen and IgE on mast cells and attraction of inflammatory cells would be relatively similar between LMW and HMW compounds. Nevertheless, there are some questions and differences. For example, it is not exactly known in which form LMW asthmagens are displayed to responsive T cells. The way an antigen or hapten is processed, is dependent on where the hapten-protein conjugate is produced. Endogenous antigens are processed inside the cell, while exogenous antigens are processed through the endosomal pathway in DC. The binding of an LMW asthmagen (or its metabolite) to some lung intracellular protein may give rise to an endogenous antigenic determinant, and this may, therefore, be presented to $CD8^+$ T cells by major histocompatibility complex (MHC) class I [19]. However, the hapten may escape endogenous processing by cells in the lung and enter the peripheral circulation to bind proteins in the circulation. Such a chemical-modified antigenic protein is then processed by professional APC, e.g., B cells, macrophages and DC, and presented to $CD4^+$ T cells on MHC class II [20].

Depending on the pathway of LMW antigen presentation (MHC class I or MHC class II), different types of immune responses might develop ($CD4^+$ or $CD8^+$), which are categorized by their dominant cytokine secretion profile into T helper (Th) type 1 (IL-2, IL-12, IFN-γ), Th2 (IL-4, IL-13, IL-5), T regulatory (Treg) (TGF-β, IL-10) and Th17 (IL-17). While previously it was suggested that Th1 and Th2 cytokines counterbalanced each other, it has become clear that both Th1 and Th2 cytokines are involved in OA caused by LMW antigens [21–23]. Th17 cells, producing IL-17 – a potent attractant of neutrophils – are the latest T cells suggested to play a role in the proinflammatory pathway of OA [24]. While Th1, Th2 and Th17 cells are involved in proinflammatory pathways, Treg cells are thought to dampen the immune (asthmatic) response, possibly explaining why the majority of individuals do not develop adverse reactions to LMW asthmagen exposure [23, 25].

Besides LMW agents that initiate an IgE-mediated asthmatic response, there are also LMW agents, such as diisocyanates and plicatic acid that do not act *via* specific IgE antibodies, even though they lead to the same phenotypical characteristics as IgE-mediated OA [26–29]. In humans, the airway inflammation process is indeed similar in both IgE- and non-IgE-dependent asthma [13, 30, 31], and is characterized by the presence of eosinophils, lymphocytes, neutrophils, mast cells, and typical features of airway remodeling [6, 31, 32]. Airway inflammation is accompanied by a wide range of proinflammatory mediators and proteins. An influx of inflammatory cells, along with proinflammatory mediators can lead to a broad variety of adverse effects, such as toxic damage, increased oxidative stress, and loss of barrier integrity, contributing to long-term airway remodeling. Although in OA to LMW asthmagens, $CD4^+$ cells are associated with eosinophilia and airway inflammation [32, 33], a role has been suggested for $CD8^+$ cells in non-IgE-dependent OA [4, 23]. Interestingly, a small but significant proportion of T lymphocytes from the peripheral blood of subjects with OA induced by red cedar produce IL-5 and IFN-γ after stimulation with the conjugate of plicatic acid and human serum albumin, which is indicative of a mixed Th1/Th2 response [34].

The fate of inhaled diisocyanates in the human body and the nature of the antigen that is eventually produced are largely unknown, as is the case for most chemicals that can induce OA [4]. Extracellular glutathione was able to prevent isocyanate induced toxicity in human epithelial cells [18]. Human monocytes exposed *in vitro* to toluene diisocyanate (TDI)-albumin conjugates, undergo activation and up-regulation of lysosomal genes, along with increased production of monocyte chemoattractant protein-1 (MCP-1), and chitinase-1 [35]. Repetitive antigenic stimulation of *in vitro* cultured PBMCs obtained from subjects with diisocyanate asthma revealed that these cells synthesized TNF-α, a non–IgE-dependent proinflammatory cytokine, and MCP-1, but not IL-4 or IL-5 [35]. These observations are consistent with the hypothesis that isocyanate-induced up-regulation of immune pattern-recognition receptors by monocytes and release of damage-associated molecular patterns from injured epithelium may be a mechanism by which isocyanates stimulate the human innate immune responses and consequently influence the hypersensitivity reactions [36].

Irritant-induced OA

Besides the allergic type of OA, there is another type of OA that is caused by exposure to airway irritants and may occur without a latency period in its most typical presentation [9]. Originally, this disease entity was termed 'reactive airway dysfunction syndrome' (RADS). A case of RADS was defined as: (1) a documented absence of preceding respiratory complaints; (2) onset of symptoms after a single exposure incident or accident; (3) exposure to a gas, smoke, fume, or vapor with irritant properties present in very high concentrations; (4) onset of symptoms within 24 h after the exposure with persistence of symptoms for at least 3 months; (5) symptoms simulate asthma with cough, wheeze, and dyspnea; (6) presence of airflow obstruction on pulmonary function tests and/or presence of nonspecific bronchial hyperresponsiveness; and (7) other pulmonary diseases ruled out. In 1989 these diagnostic criteria were modified by Tarlo and Broder, in the sense that patients may have experienced 'more than one' high-level exposure to the irritant, since in many industries accidental spills are relatively common [10]. The term RADS was progressively replaced by 'irritant-induced asthma' (IIA), but this acronym remains often cited because of its high recognition value.

Only few studies are available to characterize the histopathology of the bronchial wall of patients with IIA. In general, nonspecific inflammatory infiltrates (lymphocytes, plasma cells, neutrophils) are present, often with thickening of the connective tissue [9, 37]. Gautrin et al. [38] described desquamation of bronchial epithelium and squamous cell metaplasia, as well as fibrosis of the bronchial wall and increased basement membrane thickness in five workers, 2 years after repeated exposures to high concentrations of chlorine. In biopsies from a patient exposed to chlorine, Lemière et al. [39] saw considerable epithelial desquamation with inflammatory exudates and swelling of the subepithelial space 2 weeks after the exposure; 2 months later, biopsies showed regeneration of the epithelium by basal cells and still a pronounced inflammatory infiltrate that recovered after steroid treatment [39]. Chan-Yeung et al. [40] were the first to show the presence of eosinophils in the bronchial inflammatory infiltrate of patients that suffered from 'gassings' in a pulp mill. These scarce data on histopathology suggest that inflammatory characteristics of IIA may be less extensive than in immunologically mediated OA, but this picture is nonspecific and cannot serve to make a definite diagnosis of IIA.

Data on possible mechanisms inducing IIA are only speculative. Brooks et al. [9] proposed a 'big bang' theory in which the initial irritant exposure causes significant epithelial damage associated with activation of the non-adrenergic, non-cholinergic (NANC) nerve system *via* axon reflexes, with the onset of a neurogenic inflammation through the release of neuropeptide transmitters such as Substance P and neurokinins. This epithelial damage can lead to release of relaxing factors, along with non specific macrophage and mast cell activation, which release proinflammatory cytokines and other mediators such as leukotrienes B_4 and C_4 [41], resulting in epithelial cell desquamation, smooth muscle cell hypertrophy and matrix degranulation [1, 38].

There is increasing evidence that chronic exposure to lower levels of irritants can also induce a form of OA [9, 42]. The fact that lower levels of irritant exposure could initiate asthma requires consideration of mechanisms other than airway damage alone to induce the asthma attack. It was noteworthy that 87% of the individuals that developed IIA in a less sudden way were atopic. One theory is that atopic persons elicit a different response to irritant exposure [42]. Another theory suggests an augmentation of the sensitivity to respiratory allergens by irritants, possibly through disruption of the epithelial barrier [43]. However, so far, no evidence exists to prove these theories. Moreover, the very existence of the entity of "not so sudden IIA" is currently disputed.

Acute inhalation of irritant chemicals may lead to persisting upper airway symptoms, with complaints from nose, sinuses and larynx. This entity has been described by Meggs et al. [44] as 'reactive upper airway dysfunction syndrome' (RUDS), by analogy with its asthmatic counterpart. These authors studied patients with chronic rhinitis after a chlorine dioxide exposure. Even less is known about mechanisms causing these upper airway problems after irritant exposure, but they are thought to be similar to those causing IIA, and neurogenic inflammation in response to epithelial damage is probably the key factor. Publications on RUDS or irritant-induced rhinitis are even rarer than those of RADS and irritant-induced asthma, so that the incidence and prevalence of this condition are even more obscure.

Animal models

In comparison with occupational diseases caused by inhaling mineral dusts or fibers, there has not been a lot of experimental research using laboratory animals to unravel the pathogenesis of OA. Yet, animal models can have a valuable role in gaining more information on the complex immunological and pathophysiological mechanisms involved in the development of allergies and asthma. At present a considerable part of what we know about the pathogenesis of asthma has been derived from animal experiments [45]. However, this research has been conducted mostly with HMW agents, especially ovalbumin, and only few research groups have investigated chemical-induced asthma.

Although no mouse model is currently able to mimic the full range of clinical manifestations that constitute human asthma, a number of models are available that reproduce several features that characterize its most common phenotypes. Nevertheless, important differences in airway development and morphology exist between humans and mice, thereby preventing the direct extrapolation of data between the species. Mouse airways have fewer airway generations and do not contain smooth muscle bundles. As a consequence, mouse models cannot be considered a surrogate for human asthma but they must be viewed as an opportunity to generate and test hypotheses in a relatively simple controlled system [46, 47].

The most common mouse strain used in this research area is the BALB/c mice, which exhibits a genetically determined tendency to develop Th2-biased immune responses. However, less Th2-prone mouse strains can also develop an asthma-like response. Several protocols for the induction of asthma have been developed and published employing a wide variety of antigens, application routes, doses and sequences as well as readouts [48].

Stimulation of the cholinergic and sensory nerves

The chemicals are initially recognized by APC present in the airways. Once the chemical is taken up, the APC get activated and release proinflammatory signals that not only influence the status of other cells of the immune system but also stimulate sensory pathways that activate the central nervous system. The vagus nerve has been proposed as an immune-to-brain pathway and it has been suggested that acetylcholine may modulate the airway immune response. Cholinergic mechanisms represent the predominant constrictor neural pathway, of which airway hyperresponsiveness (AHR), an important phenotype of asthma, is a good example [49].

Scheerens et al. [50] found an involvement of sensory neuropeptides in TDI-induced AHR in mouse airways. Sensory nerves are found in abundance around pulmonary blood vessels and in the epithelium of the trachea and bronchi of many species. Scheerens et al. found that tachykinins (substance P and neurokinin A) are involved in the effector phase of TDI-induced AHR when mice were sensitized (via epicutaneous application) and intranasally challenged. Furthermore, the tachykinins did not seem to act directly on the tracheal smooth muscle but *via* the activation of other cells (T lymphocytes and mast cells). Beside the effect on AHR, substance P also plays a role in the influx of inflammatory cells, particularly neutrophils [51].

It is also important to mention that many reactive chemicals, including sensitizers such as diisocyanates, have strong irritant properties when they are used in high concentrations. The airway responses to these irritants result partly also from reflexes mediated by sensory and autonomic nerve fibers in the airways [51].

Lung function measurements

A change in breathing pattern immediately after airway exposure has been documented in various mouse models of chemical-induced asthma. Pauluhn et al. [52–54] described a decrease in breathing frequency after nose-only exposure to diphenylmethane-4,4'-diisocyanate (MDI), 1,6-hexamethylene diisocyanate (HDI) and TMA in sensitized guinea pigs and rats. Vanoirbeek et al. [55–57] showed differences in enhanced pause (Penh), a parameter representing bronchoconstriction, immediately after intranasal challenge with TDI or TMA.

Nonspecific AHR is generally measured 1 or 2 days after challenging the mice with a specific antigen. Many research groups focusing on chemical-induced asthma have found an increase in AHR to methacholine [52, 55–62]. Scheerens et al. [50] were the first to find *in vitro* AHR after carbachol exposure. As mentioned above, they found that sensory neuropeptides played an important role. Furthermore, Matheson et al. [63] and Tarkowski et al. [56] showed the absence of AHR in athymic mice and severe combined immunodeficiency (SCID) mice, respectively, suggesting an important function for T-lymphocytes in these models. Herrick et al. [64] and Matheson et al. [59] showed that both $CD4^+$ and $CD8^+$ lymphocytes are crucial in mouse models of asthma caused by HDI and MDI, respectively.

Airway inflammation

In comparison with asthma induced by HMW agents, where eosinophils and lymphocytes are the characteristic cell types present in the bronchoalveolar lavage (BAL) fluid, asthma induced by LMW agents has been associated with an influx of mainly neutrophils and eosinophils [50, 55, 56, 62, 63, 65]. The type of inflammation is also highly dependent on the duration of exposure and the route of challenge. For example, Vanoirbeek et al. [55, 60] found mainly an influx of neutrophils when TDI-dermally sensitized mice received a single intranasal challenge with TDI, whereas De Vooght et al. [62] found an influx of neutrophils as well as eosinophils, using the same dermal sensitization protocol, but altering the challenge route from intranasal instillation to oropharyngeal aspiration.

Herrick et al. [66] used HDI conjugated to mouse serum albumin (MSA) to challenge their mice. Using this complex they found an inflammation in the BAL that correlated with the phenotype of atopic asthma, i.e., an influx of eosinophils and lymphocytes.

The influx of inflammatory cells is mediated by several cytokines and chemokines. Increases of Th2 (IL-4, IL-5, IL-13) and Th1 (IFN-γ) cytokines was found in homogenates of lung tissue [59, 66]. Macrophage inflammatory protein 2 (MIP-2), a chemokine for neutrophils in mice, was found to be increased [56]. IL-1 also seems to be an important mediator in chemical-induced asthma. IL-1 stimulates the release of IL-5, which is important for the recruitment and activation of eosinophils, and induces the production of intercellular adhesion molecule-1 (ICAM-1) and vascular cell adhesion molecule-1 (VCAM-1), important for leukocyte recruitment [67]. Matrix metalloproteinase 9 (MMP-9) is the major proteinase that induces bronchial remodeling in asthma. In addition, MMP-9 as well as vascular endothelial growth factor (VEGF) induce the migration of eosinophils and neutrophils [65, 68]. Tumor necrosis factor α (TNF-α) is a major initiator and propagator of airway inflammation and promotes the migration of DC [69]. In addition, through their effect on airway inflammation, IL-1, MMP-9, VEGF and TNF-α, lead to AHR.

So far, most mouse models are based on an "acute" form of OA. The main focus has been on the inflammation found in the BAL, while structural changes of the lung and airways tissue have not often been investigated. Some degree of peribronchial and perivascular inflammation, epithelial shedding, mucus hypersecretion by proliferation of the goblet cells and some perivascular remodeling have been described in the lungs of mice with diisocyanate-induced OA [62, 66, 70].

Immunoglobulins

Both increases in specific antibodies, as well as total serum immunoglobulins (IgE and IgG) have been described in diisocyanate-treated mice. However, a consistent observation in isocyanate-induced OA is the absence of any meaningful association between these serological findings and the presence or absence of airway responses, or with airway inflammation [71].

Scheerens et al. [72] found that by altering the exposure time and/or cumulative dosage, TDI is capable of inducing different immunological reactions. When sensitizing the animals longer they were able to find specific IgE and IgG in serum, compared to a shorter protocol. Matheson et al. [58] and Herrick et al. [64] also found specific immunoglobulins (IgG) after a low-level subchronic exposure to TDI and exposure to HDI-MSA, respectively. Vanoirbeek et al. found increases in total serum IgE, IgG1 and IgG2a in TDI and TMA asthmatic mice. In isocyanate-induced OA it is known that immune responses can emerge from IgE-dependent or non-IgE-dependent mechanisms, but the functional meaning of this in animal models remains unclear and probably non-essential. It is known that immunological sensitization to LMW asthmagens is often lifelong. The only 'remedy' to avoid the symptoms of OA is removal from the exposure place [73]. If asthmatic workers can avoid contact with the causal asthmagen, improvement of AHR can occur [74]. This was confirmed in the TDI mouse model of Vanoirbeek et al. [60]. In this set of experiments, the researchers increased the time between sensitization and intranasal challenge, resulting in a decrease of the AHR and airway inflammation, regardless of the high concentrations of IgE, IgG1 and IgG2a in the serum of TDI-treated mice. This is further confirmation that immunoglobulins are present in chemical-induced asthma; however, their role in the pathophysiology of OA is uncertain at best.

Controversial issues

Neutrophils and OA

In the pathophysiology of OA due to LMW asthmagens, discussion often occurs concerning the presence and the role of neutrophils, as the main BAL inflammatory cell. In non-OA the presence of neutrophils is considered a marker of disease severity [75]; however, this is not yet established in OA. Moscato et al. [31] found that a positive response to the specific inhalation challenge (SIC) of persulfate salts was correlated with an increased sputum eosinophilia, while in symptomatic workers with a negative response to the SIC a neutrophilic inflammation was predominant. Park et al. [76] found a predominant neutrophilic inflammation in TDI-induced asthmatics, which was linked to IL-8, a chemokine involved in neutrophil attraction. This dichotomy between a predominant BAL neutrophil or eosinophil inflammation is also found in animal model of OA [52, 58, 60, 62, 66, 70]. Probably, the nature of the pulmonary inflammation in asthma is heavily dependent on the time course of the disease, the pattern of the exposure and individual susceptibility factors [28, 31, 77].

The skin and OA

In OA it is generally assumed that exposure to the respiratory tract is the key route and site for the initiation of the immune responses. Accordingly, research, regulation and prevention focus almost exclusively on airborne exposures. However, despite reductions in workplace respiratory exposures, isocyanate asthma continues to occur, and this has prompted a focus on skin as a route of exposure [78, 79]. Evidence that skin exposure may increase risk for isocyanate sensitization and asthma in humans is mainly derived from case reports and limited cross-sectional studies [78, 80, 81]. Recently, isocyanate skin exposure has been documented using newly developed qualitative and quantitative methodologies in car body shop workers and painters. The authors found substantial skin exposure to isocyanates, while these workers were occupied in a setting where airborne exposure was minimal, and despite the use of standard personal protective equipment such as gloves [81–83]. Several animal models have shown convincingly that skin exposure to chemical sensitizers (predominantly isocyanates, but also anhydrides) can induce systemic sensitization, which may result in asthma-like respiratory responses when the animal is later challenged *via* the airways [56, 64, 70]. These murine studies suggest that the occurrence of respiratory responses depend on several factors related to both the nature and timing of the sensitization and that of the challenge [55, 60, 61].

Specific antibodies and OA

Controversy still exists regarding the role of specific antibodies in asthma induced by LMW asthmagens. While some LMW asthmagens (e.g., complex platinum salts and TMA) consistently produce specific IgE antibodies, other LMW asthmagens, most notably TDI and western red cedar (plicatic acid), do not. For example, in TDI-asthmatics specific IgE antibodies are only found in 0–50% of exposed workers [84]. It has been suggested that sensitization to isocyanates can be achieved *via* other immunological mechanisms, such as direct T cell activation [20]. On the other hand, it has been suggested that IgE antibodies go undetected for largely technical and methodological reasons [4]. A technical limitation was shown by Son et al. [85], who showed that the variable results in the presence of specific IgE antibodies to TDI in serum of exposed workers depended on the heterogeneous binding of specific IgE of a TDI-asthmatic to an antigenic determinant of TDI-human serum albumin conjugate *in vitro*. This binding can differ between one individual and another. So, it remains unclear whether IgE-mediated responses contribute to the development of asthmatic symptoms in workers exposed to TDI. Not only the role of specific IgE responses, but also the role of specific IgG is under debate. After TDI exposure, specific serum IgG can persist for many years [26]. Although the sensitivity for measuring specific IgG in serum of TDI-induced asthmatics is higher than specific IgE, the sensitivity is still poor. Therefore, it is rather suggested that IgG could be used to monitor exposure to diisocyanates, rather than act as a marker of sensitization [26, 86].

Mechanisms of IIA

Little or no experimental research has been conducted to clarify the mechanisms of persistent airway hyperreactivity that occurs in some victims of a single acute inhalation injury. Morris et al. [87] showed that capsaicin treatment could reverse the respiratory effects of chlorine gas inhalation in mice, suggesting an important role of sensory receptor channels on the nerve endings in the respiratory mucosa. Martin et al. [88] described histological changes in the airways and increases in bronchial reactivity to methacholine in mice after a single inhalation of chlorine gas, but their experiments did not go beyond 7 days. Further publications by the same group point to acute immunological changes and airway remodeling [89, 90], but these studies do not yet help us understanding the determinants of RADS in humans. Both Guo et al. [91] and Venglarik et al. [92] have shown a reduction in bronchial transepithelial electric resistance in response to hypochlorite exposure. However, no phenotypic responses have been linked to this finding so far. The possible role of repeated exposures to low concentrations of occupational chemical irritants in the causation of asthma has been studied even less. An ozone-induced asthma model has been set up by the group of Pichavant et al. [93], in which iNKT cells and IL-17 seem to be important disease markers. Furthermore, findings related to co-exposures of antigens with ozone, cigarette smoke or diesel exhaust particles, involving DC priming, GM-CSF and leading to up-regulation of Th2 related cytokines, may contribute to understanding the mechanisms of IIA [94–98].

Transient receptor potential channels and IIA

As already mentioned, neural activation causes pain and irritation, neurogenic inflammation, mucus secretion, and reflex responses such as cough, sneezing, and bronchoconstriction [99, 100]. Recently, members of the transient receptor potential (TRP) superfamily of ion channels have been proposed to play a key role in the response of sensory neurons to inflammatory mediators [99, 101, 102]. The two major proinflammatory TRP ion channels in sensory neurons are TRPV1, the capsaicin receptor, and TRPA1, activated by mustard oil [99, 103]. Agonists of TRPV1 and TRPA1, such as capsaicin, acrolein, diisocyanates or chlorine, are potent tussive agents and have been associated with allergic and occupational asthma and RADS [101, 104–106]. In TRPA1$^{-/-}$ KO mice or when a TRPA1 antagonist is used in an animal model, inflammation and acute airway responses to chemical exposure are substantially decreased [104–107]. These data suggest that activation of TRPA1 and TRPV1 on airway sensory fiber terminals by hazardous irritants could evoke noxious respiratory sensation, sensitization of respiratory reflexes, and the local release of proinflammatory neuropeptides, which can lead (in the long term) to OA or IIA [99].

Putative mechanism of action

Combining all data from human and mice, sketches have been made trying to give an overview of the mechanisms of OA induced by LMW asthmagens. Keeping in mind that the skin is a relevant site for initiation of sensitization, Figure 1A gives an overview of the sequential events that presumably take place after dermal contact with LMW sensitizers that could lead to sensitization. When applied on the skin, LMW sensitizers bind to proteins (e.g., keratine) [16] and form hapten-protein complexes. Langerhans cells in the epidermis internalize these hapten-protein complexes. The activated Langerhans cells mature and migrate to the draining lymph nodes, while processing the protein complex. The processed protein complex is

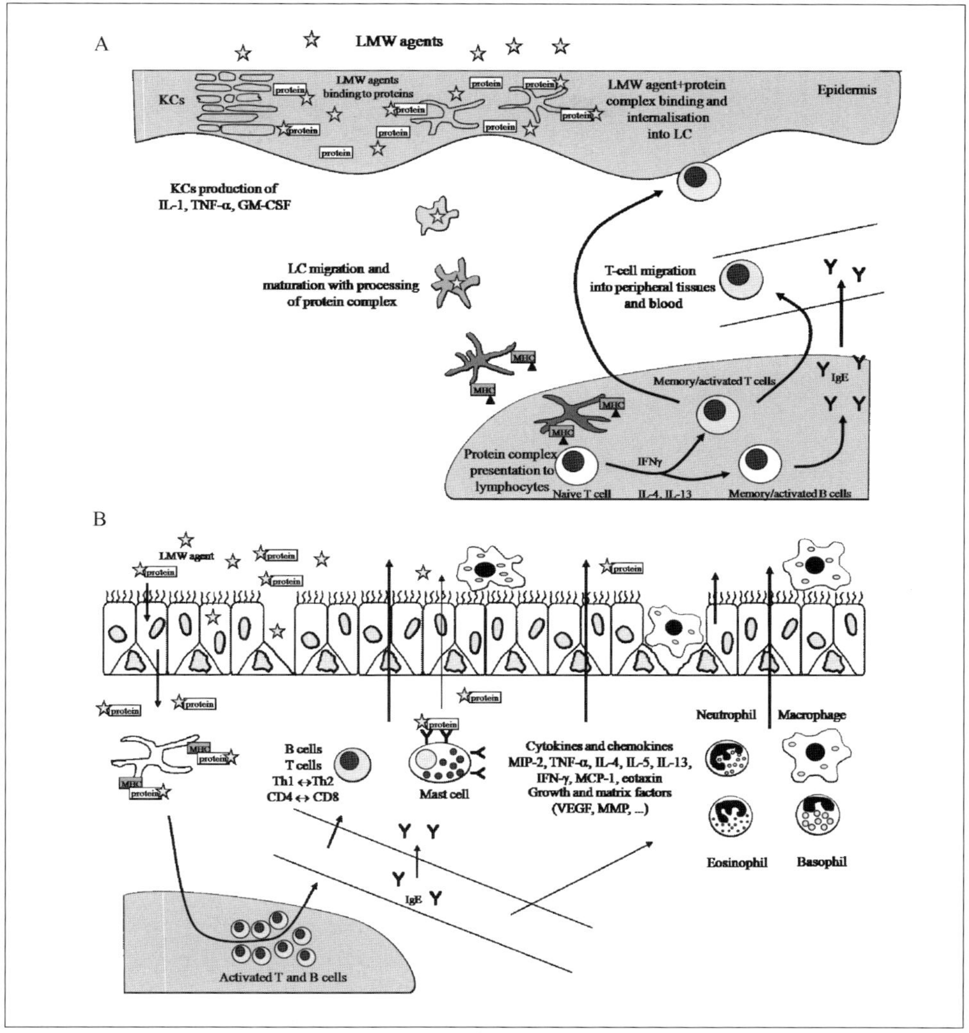

Figure 1.
(A) Hypothetical scheme to describe the dermal sensitization phase. (B) Hypothetical model of the immunopathogenesis of asthma induced by LMW agents. These two models give an overview of findings in the literature. APC, antigen presenting cell; GM-CSF, granulocyte-macrophage colony stimulating factor IFN, interferon; IgE, immunoglobulin E; IL, interleukin; KC, keratinocyte; LC, Langerhans cells; LMW, low-molecular-weight; MHC, major histocompatibility complex; MIP, macrophage inflammatory protein; MMP, matrix metalloproteinase; MCP, monocyte chemotactic protein; TNF, tumor necrosis factor; VEGF, vascular endothelial growth factor. Figure adapted and modified from [71, 108, 109].

presented to naïve T cells *via* the MHC, hereby activating the T cells. T cells differentiate to both memory Th1 (*via* IL-12) and Th2 (*via* IL-4) cells. IL-4 and IL-13 released from Th2 cells also stimulate B cells to produce IgE, which is released into the blood. Activated and memory T cells (Th1 and Th2) and B cells migrate from the local draining lymph nodes to the peripheral tissues and the blood [108, 109].

Subsequently, Figure 1B illustrates the possible pathogenic cascade leading to LMW asthmagen-induced OA. The primary event in this process, after the LMW asthmagens have reached the respiratory mucosa, is the conjugation of asthmagens with proteins in the airways, such as albumin and possibly other epithelial cell proteins (e.g., tubulin on top of the cilia and actin) [16, 17, 110]. The antigenic epitopes resulting from the interaction of LMW asthmagens with the proteins will lead to airway inflammation, but this remains poorly characterized. Probably the antigenic epitopes of the protein-hapten complex will be presented to the Th1, Th2 and B cells by APC. IgE from the B cells will cross-link the protein-hapten complex with mast cells that release their mediators (e.g., histamine) and cause an acute asthmatic response. Moreover, *via* the T cells several cytokines and chemokines get released, which mediate several cellular responses and activate neutrophils, eosinophils and basophils, leading to a chronic state of asthma [20, 71, 79, 109, 111].

Admittedly, in this schematic overview we only focused on the well-known allergic pathway of OA and we did not included the neurogenic mechanisms of action (TRP-receptors, substance P, neurokinines), which recently have been suggested to play a (important) role in both IIA and OA. Multiple questions remain to be answered, including the determination of relevant routes of exposure, better characterization of the immune response, the inflammatory cells involved and mediators responsible for LMW asthmagen-induced sensitization and OA, along with the identification of the genetic factors that regulate airway inflammation. Although the mouse models of LMW asthmagen-induced asthma share features common with human chemical-induced OA, none of them perfectly replicates real-life human exposures or the disease in humans. Nevertheless, good models are important to protect workers from compounds that act as respiratory sensitizers, which can lead to asthma after repeated exposures.

References

1 Bernstein IL, Chan-Yeung M, Malo JL, Bernstein DI. *Asthma in the Workplace*, 2 edn. Marcel Dekker, New York 1999

2 Bardana EJ, Jr. 10. Occupational asthma. *J Allergy Clin Immunol* 2008; 121(2 Suppl): S408–S411

3 Chan-Yeung M, Malo JL. Occupational asthma. *N Engl J Med* 1995; 333(2): 107–12

4 Maestrelli P, Boschetto P, Fabbri LM, Mapp CE. Mechanisms of occupational asthma. *J Allergy Clin Immunol* 2009; 123(3): 531–42

5 Bardana EJ, Jr. Occupational asthma and allergies. *J Allergy Clin Immunol* 2003; 111(2 Suppl): S530–S539

6 Maestrelli P, Saetta M, Mapp C, Fabbri LM. Mechanisms of occupational asthma. *Clin Exp Allergy* 1997; 27 (Suppl 1): 47–54

7 Chan-Yeung M, Malo JL, Tarlo SM, Bernstein L, Gautrin D, Mapp C et al. Proceedings of the first Jack Pepys Occupational Asthma Symposium. *Am J Respir Crit Care Med* 2003; 167(3): 450–71

8 Lombardo LJ, Balmes JR. Occupational asthma: A review. *Environ Health Perspect* 2000; 108(Suppl 4): 697–704

9 Brooks SM, Weiss MA, Bernstein IL. Reactive airways dysfunction syndrome (RADS). Persistent asthma syndrome after high level irritant exposures. *Chest* 1985; 88(3): 376–84

10 Tarlo SM, Broder I. Irritant-induced occupational asthma. *Chest* 1989; 96(2): 297–300

11 Banauch GI, Dhala A, Alleyne D, Alva R, Santhyadka G, Krasko A et al. Bronchial hyperreactivity and other inhalation lung injuries in rescue/recovery workers after the World Trade Center collapse. *Crit Care Med* 2005; 33(1 Suppl): S102–S106

12 Tarlo SM. Recent advances in occupational asthma. *Curr Opin Pulm Med* 2000; 6(2): 145–50

13 Mapp C, Boschetto P, Miotto D, De Rosa E, Fabbri LM. Mechanisms of occupational asthma. *Ann Allergy Asthma Immunol* 1999; 83(6 Pt 2): 645–64

14 Baur X, Czuppon A. Diagnostic validation of specific IgE antibody concentrations, skin prick testing, and challenge tests in chemical workers with symptoms of sensitivity to different anhydrides. *J Allergy Clin Immunol* 1995; 96(4): 489–94

15 Wisnewski AV, Redlich CA. Recent developments in diisocyanate asthma. *Curr Opin Allergy Clin Immunol* 2001; 1(2): 169–75

16 Wisnewski AV, Srivastava R, Herick C, Xu L, Lemus R, Cain H et al. Identification of human lung and skin proteins conjugated with hexamethylene diisocyanate *in vitro* and *in vivo*. *Am J Respir Crit Care Med* 2000; 162(6): 2330–6

17 Wisnewski AV, Lemus R, Karol MH, Redlich CA. Isocyanate-conjugated human lung epithelial cell proteins: A link between exposure and asthma? *J Allergy Clin Immunol* 1999; 104(2 Pt 1): 341–7

18 Wisnewski AV, Liu Q, Liu J, Redlich CA. Glutathione protects human airway proteins and epithelial cells from isocyanates. *Clin Exp Allergy* 2005; 35(3): 352–7

19 Heath WR, Carbone FR. Cross-presentation, dendritic cells, tolerance and immunity. *Annu Rev Immunol* 2001; 19: 47–64

20 Lutz W, Palczynski C. Advances in molecular immunotoxicology of occupational asthma induced by low molecular weight chemicals. *Int J Occup Med Environ Health* 2003; 16(4): 285–99

21 Karol MH. Respiratory allergy: What are the uncertainties? *Toxicology* 2002; 181–182: 305–10

22 Wisnewski AV, Herrick CA, Liu Q, Chen L, Bottomly K, Redlich CA. Human gamma/delta T-cell proliferation and IFN-gamma production induced by hexamethylene diisocyanate. *J Allergy Clin Immunol* 2003; 112(3): 538–46

23 Mamessier E, Milhe F, Guillot C, Birnbaum J, Dupuy P, Lorec AM et al. T-cell activation in occupational asthma and rhinitis. *Allergy* 2007; 62(2): 162–9

24 Ivanov S, Palmberg L, Venge P, Larsson K, Linden A. Interleukin-17A mRNA and protein expression within cells from the human bronchoalveolar space after exposure to organic dust. *Respir Res* 2005; 6: 44

25 Naisbitt DJ, Williams DP, Pirmohamed M, Kitteringham NR, Park BK. Reactive metabolites and their role in drug reactions. *Curr Opin Allergy Clin Immunol* 2001; 1(4): 317–25

26 Park HS, Kim HY, Nahm DH, Son JW, Kim YY. Specific IgG, but not specific IgE, antibodies to toluene diisocyanate-human serum albumin conjugate are associated with toluene diisocyanate bronchoprovocation test results. *J Allergy Clin Immunol* 1999; 104(4 Pt 1): 847–51

27 Karol MH, Tollerud DJ, Campbell TP, Fabbri L, Maestrelli P, Saetta M et al. Predictive value of airways hyperresponsiveness and circulating IgE for identifying types of responses to toluene diisocyanate inhalation challenge. *Am J Respir Crit Care Med* 1994; 149(3 Pt 1): 611–5

28 Anees W, Huggins V, Pavord ID, Robertson AS, Burge PS. Occupational asthma due to low molecular weight agents: Eosinophilic and non-eosinophilic variants. *Thorax* 2002; 57(3): 231–6

29 Chan-Yeung M, Malo JL. Aetiological agents in occupational asthma. *Eur Respir J* 1994; 7(2): 346–71

30 Turato G, Saetta M. Why does airway obstruction persist in asthma due to low-molecular-weight agents? A Pathologistis view. *Occup Med* 2000; 15(2): 445–54

31 Moscato G, Pignatti P, Yacoub MR, Romano C, Spezia S, Perfetti L. Occupational asthma and occupational rhinitis in hairdressers. *Chest* 2005; 128(5): 3590–8

32 Frew AJ, Chan H, Lam S, Chan-Yeung M. Bronchial inflammation in occupational asthma due to western red cedar. *Am J Respir Crit Care Med* 1995; 151(2 Pt 1): 340–4

33 Yawalkar N, Helbling A, Pichler CE, Zala L, Pichler WJ. T cell involvement in persulfate triggered occupational contact dermatitis and asthma. *Ann Allergy Asthma Immunol* 1999; 82(4): 401–4

34 Frew A, Chang JH, Chan H, Quirce S, Noertjojo K, Keown P et al. T-lymphocyte responses to plicatic acid-human serum albumin conjugate in occupational asthma caused by western red cedar. *J Allergy Clin Immunol* 1998; 101(6 Pt 1): 841–7

35 Lummus ZL, Alam R, Bernstein JA, Bernstein DI. Diisocyanate antigen-enhanced production of monocyte chemoattractant protein-1, IL-8, and tumor necrosis factor-alpha by peripheral mononuclear cells of workers with occupational asthma. *J Allergy Clin Immunol* 1998; 102(2): 265–74

36 Wisnewski AV, Liu Q, Liu J, Redlich CA. Human innate immune responses to hex-

amethylene diisocyanate (HDI) and HDI-albumin conjugates. *Clin Exp Allergy* 2008; 38(6): 957–67

37 Deschamps D, Rosenberg N, Soler P, Maillard G, Fournier E, Salson D et al. Persistent asthma after accidental exposure to ethylene oxide. *Br J Ind Med* 1992; 49(7): 523–5

38 Gautrin D, Boulet LP, Boutet M, Dugas M, Bherer L, L'Archeveque J et al. Is reactive airways dysfunction syndrome a variant of occupational asthma? *J Allergy Clin Immunol* 1994; 93(1 Pt 1): 12–22

39 Lemiere C, Malo JL, Boutet M. Reactive airways dysfunction syndrome due to chlorine: Sequential bronchial biopsies and functional assessment. *Eur Respir J* 1997; 10(1): 241–4

40 Chan-Yeung M, Lam S, Kennedy SM, Frew AJ. Persistent asthma after repeated exposure to high concentrations of gases in pulp mills. *Am J Respir Crit Care Med* 1994; 149(6): 1676–80

41 Jame AJ, Lackie PM, Cazaly AM, Sayers I, Penrose JF, Holgate ST et al. Human bronchial epithelial cells express an active and inducible biosynthetic pathway for leukotrienes B4 and C4. *Clin Exp Allergy* 2007; 37(6): 880–92

42 Brooks SM, Hammad Y, Richards I, Giovinco-Barbas J, Jenkins K. The spectrum of irritant-induced asthma: Sudden and not-so-sudden onset and the role of allergy. *Chest* 1998; 113(1): 42–9

43 Jorres R, Nowak D, Magnussen H. The effect of ozone exposure on allergen responsiveness in subjects with asthma or rhinitis. *Am J Respir Crit Care Med* 1996; 153(1): 56–64

44 Meggs WJ, Elsheik T, Metzger WJ, Albernaz M, Bloch RM. Nasal pathology and ultrastructure in patients with chronic airway inflammation (RADS and RUDS) following an irritant exposure. *J Toxicol Clin Toxicol* 1996; 34(4): 383–96

45 Irvin CG. Using the mouse to model asthma: The cup is half full and then some. *Clin Exp Allergy* 2008; 38(5): 701–3

46 Willis-Owen SA, Valdar W. Deciphering gene-environment interactions through mouse models of allergic asthma. *J Allergy Clin Immunol* 2009; 123(1): 14–23

47 Wenzel S, Holgate ST. The mouse trap: It still yields few answers in asthma. *Am J Respir Crit Care Med* 2006; 174(11): 1173–6

48 Schroder NW, Maurer M. The role of innate immunity in asthma: Leads and lessons from mouse models. *Allergy* 2007; 62(6): 579–90

49 Lutz W, Sulkowski WJ. Vagus nerve participates in regulation of the airways: Inflammatory response and hyperreactivity induced by occupational asthmogens. *Int J Occup Med Environ Health* 2004; 17(4): 417–31

50 Scheerens H, Buckley TL, Muis T, Van Loveren H, Nijkamp FP. The involvement of sensory neuropeptides in toluene diisocyanate-induced tracheal hyperreactivity in the mouse airways. *Br J Pharmacol* 1996; 119(8): 1665–71

51 Hunter DD, Satterfield BE, Huang J, Fedan JS, Dey RD. Toluene diisocyanate enhances substance P in sensory neurons innervating the nasal mucosa. *Am J Respir Crit Care Med* 2000; 161(2 Pt 1): 543–9

52 Pauluhn J, Woolhiser MR, Bloemen L. Repeated inhalation challenge with diphenylmethane-4,4'-diisocyanate in brown Norway rats leads to a time-related increase of neutrophils in bronchoalveolar lavage after topical induction. *Inhal Toxicol* 2005; 17(2): 67–78

53 Pauluhn J, Eidmann P, Mohr U. Respiratory hypersensitivity in guinea pigs sensitized to 1,6–hexamethylene diisocyanate (HDI): Comparison of results obtained with the monomer and homopolymers of HDI. *Toxicology* 2002; 171(2–3): 147–60

54 Pauluhn J. Respiratory hypersensitivity to trimellitic anhydride in Brown Norway rats: Analysis of dose-response following topical induction and time course following repeated inhalation challenge. *Toxicology* 2003; 194(1–2): 1–17

55 Vanoirbeek JA, Tarkowski M, Ceuppens JL, Verbeken EK, Nemery B, Hoet PH. Respiratory response to toluene diisocyanate depends on prior frequency and concentration of dermal sensitization in mice. *Toxicol Sci* 2004; 80(2): 310–21

56 Tarkowski M, Vanoirbeek JA, Vanhooren HM, De Vooght V, Mercier CM, Ceuppens J et al. Immunological determinants of ventilatory changes induced in mice by dermal sensitization and respiratory challenge with toluene diisocyanate. *Am J Physiol Lung Cell Mol Physiol* 2007; 292(1): L207–L214

57 Vanoirbeek JA, Tarkowski M, Vanhooren HM, De Vooght V, Nemery B, Hoet PH. Validation of a mouse model of chemical-induced asthma using trimellitic anhydride, a respiratory sensitizer, and dinitrochlorobenzene, a dermal sensitizer. *J Allergy Clin Immunol* 2006; 117(5): 1090–7

58 Matheson JM, Johnson VJ, Vallyathan V, Luster MI. Exposure and immunological determinants in a murine model for toluene diisocyanate (TDI) asthma. *Toxicol Sci* 2005; 84(1): 88–98

59 Matheson JM, Johnson VJ, Luster MI. Immune mediators in a murine model for occupational asthma: Studies with toluene diisocyanate. *Toxicol Sci* 2005; 84(1): 99–109

60 Vanoirbeek JA, De V, V, Vanhooren HM, Nawrot TS, Nemery B, Hoet PH. How long do the systemic and ventilatory responses to toluene diisocyanate persist in dermally sensitized mice? *J Allergy Clin Immunol* 2008; 121(2): 456–63

61 Vanoirbeek JA, De V, V, Nemery B, Hoet PH. Multiple challenges in a mouse model of chemical-induced asthma lead to tolerance: Ventilatory and inflammatory responses are blunted, immunologic humoral responses are not. *Toxicology* 2009; 257(3): 144–52

62 De Vooght V, Vanoirbeek JA, Haenen S, Verbeken E, Nemery B, Hoet PH. Oropharyngeal aspiration: An alternative route for challenging in a mouse model of chemical-induced asthma. *Toxicology* 2009; 259(1–2): 84–9

63 Matheson JM, Lange RW, Lemus R, Karol MH, Luster MI. Importance of inflammatory and immune components in a mouse model of airway reactivity to toluene diisocyanate (TDI). *Clin Exp Allergy* 2001; 31(7): 1067–76

64 Herrick CA, Das J, Xu L, Wisnewski AV, Redlich CA, Bottomly K. Differential roles for CD4 and CD8 T cells after diisocyanate sensitization: Genetic control of TH2-induced lung inflammation. *J Allergy Clin Immunol* 2003; 111(5): 1087–94

65 Lee YC, Song CS, Lee HB, Oh JL, Rhee YK, Park HS et al. A murine model of toluene

diisocyanate-induced asthma can be treated with matrix metalloproteinase inhibitor. *J Allergy Clin Immunol* 2001; 108(6): 1021–6
66 Herrick CA, Xu L, Wisnewski AV, Das J, Redlich CA, Bottomly K. A novel mouse model of diisocyanate-induced asthma showing allergic- type inflammation in the lung after inhaled antigen challenge. *J Allergy Clin Immunol* 2002; 109(5 Pt 1): 873–8
67 Johnson VJ, Yucesoy B, Luster MI. Prevention of IL-1 signaling attenuates airway hyperresponsiveness and inflammation in a murine model of toluene diisocyanate-induced asthma. *J Allergy Clin Immunol* 2005; 116(4): 851–8
68 Lee YC, Kwak YG, Song CH. Contribution of vascular endothelial growth factor to airway hyperresponsiveness and inflammation in a murine model of toluene diisocyanate-induced asthma. *J Immunol* 2002; 168(7): 3595–600
69 Matheson JM, Lemus R, Lange RW, Karol MH, Luster MI. Role of tumor necrosis factor in toluene diisocyanate asthma. *Am J Respir Cell Mol Biol* 2002; 27(4): 396–405
70 Ban M, Morel G, Langonne I, Huguet N, Pepin E, Binet S. TDI can induce respiratory allergy with Th2–dominated response in mice. *Toxicology* 2006; 218(1): 39–47
71 Redlich CA, Wisnewski AV, Gordon T. Mouse models of diisocyanate asthma. *Am J Respir Cell Mol Biol* 2002; 27(4): 385–90
72 Scheerens H, Buckley TL, Muis TL, Garssen J, Dormans J, Nijkamp FP et al. Long-term topical exposure to toluene diisocyanate in mice leads to antibody production and *in vivo* airway hyperresponsiveness three hours after intranasal challenge. *Am J Respir Crit Care Med* 1999; 159(4 Pt 1): 1074–80
73 Lemiere C, Cartier A, Malo JL, Lehrer SB. Persistent specific bronchial reactivity to occupational agents in workers with normal nonspecific bronchial reactivity. *Am J Respir Crit Care Med* 2000; 162(3 Pt 1): 976–80
74 Lemiere C. Persistence of bronchial reactivity to occupational agents after removal from exposure and identification of associated factors. *Ann Allergy Asthma Immunol* 2003; 90(5 Suppl 2): 52–5
75 Jatakanon A, Uasuf C, Maziak W, Lim S, Chung KF, Barnes PJ. Neutrophilic inflammation in severe persistent asthma. *Am J Respir Crit Care Med* 1999; 160(5 Pt 1): 1532–9
76 Park H, Jung K, Kim H, Nahm D, Kang K. Neutrophil activation following TDI bronchial challenges to the airway secretion from subjects with TDI-induced asthma. *Clin Exp Allergy* 1999; 29(10): 1395–401
77 Lemiere C, Romeo P, Chaboillez S, Tremblay C, Malo JL. Airway inflammation and functional changes after exposure to different concentrations of isocyanates. *J Allergy Clin Immunol* 2002; 110(4): 641–6
78 Bello D, Herrick CA, Smith TJ, Woskie SR, Streicher RP, Cullen MR et al. Skin exposure to isocyanates: Reasons for concern. *Environ Health Perspect* 2007; 115(3): 328–35
79 Redlich CA, Herrick CA. Lung/skin connections in occupational lung disease. *Curr Opin Allergy Clin Immunol* 2008; 8(2): 115–9
80 Petsonk EL, Wang ML, Lewis DM, Siegel PD, Husberg BJ. Asthma-like symptoms in

wood product plant workers exposed to methylene diphenyl diisocyanate. *Chest* 2000; 118(4): 1183–93

81 Pronk A, Yu F, Vlaanderen J, Tielemans E, Preller L, Bobeldijk I et al. Dermal, inhalation, and internal exposure to 1,6–HDI and its oligomers in car body repair shop workers and industrial spray painters. *Occup Environ Med* 2006; 63(9): 624–31

82 Bello D, Redlich CA, Stowe MH, Sparer J, Woskie SR, Streicher RP et al. Skin exposure to aliphatic polyisocyanates in the auto body repair and refinishing industry: II. A quantitative assessment. *Ann Occup Hyg* 2008; 52(2): 117–24

83 Liu Y, Stowe MH, Bello D, Sparer J, Gore RJ, Cullen MR et al. Skin exposure to aliphatic polyisocyanates in the auto body repair and refinishing industry: III. A personal exposure algorithm. *Ann Occup Hyg* 2009; 53(1): 33–40

84 Mapp CE, Boschetto P, Maestrelli P, Fabbri LM. Occupational asthma. *Am J Respir Crit Care Med* 2005; 172(3): 280–305

85 Son M, Lee M, Kim YT, Youn JK, Park H. Heterogeneity of IgE response to TDI-HSA conjugates by ELISA in toluene diisocyanate (TDI)-induced occupational asthma (OA) patients. *J Korean Med Sci* 1998; 13(2): 147–52

86 Pronk A, Preller L, Raulf-Heimsoth M, Jonkers IC, Lammers JW, Wouters IM et al. Respiratory symptoms, sensitization, and exposure response relationships in spray painters exposed to isocyanates. *Am J Respir Crit Care Med* 2007; 176(11): 1090–7

87 Morris JB, Wilkie WS, Shusterman DJ. Acute respiratory responses of the mouse to chlorine. *Toxicol Sci* 2005; 83(2): 380–7

88 Martin JG, Campbell HR, Iijima H, Gautrin D, Malo JL, Eidelman DH et al. Chlorine-induced injury to the airways in mice. *Am J Respir Crit Care Med* 2003; 168(5): 568–74

89 Koohsari H, Tamaoka M, Campbell HR, Martin JG. The role of gamma delta T cells in airway epithelial injury and bronchial responsiveness after chlorine gas exposure in mice. *Respir Res* 2007; 8: 21

90 Tuck SA, Ramos-Barbon D, Campbell H, McGovern T, Karmouty-Quintana H, Martin JG. Time course of airway remodelling after an acute chlorine gas exposure in mice. *Respir Res* 2008; 9: 61

91 Guo Y, Krumwiede M, White JG, Wangensteen OD. HOCl effects on the tight junctions of rabbit tracheal epithelium. *Am J Physiol* 1996; 270(2 Pt 1): L224–L231

92 Venglarik CJ, Giron-Calle J, Wigley AF, Malle E, Watanabe N, Forman HJ. Hypochlorous acid alters bronchial epithelial cell membrane properties and prevention by extracellular glutathione. *J Appl Physiol* 2003; 95(6): 2444–52

93 Pichavant M, Goya S, Meyer EH, Johnston RA, Kim HY, Matangkasombut P et al. Ozone exposure in a mouse model induces airway hyperreactivity that requires the presence of natural killer T cells and IL-17. *J Exp Med* 2008; 205(2): 385–93

94 Kierstein S, Krytska K, Sharma S, Amrani Y, Salmon M, Panettieri RA, Jr. et al. Ozone inhalation induces exacerbation of eosinophilic airway inflammation and hyperresponsiveness in allergen-sensitized mice. *Allergy* 2008; 63(4): 438–46

95 Samuelsen M, Nygaard UC, Lovik M. Allergy adjuvant effect of particles from wood smoke and road traffic. *Toxicology* 2008; 246(2–3): 124–31
96 Liu J, Ballaney M, Al-alem U, Quan C, Jin X, Perera F et al. Combined inhaled diesel exhaust particles and allergen exposure alter methylation of T helper genes and IgE production *in vivo*. *Toxicol Sci* 2008; 102(1): 76–81
97 Trimble NJ, Botelho FM, Bauer CM, Fattouh R, Stampfli MR. Adjuvant and anti-inflammatory properties of cigarette smoke in murine allergic airway inflammation. *Am J Respir Cell Mol Biol* 2009; 40(1): 38–46
98 Robays LJ, Lanckacker EA, Moerloose KB, Maes T, Bracke KR, Brusselle GG et al. Concomitant inhalation of cigarette smoke and aerosolized protein activates airway dendritic cells and induces allergic airway inflammation in a TLR-independent way. *J Immunol* 2009; 183(4): 2758–66
99 Bessac BF, Jordt SE. Breathtaking TRP channels: TRPA1 and TRPV1 in airway chemosensation and reflex control. *Physiology (Bethesda)* 2008; 23: 360–70
100 Nassenstein C, Kwong K, Taylor-Clark T, Kollarik M, Macglashan DM, Braun A et al. Expression and function of the ion channel TRPA1 in vagal afferent nerves innervating mouse lungs. *J Physiol* 2008; 586(6): 1595–604
101 Caterina MJ, Leffler A, Malmberg AB, Martin WJ, Trafton J, Petersen-Zeitz KR et al. Impaired nociception and pain sensation in mice lacking the capsaicin receptor. *Science* 2000; 288(5464): 306–13
102 Bautista DM, Jordt SE, Nikai T, Tsuruda PR, Read AJ, Poblete J et al. TRPA1 mediates the inflammatory actions of environmental irritants and proalgesic agents. *Cell* 2006; 124(6): 1269–82
103 Jordt SE, Bautista DM, Chuang HH, McKemy DD, Zygmunt PM, Hogestatt ED et al. Mustard oils and cannabinoids excite sensory nerve fibres through the TRP channel ANKTM1. *Nature* 2004; 427(6971): 260–5
104 Bessac BF, Sivula M, von Hehn CA, Caceres AI, Escalera J, Jordt SE. Transient receptor potential ankyrin 1 antagonists block the noxious effects of toxic industrial isocyanates and tear gases. *FASEB J* 2009; 23(4): 1102–14
105 Taylor-Clark TE, Kiros F, Carr MJ, McAlexander MA. Transient receptor potential ankyrin 1 mediates toluene diisocyanate-evoked respiratory irritation. *Am J Respir Cell Mol Biol* 2009; 40(6): 756–62
106 Bessac BF, Sivula M, von Hehn CA, Escalera J, Cohn L, Jordt SE. TRPA1 is a major oxidant sensor in murine airway sensory neurons. *J Clin Invest* 2008; 118(5): 1899–910
107 Caceres AI, Brackmann M, Elia MD, Bessac BF, del CD, D'Amours M et al. A sensory neuronal ion channel essential for airway inflammation and hyperreactivity in asthma. *Proc Natl Acad Sci USA* 2009; 106(22): 9099–104
108 Grabbe S, Schwarz T. Immunoregulatory mechanisms involved in elicitation of allergic contact hypersensitivity. *Immunol Today* 1998; 19(1): 37–44
109 Novak N, Allam JP, Betten H, Haberstok J, Bieber T. The role of antigen presenting cells at distinct anatomic sites: They accelerate and they slow down allergies. *Allergy* 2004; 59(1): 5–14

110 Wisnewski AV, Liu Q, Miller JJ, Magoski N, Redlich CA. Effects of hexamethylene diisocyanate exposure on human airway epithelial cells: *In vitro* cellular and molecular studies. *Environ Health Perspect* 2002; 110(9): 901–7
111 Liu Q, Wisnewski AV. Recent developments in diisocyanate asthma. *Ann Allergy Asthma Immunol* 2003; 90(5 Suppl 2): 35–41

Asthma-like diseases in agriculture

Torben Sigsgaard[1], *Øyvind Omland*[1,2] *and Peter S. Thorne*[3]

[1]School of Public Health, Department of Environmental and Occupational Medicine, Aarhus University, Denmark
[2]Department of Occupational and Environmental Medicine Aalborg, Aarhus University Hospital, Denmark
[3]Environmental Health Sciences Research Center, University of Iowa, Iowa City, USA

Abstract

Although many studies on asthma have been conducted in farming populations, no longitudinal studies have been published so far. Smoking, work in pig barns, and crop farming together with exposure to endotoxin and quaternary ammonium have been described as environmental risk factors for self-reported asthma and/or wheeze in cross-sectional studies. The prevalence of self-reported asthma has been found to range from 0.7% in female greenhouse workers to 21% in Danish smoking female farming students. Exposure in farming is diverse, but dominated by organic dust containing high amounts of compounds known to trigger the innate immune system. This is confirmed by a wide range of human experimentation where naïve persons have been introduced to swine confinements. Cross-sectional data suggest a protective effect of farming on allergy. However, differences in the diagnostic procedure and the predominantly wheezy asthma type in farming concomitant with a lower rate of allergic asthma makes the comparison difficult. Furthermore, healthy worker selection, misclassification, age differences, difference in time of study and small study populations, resulting in low statistical power, might be factors explaining the findings. Well-designed longitudinal studies of the incidence of carefully defined phenotypes of asthma and risk factors are needed to clarify the risk of asthma, or wheezy phenotypes related to farming.

Introduction

Agricultural work represents a major hazard for respiratory disease. Both asthma and chronic obstructive pulmonary disease (COPD) have been reported related to farming [1, 2]. While farm workers have inhalation exposures to pesticides, diesel particulates and toxic vapors, the major exposure is organic dust composed of mould hyphal fragments and spores, bacteria, endotoxins, glucans, mite allergens, animal-derived material like dander, hair, bristle, urine, and feces together with animal feeds. The vast majority of studies of asthma in agriculture have been performed without agent-specific exposure assessment, and only a few studies have included exposure assessment as part of the design.

Occupational Asthma, edited by Torben Sigsgaard and Dick Heederik

Respiratory symptoms in agriculture

Prevalent work-related lung symptoms in farming are wheeze, cough, and dyspnea, and these are often much more frequent than among control subjects or among random population samples [3–6]. However, these symptoms are nonspecific and might reflect acute lung irritation as well as symptoms associated with respiratory disease. The clinical picture of obstructive lung diseases in agriculture is diverse with major symptoms of asthma, COPD (or both), bronchial hyperresponsiveness and increased yearly loss in FEV_1 associated with few or any respiratory symptoms. The designation of asthma-like syndrome in agriculture has been introduced from studies mainly in the U.S. of highly exposed swine confinement workers [6, 7]. However, farming is probably one of the exposure situations with the most diverse range of asthma phenotypes [8], ranging from clearly IgE-dependent asthma with eosinophilic influx related to allergen exposure (e.g., enzymes or cow dander or horse hair) to non-IgE-dependent asthma dominated by neutrophilic influx and wheezing [9]. The neutrophilic phenotype is characterized by a self-limited inflammatory event that might or might not involve persistent airway hyperresponsiveness [10]. The end stage presents as respiratory symptoms, bronchial hyperresponsiveness, and accelerated lung function decline in the absence of sensitization against swine feed and food allergens [10].

These features have been confounding research into asthma in farming, and only recently has the discussion of asthma phenotypes been addressed by the scientific community [11–13].

Studies of asthma-like symptoms in agriculture

In this chapter we apply the term "asthma-like diseases" as a questionnaire-defined outcome of "asthma" or "asthma-like symptoms" in epidemiological studies in agriculture. No longitudinal studies on incidence of asthma in farming populations have been published and rates of asthma incidence associated with farming are based on data from surveillance systems for occupational diseases including asthma. These systems are mainly made for insurance and compensation purposes for the workforce [14]. In the available data sources there are differences in the definition of occupational asthma (OA) between countries and heterogeneity in classification of occupation. Some surveillance programs are without information as to whether farming is classified as an occupation. Due to weakness in coverage and case ascertainment there might, therefore, be a general tendency in underreporting of asthma in farming. From those surveillance systems in which data from farming occupation are present, the incidence figures from Finland [14] are by far the highest. The mean annual incidence rate was 174 cases/10^6 employed workers and the mean annual incidence rate for male farmers was 1200 and for female farmers 1910. These high figures in the farming population are probably due to the custom in the Finnish farming to brush their cows daily. Data from Germany [15] arise from the worker compensation system. The annual mean incidence rate was 51 cases/10^6 employed workers, and in farmers the figure was 113 cases/10^6 employed workers. Swedish surveillance data are based on self-reported asthma and here the mean annual incidence rate was 80 cases /10^6 employed workers, while in male farmers and in female farmers it was 170 and 203 cases/10^6 employed workers, respectively [16]. By far the lowest data on incidence of OA has been reported from USA, the state of Michigan [17]. These data arise from physicians' reports, compensation claims and hospitals. The annual mean incidence rate was 30 cases/10^6 employed workers and in agricultural production the figure was 3 cases/10^6 employed workers.

More than 30 cross-sectional studies of the prevalence of asthma-like symptoms in agriculture have been published, and in 18 the prevalence data have been related to the prevalence in a non-exposed control group (Tab. 1) or associated with the prevalence in the general population or a random sample of the general population (Tab. 2).

The mean prevalence of asthma in a representative sample of 1685 Danish farmers [3] was 7.7%, lowest (3.6%) among farmers aged 30–49 and highest (11.8%) among farmers aged 50–69 years. The prevalence of asthma was highest among pig farmers (10.9%). Age (OR 5.8, 95% CI 2.8–12.2) and pig farming (OR 2.0, 95% CI 2.0–3.5) were risk factors for self-reported asthma. The prevalence of asthma among farmers was the same as in a representative sample of the Danish populations aged 30–49 years, but significantly higher among farmers aged 50–69 years (OR 2.25, $p<0.001$). The prevalence of current asthma in 1706 farmers from New Zealand [18] was high (11.8%), although lower than the prevalence of asthma measured in the general population (15%). Female farmers had an increased risk for asthma (OR 1.8, 95% CI 1.3–2.5). High prevalence of asthma (18.3%) was also found among 904 randomly selected Swiss farmers [19], but no difference was observed in the prevalence of asthma attack between farmers (2.1%) and a random sample of the Swiss population (3.1%). Current (OR 2.14, 95% CI 1.43–3.19) and former smoking (OR 2.05, 95% CI 1.34–3.14) were risk factors for asthma. The prevalence of asthma was 2.8% (95% CI 2.4–3.2) in a random sample of 7496 European farmers from Denmark, Northern Germany, Switzerland and Spain [20]. In an American rural population, farmers had an asthma prevalence of 9.8% in females and 3.8% in males: the OR for 'ever farmed' *versus* 'never farmed' was 0.77 (95% CI 0.48–1.24) [21]. The prevalence of asthma among the farmers aged 20–44 years (1.3%, 95% CI 0.9–1.7) was significantly lower than in an age-matched sample of the general European population (ECRHS) (3.2%, 95% CI 2.9–3.9; $p=0.001$). In Norway [22] the asthma prevalence among a random sample of 2106 farmers was 4.0%, significantly lower than among a random sample of 351 rural (5.7%) and 727 urban (7.6%) controls. Recent data from The Netherlands [23] have found a significantly lower

Table 1. Cross-sectional studies of the prevalence of asthma-like symptoms in agriculture and in the general population.

Ref.	Year	Country	No. of subjects	Asthma prevalence among farmers	Prevalence in agriculture vs general population	Environmental risk factors
[3]	1988	Denmark	1685	7.7 11.8 age 50–69 3.6 age 30–49	↑ subjects aged 50–69 OR 2.25 N.D. for aged 30–49	Pig farming OR 2.0
[18]	1999	New Zealand	1706	11.8	N.D.	Female OR 1.8
[19]	2001	Switzerland	904	18.3	N.D.	Smoking OR 2.1
[20]	2001	Denmark, Germany, Sweden, Spain	7496	1.3	Sign lower than controls	
[21]	2002	USA	574+1056	3.8 males 9.5 females	Lower for males N.D. for females	Smoking OR 1.1
[22]	2004	Norway	2106+1078s	4.0	Sign lower than controls, both atopic and non-atopic	
[23]	2007	Netherlands	1205 conv. 593 organic 2679s	5.2 conv. 2.9 organic	Sign. Lower than controls	

s, sample of the general population; conv., conventional farmers; organic, organic farmers; N.D., no difference.

Table 2. Cross-sectional studies of the prevalence of asthma-like symptoms in agriculture and in controls.

Ref.	Year	Country	No. of subjects	Asthma prevalence	Prevalence in agriculture vs controls	Environmental risk factors
[24]	1997	DK	1691 + 407c	Smo 11.3/13.2 Non sm 5.3/5.9	N.D.	Smoking sign ↑
[25]	1999	DK	1901 + 407c	5.4–21.0	N.D.	Smoking OR 1.7
[26]	2001	Croatia	236 + 165c	0.7–7.7	N.D.	
[27]	2001	Croatia	814 + 635c	0.7–7.7	N.D.	
[28]	1999	NL	239 + 311c	5.9	N.D.	Quaternary ammonium OR 9.4
[29]	1998	Fr	265 + 149c	5.3	N.D.	
[30]	1993	Croatia	167 + 81c	0.7–6.3	N.D.	
[31]	1998	South Africa	134 + 122c	4–13	Sign. higher	
[32]	2005	Gr	122 + 100c	6.7	N.D.	
[33]	2005	US	1140 + 10132c	7.73	Sign. higher	Farming OR 1.54
[34]	2007	NZ	4288 + 1328c	14.3–15.6	Sign. lower	

c, controls; Sign., significantly; N.D., no difference.

prevalence of asthma-like symptoms among both conventional farmer (5.2%) and organic farmers (3.9%) compared a random sample of the general population (7.6%).

In a Danish study of 1901 farming students, of whom 210 were females, and in 407 rural controls the prevalence of asthma-like symptoms was between 5.4% and 21%, but no difference was observed between farming students and controls [25]. Asthma in the mother (OR 3.4, 95% CI 2.1–5.7), sex [OR (males) 0.5, 95% CI 0.3–0.8], and smoking (OR 1.7, 95% CI 1.2–2.4) were factors significantly associated with asthma. Data of the prevalence of OA from two studies in farm workers in Croatia [26, 27] showed no differences (0–7.7%) among the 236 livestock and the 814 crop farm workers and food packing controls, for either smokers or non smokers. Vogelzang et al. [35] found in a study of 239 pig farmers and 311 rural controls the same prevalence of asthma in the two groups (5.9%) *versus* (5.5%). In pig farmers the use of disinfectants (quaternary ammonium compounds) (OR 9.4, 95% CI 1.6–57.2) and aspects of disinfecting procedure were associated with the prevalence of asthma. Atopy was significantly less prevalent in pig farmers (4.6%) compared to controls (14.6%) and pig farmers had significantly fewer symptoms of allergy in childhood (9.9%) than controls (17.2%). Atopy in childhood was strongly associated with the prevalence of asthma symptoms (OR 4.1, 95% CI 2.2–7.7). Cross-sectional data from a French study of 265 dairy farmers and 149 non-exposed controls [29] revealed the same cumulative prevalence of self-reported asthma and of current asthma in farmers and in controls; 5.3% and 1.5%, respectively, *versus* 3.4% and 1.3%. Prevalence data of asthma in non-animal farming occupation has been analyzed among 135 female and 32 male greenhouse workers [30]. No significant increase in the prevalence of asthma was observed compared to non-exposed 51 female and 30 male controls, either for males (6.3% vs 0%) or for females (0.7% vs 0%). Among 134 South African poultry workers, the prevalence of asthma was significantly higher (4–11%) than among 122 controls [31], while the prevalence of asthma was elevated but not significantly higher (6.7%) among 120 grape farmers from Crete compared to 100 controls (2.0%) [32]. Among 1140 male New York dairy farmers [33], the prevalence of asthma was 7.73% and significantly higher than among 10 132 male non-farmers (5.03%). New Zealand data involving 4288 farmers and 1328 controls found a significantly lower prevalence of "asthma ever" among dairy farmers (14.8%) and sheep and beef farmers (15.6%) compared to non-farming controls (23.3%) [18].

Exposures in agriculture

Exposures in agriculture are varied and dependent upon whether the operation is producing row crops, livestock or fruits, nuts and vegetables. Common exposures may include diesel exhaust, fuel vapors, pesticides and disinfectants, and welding fumes. Crop production generally includes exposures to fertilizers such as anhydrous ammonia, while livestock production usually is associated with exposures to hydrogen sulfide, ammonia, and a multitude of odorous sulfur- and nitrogen-containing vapors [36]. Among the most potent odorous compounds are the organic acids, including acetic, butyric, caproic, propionic, and valeric acids; nitrogen-containing compounds such as ammonia, methyl amines, methyl pyrazines, skatoles and indoles; and sulfur-containing compounds such as hydrogen sulfide and dimethyl sulfide [37]. These odors smell like rotten eggs (hydrogen sulfide, dimethyl sulfide) or rancid butter (butyric acid, isobutyric acid) or have a putrid-fecal smell (indole, skatole, valeric and isovaleric acid).

Organic dust is a catchall term for the array of bioaerosols that arise in agriculture and downstream manufacturing that produces value-added food products, animal feed, seeds, ethanol, biomass, and compost. Toxicologically important components of organic dust include pathogenic microorganisms; microbial, plant and animal allergens; and microbial-associated molecular patterns (MAMPs) including endotoxin, β-glucans, and CpG DNA (Fig. 1).

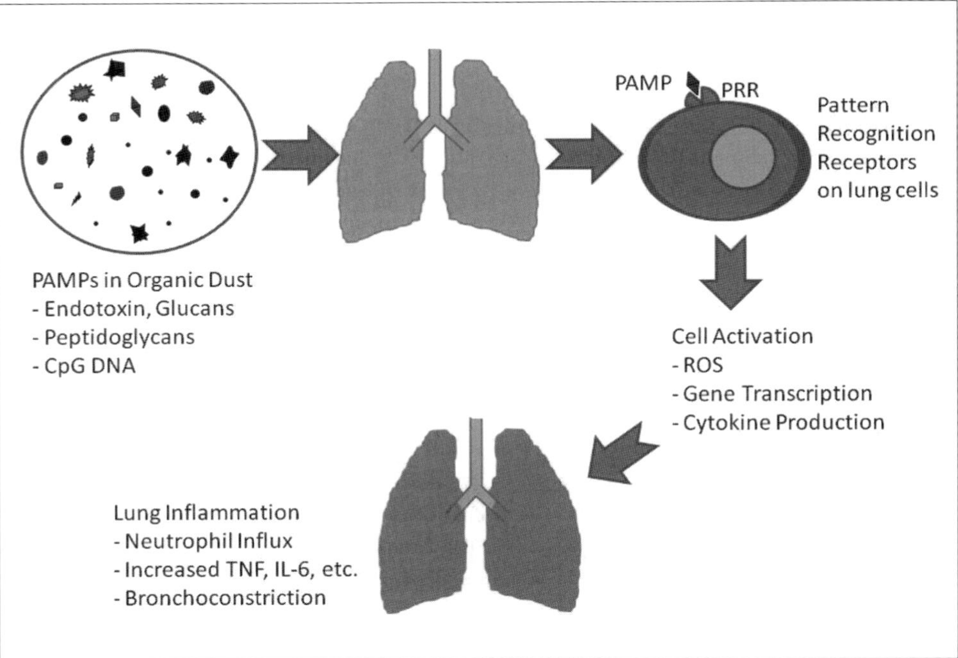

Figure 1.
The role of pathogen-associated molecular patterns (MAMPs) and pattern recognition receptors in organic dust exposure.

Pathogenic bioaerosols from livestock facilities are responsible for cases of infectious disease that extend beyond zoonoses typically seen only among farmers and veterinarians. The use of antimicrobials as growth promotants in livestock production has led to increased antimicrobial resistance of bacteria in swine and calf barn effluents to medically important antibiotics. In the U.S. over 300 scientific, medical, and advocacy organizations have called for legislation to eliminate the non-therapeutic use of antimicrobial agents (Pew Commission on Industrial Farm Animal Production 2008). Methicillin-resistant *Staphylococcus aureus* (MRSA) is an emerging concern that has been linked to excessive use of antibiotics [38]. Multidrug-resistant culturable bacteria were measured in bioaerosols 150 m downwind of a swine operation with the finding that over 80% of the organisms were resistant to two or more classes of antibiotics [39]. Another infectious disease concern is that conditions inside industrialized livestock facilities will give rise to a pandemic strain of influenza [40]. Past outbreaks in Asia and recent cases in Southern California demonstrate the significance of this threat (CDC 2009). The two cases of infection with swine influenza A (H1N1) virus in the San Diego area occurred in unrelated children living in adjacent counties neither of whom had contact with pigs. The influenza virus they carried was resistant to two antiviral agents used to treat flu and contained gene segments that had not previously been observed in humans or swine. It is presumed that they both contracted influenza *via* human-to-human transmission.

Allergenic components of organic dust include thermophilic bacteria such as *Saccharopolyspora rectivirgula* and *Thermoactinomyces vulgaris* that are responsible for allergic alveolitis (also called hypersensitivity pneumonitis). Grain storage mites, animal danders, plant pollens, enzymes and possibly antibiotics added to animal feed can act as allergens, leading to allergic rhinitis and allergic asthma in some workers.

The constituents of organic dust posing the greatest health burden are arguably the MAMPs of which endotoxin has been studied the most. Endotoxin is an amphiphilic molecule of bacterial cell walls that induces innate immune responses in an amplifying cascade [41], leading to recruitment of neutrophils and macrophages to the lung. Endotoxin exposures in agriculture have been extensively studied and representative exposure data are presented in Table 3.

In recent work, Spaan et al. [42] have carefully evaluated methods for analyzing endotoxin with an eye toward recommending a fully specified standard method. Identical inhalable dust samples were collected to investigate the effects of filter type (glass fiber or Teflon), transport conditions (with/without desiccant), sample storage (–20° or 4°C), extraction solution [pyrogen-free water (PFW) or PFW plus 0.05% Tween 20], extract storage (–20° or 4°C), and assay solution (PFW or PFW plus 0.05% Tween 20) on endotoxin concentration [42]. No differences in endotoxin concentration were attributable to transport conditions or storage temperature of extracts. Extraction in PFW plus 0.05% Tween 20 resulted in 2.1-fold higher estimated endotoxin concentrations. Sampling on glass-fiber filters and storage of sam-

Table 3. Airborne endotoxin exposure values in agricultural operations.

Operation	Air sample	No. of samples	GM endotoxin concentration, EU/m^3	Reference
Livestock operations				
Dairy	Personal – inhalable Area – respirable	194 216	64 17	Kullman et al. 1998 [98]
Swine	Personal – inhalable	350	920	Preller et al. 1995 [99]
Swine	Area – total	81	8290	Thorne et al.1997 [100]
Swine	Area – total	21	3927	Duchaine et al. 2001 [101]
Swine conventional confinements Swine hoop barns	Area – inhalable	40 30	3100 3250	Thorne et al. 2009 [100]
Poultry	Area – total	81	1340	Thorne et al. 1997 [102]
Chicken Dairy Cattle feedlot Horse Swine Turkey	Area – inhalable	200 81 120 118 198 191	5000 35 150 1000 9000 2000	Saito et al. 2009 [44]
Other agriculture				
Animal feed manufacturers	Personal – inhalable Area – inhalable	530 79	12–285 19	Smid et al. 1992 [103]
Grain elevators	Personal – total Personal – respirable	410 410	2860 83.2	Schwartz et al. 1995 [104]
Potato processing	Personal – inhalable Area – inhalable	195 68	9–102 1–000	Zock et al. 1998 [105]
Soybean harvesting (closed tractors)	Personal – total	32	56	Roy & Thorne, 2003 [106]
Agricultural seed processing industry	Personal – inhalable	100	1800	Smit et al. 2006 [107]

GM, geometric mean.

ples in the freezer produced 1.3-fold and 1.1-fold higher endotoxin concentrations, respectively. This study found that there were important gaps in the specification of the CEN protocol and suggested parameters needed to fully specify a standardized protocol. In a second manuscript, Spaan et al. [43] compared four extraction media: PFW, PFW-Tween 20, PFW-Tris, and PFW-triethylamine-phosphate (TAP) to determine which performed best in the LAL assay and extracted the most endotoxin. PFW-Tris produced similar results to the PFW alone. PFW-TAP showed lower yields and a deviant calibration curve. Tween in the extraction medium resulted in significantly higher endotoxin yields from all dust types, independent of the effect of Tween in the assay. Among these four media, only Tween reproducibly enhanced the efficiency of endotoxin extraction from airborne dust samples.

A recent study evaluated endotoxin exposure assessment in six types of livestock operations using four types of air samplers in two regions of the U.S. [44]. This study demonstrated excellent agreement in 906 samples between analysis of endotoxin using the kinetic chromogenic LAL assay and the recombinant factor C assay with a correlation coefficient of $r=0.91$ ($p<0.01$) and the relationship overlaying the line of identity.

The other MAMP for which there has been exposure assessment in agriculture, albeit limited, is fungal β-glucans. These polysaccharide components of fungal cell walls can be measured using the Factor G pathway of the LAL assay [45] or by single-antibody ELISA [46, 47] or sandwich ELISA [48, 49]. Most studies that have measured glucans were focused on mold exposures in the indoor environment.

Human experiments

The first systematic studies of farming responses in humans were performed at the University of Iowa using extracts of corn dust (CDE) and LPS [50–53]. This research initiated the human experimental approach to the basic mechanism of the innate immune system on acute respiratory inflammation. The results showed that neutrophils increased in nasal lavage from 17×10^3 to 40×10^3 cells/ml in grain workers exposed to 2372 EU LPS/m^3 compared to postal workers exposed to 4 EU/m^3. However, no association was found to the LPS concentration among grain workers [52]. A study with an inhalation of aerosolized CDE confirmed the inflammation related to CDE. This initiated a series of experiments on the kinetics of the human and the mouse reaction to CDE. The response in humans was shown to start immediately after inhalation and last 2 days for bronchoconstriction, 4 days for neutrophilic influx, and 7 days for the increase in proinflammatory cytokines IL-1β IL-6 and IL-8. These changes were mirrored in the mouse model, although within a shorter period, leading to the conclusion that the mouse model would be an appropriate model to study grain dust-induced inflammation [53]. No increase in the reaction was found in atopic subjects compared to non-atopic subjects. In a study of grain workers with bronchial hyperresponsiveness (BHR), it was shown that those workers with BHR had a greater decline in FEV_1 compared to "normal" workers. Surprisingly, this was not reflected in any differences in the bronchoalveolar lavage (BAL) fluid sampled 4 h after the exposure to 0.16 μg/kg nebulized endotoxin in CDE [52].

Swine

In farming, the first studies to suggest that LPS is the causative agent were from the Sweden and the Netherlands, and showed that endotoxin exposure was related to symptoms and FEV_1 in pig farmers [54, 55]. These initial studies have been followed by a range of quasi experiments in which the farming environment has been used to study the effect of the innate immune system. A group from Stockholm has been especially active in this field. Their work has elucidated the time course of the inflammatory events occurring after an acute exposure to organic dust [56–61]. In one study, this group showed that the acute changes they had observed in non-farmers were attenuated or totally abolished in healthy farmers adapted to the environment, and speculated on which mechanisms might be responsible for such an adaptive mechanism [62].

In a study of farmers experiencing asthma-like symptoms during work in swine confinement buildings and controls, it was shown that inflammatory responses in a work-like environment with low concentrations of LPS (0.5 μg/m3) and dust (4 mg/m^3) are similar to responses found after exposure to higher concentrations often used in experimental situations. Acute neutrophilic inflammatory responses and increases in BAL IL-6 and IL-8 were found; however, this response was attenuated among farmers who had already experienced asthma-like symptoms during exposure in swine confinement buildings [63]. In the same experiment, differences in complement response were found that may compensate for variation in the inflammatory response [64].

Laboratory animal-exposure studies

Inhalation experiments using guinea pigs, rats and mice have been extremely informative for identifying inflammatory agents in organic dust, establishing their potency and elucidating their mechanistic underpinnings. Studies in the 1980s in guinea pigs investigated the pulmonary effects of cotton dust and demonstrated that the effects on breathing patterns and production of fever were due to the endotoxin content. In more recent work, mice have been the animal model of choice due to the availability of inbred strains and knockout mice with specific characteristics or gene deletions [65]. Murine studies in the 1990s demonstrated that endotoxin was the principal inflammatory agent in extracts of organic dust recovered from the air handling system of grain elevators handling corn (CDE). Inhalation-exposed mice developed a dose-dependent influx of monocytes and neutrophils to the lung and increases in TNF-α and IL-6 [36, 53, 66]. C3H/Hej mice bearing a mutation in the TLR4 gene exhibited a blunted response to a semi-purified endotoxin preparation [67] with a 1000-fold lower neutrophilic response than C3HeBFej normoresponsive mice [68].

Endotoxin exposure studies in mice of different strains have demonstrated a wide range of inflammatory responsiveness [69]. Among inbred strains without recognized genetic defects in endotoxin response genes, there was a 3-fold range of neutrophilic response between the least responsive to the strongest responder. Among mutant strains there was a 50-fold range. These studies used the Sigma *E. coli* 0111:B4 preparation of endotoxin which is believed to contain other MAMPs.

Recent murine studies [41], informed by previous *in vitro* studies [70–72], have shown that responsiveness to highly purified endotoxin requires functional CD14, MD-2 and TLR4 [41]. MD-2 knockout mice do not mount an inflammatory response when exposed to purified endotoxin, but the response can be reconstituted if the same amount of endotoxin is delivered to the lung as a monomeric complex of endotoxin and recombinant MD-2 [41]. Lung exposure to mutant penta-acylated endotoxin produces a blunted inflammatory response as compared with treatment with wild-type, hexa-acylated endotoxin. Treatment of CD14 knockout mice with endotoxin is also blunted but can be restored by treating with endotoxin:MD-2 complex.

Simultaneous exposures to endotoxin and allergens in lab animals have produced conflicting results. Studies using ovalbumin as the allergen found that concomitant endotoxin exposure suppressed the development of allergy [73, 74], while studies that used environmental allergens such as *Aspergillus flavus*, cat dander or cockroach allergen observed amplification of antibody production and pulmonary hypersensitivity [75–77]. In a neonatal exposure model, mice inhaling endotoxin (300 EU/day) and cockroach allergen (10 ng/day) on days 2–21 of life demonstrated increased pulmonary inflammation, increased total and specific IgE production, and lung remodeling compared to mice that inhaled endotoxin alone or allergen alone [77]. The inflammatory response measured in lung lavage fluid was marked by an influx of neutrophils and cytokines (TNF-α, IL-6, MIP-1α, KC, RANTES, G-CSF, and IL-12p40) that were 4–18-fold higher than observed in the mice treated with endotoxin only. These data illustrate that the complex mixtures we encounter in complex settings such as agricultural environments can be synergistic, and therefore need to be studied as mixtures rather than one compound at a time.

The modification of disease by farming exposure

It has been known for some time that being brought up at a farm decreases the allergic manifestations among the children concomitantly with an increased risk of wheezing among the children associated to high concentrations of endotoxin [78–80], with an effect still detectable during young adulthood [81]. Recently, it has been shown that this effect is still observable even later in adulthood. Studies in a rural community in Norway [82] have shown that farmers have a lower prevalence of atopic diseases including asthma. However, they have a higher prevalence of inflammatory wheeze associated with endotoxin exposure.

Studies of agricultural workers from New Zealand [83] and The Netherlands [23, 84] have demonstrated that being brought up on a farm has a bearing on the subsequent reaction to agricultural exposures. This was most clearly demonstrated in a recent study of Dutch agricultural workers, where Smit et al. [84] showed that the place of upbringing was an effect modifier for the association between wheeze and endotoxin exposure (Fig. 2).

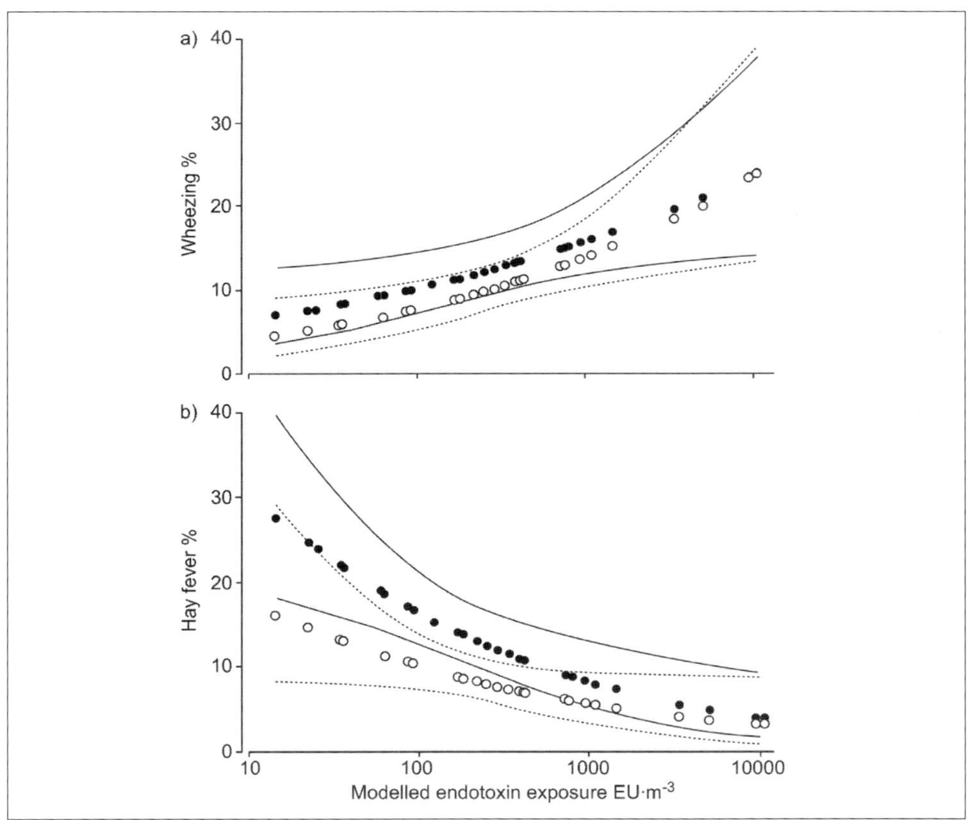

Figure 2.
The association between hay fever, wheezing prevalence and endotoxin exposure stratified for place of upbringing. From [84].

Susceptibility factors

There is a great variability in the individual response to organic dusts. Almost 50% of Caucasians respond to LPS exposure [85], and people with α-1-antitrypsin deficiency are hyperresponsive to organic dust exposure [86, 87].

Atopy has been proposed as one of the factors associated with increased susceptibility to organic dusts. The evidence is scarce; however, people with mild asthma or with BHR do have an increased reactivity towards LPS exposure [88, 89] and garbage workers with OA of the neutrophil type are not able to recruit PMNs in the nose as readily as workers without OA after nasal installation of LPS [90]. Furthermore, atopic subjects seem to react differently to LPS in the whole blood assay [91].

A few studies have shown α-1-antitrypsin to be a risk factor for respiratory symptoms among workers exposed to organic dusts such as cotton dust and grain dust [86, 92]. CD14 polymorphisms have been studied as a risk factor for OA; however, the data are conflicting regarding the possible effect of such polymorphisms, which might relate to differences in the techniques used for LPS analysis or to different study designs. The first polymorphism related to LPS susceptibility was demonstrated in a study by Arbour et al. [93] who found that a few co-segregating mutations in the TLR4 gene were responsible for LPS hyporesponsiveness in humans. The allele frequency was around 8% in the Iowa population, and, hence, it cannot explain the high number of non-responders reported by Castellan et al. [85] in the cotton-exposure study. TLR4 polymorphisms have not been associated with asthma in studies of populations [94], and it has not been possible to demonstrate any association with the protective effect on atopy that is seen among farmers' children [95]. TLR4 is one factor in a complex and long response pathway, which may accumulate mutations in other components of the pathway [96].

In Germany, a study of atopy among children from farms and non-farms has demonstrated that the protective effect of being raised on a farm was abolished if the children had a mutation in the TLR2 gene. Although TLR2 was previously thought to play a role in LPS recognition, other receptors like β-glucans and peptidoglycans are now considered as candidates for agents responsible for the protection against atopy, such as that observed among the farmers' children [95].

Very recently, a polymorphism in TLR10 has been shown to be a risk factor for asthma, consistent within different samples of the American population. Whether this will have any implications for persons exposed to organic dust is presently unknown, since the ligand for TLR10 is not known [97].

References

1 Monso E, Schenker M, Radon K, Riu E, Magarolas R, McCurdy S et al. Region-related risk factors for respiratory symptoms in European and Californian farmers. *Eur Respir J* 2003; 21(2): 323–331

2 Monso E, Riu E, Radon K, Magarolas R, Danuser B, Iversen M et al. Chronic obstructive pulmonary disease in never-smoking animal farmers working inside confinement buildings. *Am J Ind Med* 2004; 46(4): 357–362

3 Iversen M, Dahl R, Korsgaard J, Hallas T, Jensen EJ. Respiratory symptoms in Danish farmers: An epidemiological study of risk factors. *Thorax* 1988; 43: 872–877

4 Dalphin JC, Debieuvre D, Pernet D, Maheu MF, Polio JC, Toson B et al. Prevalence and risk factors for chronic bronchitis and farmer's lung in French dairy farmers. *Br J Ind Med* 1993; 50(10): 941–944

5 Terho EO. Work-related respiratory disorders among Finnish farmers. *Am J Ind Med* 1990; 18(3): 269–272

6 Senthilselvan A, Chenard L, Ulmer K, Gibson-Burlinguette N, Leuschen C, Dosman JA. Excess respiratory symptoms in full-time male and female workers in large-scale swine operations. *Chest* 2007; 131(4): 1197–1204

7 Von Essen SG, Scheppers LA, Robbins RA, Donham KJ. Respiratory tract inflammation in swine confinement workers studied using induced sputum and exhaled nitric oxide. *J Toxicol Clin Toxicol* 1998; 36(6): 557–565

8 Dalphin JC. [In the agricultural environment there is asthma and asthma... or the paradox of agricultural asthma]. *Rev Mal Respir* 2007; 24(9): 1083–1086

9 Tutluoglu B, Atis S, Anakkaya AN, Altug E, Tosun GA, Yaman M. Sensitization to horse hair, symptoms and lung function in grooms. *Clin Exp Allergy* 2002; 32(8): 1170–1173

10 Heederik D, Sigsgaard T. Respiratory allergy in agricultural workers: Recent developments. *Curr Opin Allergy Clin Immunol* 2005; 5(2): 129–134

11 A plea to abandon asthma as a disease concept. *Lancet* 2006; 368(9537): 705

12 Douwes J, Gibson P, Pekkanen J, Pearce N. Non-eosinophilic asthma: Importance and possible mechanisms. *Thorax* 2002; 57(7): 643–648

13 Wenzel SE. Asthma: Defining of the persistent adult phenotypes. *Lancet* 2006; 368(9537): 804–813

14 Karjalainen A, Kurppa K, Virtanen S, Keskinen H, Nordman H. Incidence of occupational asthma by occupation and industry in Finland. *Am J Ind Med* 2000; 37(5): 451–458

15 Baur X, Degens P, Weber K. Occupational obstructive airway diseases in Germany. *Am J Ind Med* 1998; 33(5): 454–462

16 Toren K. Self reported rate of occupational asthma in Sweden 1990–2. *Occup Environ Med* 1996; 53(11): 757–761

17 Rosenman KD, Reilly MJ, Kalinowski DJ. A state-based surveillance system for work-related asthma. *J Occup Environ Med* 1997; 39(5): 415–425

18 Kimbell-Dunn M, Bradshaw L, Slater T, Erkinjuntti-Pekkanen R, Fishwick D, Pearce N. Asthma and allergy in New Zealand farmers. *Am J Ind Med* 1999; 35(1): 51–57

19 Danuser B, Weber C, Kunzli N, Schindler C, Nowak D. Respiratory symptoms in Swiss farmers: An epidemiological study of risk factors. *Am J Ind Med* 2001; 39(4): 410–418

20 Radon K, Danuser B, Iversen M, Jorres R, Monso E, Opravil U et al. Respiratory symptoms in European animal farmers. *Eur Respir J* 2001; 17(4): 747–754
21 Merchant JA, Stromquist AM, Kelly KM, Zwerling C, Reynolds SJ, Burmeister L. Chronic disease and injury in an agricultural county: The Keokuk County Rural Health Cohort Study. *J Rural Health* 2002; 18: 521–535
22 Eduard W, Omenaas E, Bakke PS, Douwes J, Heederik D. Atopic and non-atopic asthma in a farming and a general population. *Am J Ind Med* 2004; 46(4): 396–399
23 Smit LA, Zuurbier M, Doekes G, Wouters IM, Heederik D, Douwes J. Hay fever and asthma symptoms in conventional and organic farmers in The Netherlands. *Occup Environ Med* 2007; 64(2): 101–107
24 Sigsgaard T, Hjort C, Omland Ø, Miller MR, Pedersen OF. Respiratory health and allergy among young farmers and non-farming rural males. *J Agromed* 1997; 4: 63–78
25 Omland O, Sigsgaard T, Hjort C, Pedersen OF, Miller MR. Lung status in young Danish rurals: The effect of farming exposure on asthma-like symptoms and lung function. *Eur Respir J* 1999; 13(1): 31–37
26 Mustajbegovic J, Zuskin E, Schachter EN, Kern J, Vrcic-Keglevic M, Vitale K et al. Respiratory findings in livestock farmworkers. *J Occup Environ Med* 2001; 43(6): 576–584
27 Kern J, Mustajbegovic J, Schachter EN, Zuskin E, Vrcic-Keglevic M, Ebling Z et al. Respiratory findings in farmworkers. *J Occup Environ Med* 2001; 43(10): 905–913
28 Vogelzang PF, van der Gulden JW, Tielen MJ, Folgering H, van Schayck CP. Health-based selection for asthma, but not for chronic bronchitis, in pig farmers: An evidence-based hypothesis. *Eur Respir J* 1999; 13(1): 187–189
29 Dalphin JC, Dubiez A, Monnet E, Gora D, Westeel V, Pernet D et al. Prevalence of asthma and respiratory symptoms in dairy farmers in the French province of the Doubs. *Am J Respir Crit Care Med* 1998; 158(5 Pt 1): 1493–1498
30 Zuskin E, Schachter EN, Mustajbegovic J. Respiratory function in greenhouse workers. *Int Arch Occup Environ Health* 1993; 64: 521–526
31 Rees D, Nelson G, Kielkowski D, Wasserfall C, da Costa A. Respiratory health and immunological profile of poultry workers. *S Afr Med J* 1998; 88(9): 1110–1117
32 Chatzi L, Prokopakis E, Tzanakis N, Alegakis A, Bizakis I, Siafakas N et al. Allergic rhinitis, asthma, and atopy among grape farmers in a rural population in Crete, Greece. *Chest* 2005; 127(1): 372–378
33 Jenkins PL, Earle-Richardson G, Bell EM, May JJ, Green A. Chronic disease risk in central New York dairy farmers: Results from a large health survey 1989–1999. *Am J Ind Med* 2005; 47(1): 20–26
34 Douwes J, Travier N, Huang K, Cheng S, McKenzie J, Le GG et al. Lifelong farm exposure may strongly reduce the risk of asthma in adults. *Allergy* 2007; 62(10): 1158–1165
35 Vogelzang PFJ, van der Gulden JWJ, Preller L, Tielen MJM, van Schayck CP, Folgering H. Bronchial hyperresponsiveness and exposure in pig farmers. *Int Arch Occup Environ Health* 1997; 70: 327–333

36 Thorne PS, Ansley AC, Perry SS. Concentrations of bioaerosols, odors, and hydrogen sulfide inside and downwind from two types of swine livestock operations. *J Occup Environ Hyg* 2009; 6(4): 211–220
37 Schiffman SS, Bennett J.L., Raymer JH. Quantification of odors and odorants from swine operatins in North Carolina. *Agric Forest Meteorol* 2001; 108: 213–240
38 Gilchrist MJ, Greko C, Wallinga DB, Beran GW, Riley DG, Thorne PS. The potential role of concentrated animal feeding operations in infectious disease epidemics and antibiotic resistance. *Environ Health Perspect* 2007; 115(2): 313–316
39 Gibbs SG, Green CF, Tarwater PM, Mota LC, Mena KD, Scarpino PV. Isolation of antibiotic-resistant bacteria from the air plume downwind of a swine confined or concentrated animal feeding operation. *Environ Health Perspect* 2006; 114(7): 1032–1037
40 Webster R, Hulse D. Controlling avian flu at the source. *Nature* 2005; 435(7041): 415–416
41 Hadina S, Weiss JP, McCray PB Jr, Kulhankova K, Thorne PS. MD-2–dependent pulmonary immune responses to inhaled lipooligosaccharides: Effect of acylation state. *Am J Respir Cell Mol Biol* 2008; 38(6): 647–654
42 Spaan S, Heederik DJ, Thorne PS, Wouters IM. Optimization of airborne endotoxin exposure assessment: Effects of filter type, transport conditions, extraction solutions, and storage of samples and extracts. *Appl Environ Microbiol* 2007; 73(19): 6134–6143
43 Spaan S, Doekes G, Heederik D, Thorne PS, Wouters IM. Effect of extraction and assay media on analysis of airborne endotoxin. *Appl Environ Microbiol* 2008; 74(12): 3804–3811
44 Saito R, Cranmer BK, Tessari JD, Larsson L, Mehaffy JM, Keefe TJ et al. Recombinant factor C (rFC) assay and gas chromatography/mass spectrometry (GC/MS) analysis of endotoxin variability in four agricultural dusts. *Ann Occup Hyg* 2009; 53(7): 713–722
45 Tamura H, Arimoto Y, Tanaka S, Yoshida M, Obayashi T, Kawai T. Automated kinetic assay for endotoxin and (1→3)-beta-D-glucan in human blood. *Clin Chim Acta* 1994; 226(1): 109–112
46 Douwes J, Doekes G, Montijn R, Heederik D, Brunekreef B. Measurement of beta(1→3)-glucans in occupational and home environments with an inhibition enzyme immunoassay. *Appl Environ Microbiol* 1996; 62(9): 3176–3182
47 Milton DK, Alwis KU, Fisette L, Muilenberg M. Enzyme-linked immunosorbent assay specific for (1→6) branched, (1→3)-beta-D-glucan detection in environmental samples. *Appl Environ Microbiol* 2001; 67(12): 5420–5424
48 Sander I, Fleischer C, Borowitzki G, Bruning T, Raulf-Heimsoth M. Development of a two-site enzyme immunoassay based on monoclonal antibodies to measure airborne exposure to (1→3)-beta-D-glucan. *J Immunol Methods* 2008; 337(1): 55–62
49 Blanc PD, Eisner MD, Katz PP, Yen IH, Archea C, Earnest G et al. Impact of the home indoor environment on adult asthma and rhinitis. *J Occup Environ Med* 2005; 47(4): 362–372

50 Schwartz J, Morris R. Air pollution and hospital admissions for cardiovasclar disease in Detroit, Michigan. *Am J Epidemiol* 1995; 142: 23–35

51 Jagielo PJ, Thorne PS, Watt JL, Fress KL, Quinn TJ, Schwartz DA. Grain dust and endotoxin inhalation challenges produce similar inflammatory response in normal subjects. *Chest* 1996; 110: 263–270

52 Blaski CA, Clapp WD, Thorne PS, Quinn TJ, Watt JL, Fress KL et al. The role of atopy in grain dust-induced airway disease. *Am J Respir Crit Care Med* 1996; 154: 334–340

53 Deetz DC, Jagielo PJ, Quinn TJ, Thorne PS, Bleuer SA, Schwartz DA. The kinetics of grain dust-induced inflammation of the lower respiratory tract. *Am J Respir Crit Care Med* 1997; 155: 254–259

54 Rylander R, Peterson Y, Donham KJ. Health effects of organic dust in the farm environment. *Am J Ind Med* 1986; 10: 199–200

55 Heederik D, van ZR, Brouwer R. Across-shift lung function changes among pig farmers. *Am J Ind Med* 1990; 17(1): 57–58

56 Muller-Suur C, Larsson K, Malmberg P, Larsson PH. Increased number of activated lymphocytes in human lung following swine dust inhalation. *Eur Respir J* 1997; 10(2): 376–380

57 Zhiping W, Malmberg P, Larsson BM, Larsson KA, Larsson L, Saraf A. Exposure to bacteria in swine-house dust and acute inflammatory reactions in humans. *Am J Respir Crit Care Med* 1996; 154: 1261–1266

58 Wang Z, Larsson KA, Palmberg L, Malmberg P, Larsson P, Larsson L. Inhalation of swine dust induces cytokine release in the upper and lower airways. *Eur Respir J* 1997; 10: 381–387

59 Larsson KA, Eklund AG, Hansson L-O, Isaksson B-M, Malmberg PO. Swine dust causes intensive airways inflammation in healthy subjects. *Am J Respir Crit Care Med* 1994; 150: 973–977

60 Malmberg P, Larsson K. Acute exposure to to swine dust causes bronchial hyperresponsiveness in healthy subjects. *Eur Respir J* 1993; 6: 400–404

61 O'Sullivan S, Dahlén S-E, Larsson KA, Larsson BM, Malmberg P, Kumlin M et al. Exposure of healthy volunteers to swine house dust increases formation of leucotrienes, prostaglandin D-2 and bronchial responsiveness to methacholine. *Thorax* 1998; 53: 1041–1044

62 Palmberg L, Larssson BM, Malmberg P, Larsson K. Airway responses of healthy farmers and nonfarmers to exposure in a swine confinement building. *Scand J Work Environ Health* 2002; 28(4): 256–263

63 Hoffmann HJ, Iversen M, Sigsgaard T, Omland O, Takai H, Bonefeld-Jorgensen E et al. A single exposure to organic dust of non-naive non-exposed volunteers induces long-lasting symptoms of endotoxin tolerance. *Int Arch Allergy Immunol* 2005; 138(2): 121–126

64 Hoffmann HJ, Iversen M, Brandslund I, Sigsgaard T, Omland O, Oxvig C et al. Plasma C3d levels of young farmers correlate with respirable dust exposure levels during normal work in swine confinement buildings. *Ann Agric Environ Med* 2003; 10(1): 53–60

65 Thorne PS. Inhalation toxicology models of endotoxin- and bioaerosol-induced inflammation. *Toxicology* 2000; 152(1–3): 13–23

66 Jagielo PJ, Thorne PS, Watt JL, Frees KL, Quinn TJ, Schwartz DA. Grain dust and endotoxin inhalation challenges produce similar inflammatory responses in normal subjects. *Chest* 1996; 110(1): 263–270

67 Schwartz DA, Thorne PS, Jagielo PJ, White GE, Bleuer SA, Frees KL. Endotoxin responsiveness and grain dust-induced inflammation in the lower respiratory tract. *Am J Physiol* 1994; 267(5 Pt 1): L609–L617

68 Thorne PS, McCray PB, Howe TS, O'Neill MA. Early-onset inflammatory responses *in vivo* to adenoviral vectors in the presence or absence of lipopolysaccharide-induced inflammation. *Am J Respir Cell Mol Biol* 1999; 20(6): 1155–1164

69 Lorenz E, Jones M, Wohlford-Lenane C, Meyer N, Frees KL, Arbour NC et al. Genes other than TLR4 are involved in the response to inhaled LPS. *Am J Physiol Lung Cell Mol Physiol* 2001; 281(5): L1106–L1114

70 Gioannini TL, Weiss JP. Regulation of interactions of Gram-negative bacterial endotoxins with mammalian cells. *Immunol Res* 2007; 39(1–3): 249–260

71 Gioannini TL, Teghanemt A, Zhang D, Coussens NP, Dockstader W, Ramaswamy S et al. Isolation of an endotoxin-MD-2 complex that produces Toll-like receptor 4–dependent cell activation at picomolar concentrations. *Proc Natl Acad Sci USA* 2004; 101(12): 4186–4191

72 Jia HP, Kline JN, Penisten A, Apicella MA, Gioannini TL, Weiss J et al. Endotoxin responsiveness of human airway epithelia is limited by low expression of MD-2. *Am J Physiol Lung Cell Mol Physiol* 2004; 287(2): L428–L437

73 Delayre-Orthez C, Becker J, de BF, Frossard N, Pons F. Exposure to endotoxins during sensitization prevents further endotoxin-induced exacerbation of airway inflammation in a mouse model of allergic asthma. *Int Arch Allergy Immunol* 2005; 138(4): 298–304

74 Watanabe J, Miyazaki Y, Zimmerman GA, Albertine KH, McIntyre TM. Endotoxin contamination of ovalbumin suppresses murine immunologic responses and development of airway hyper-reactivity. *J Biol Chem* 2003; 278(43): 42361–42368

75 Ormstad H, Groeng EC, Duffort O, Lovik M. The effect of endotoxin on the production of IgE, IgG1 and IgG2a antibodies against the cat allergen Fel d 1 in mice. *Toxicology* 2003; 188(2–3): 309–318

76 Pirie RS, Dixon PM, McGorum BC. Endotoxin contamination contributes to the pulmonary inflammatory and functional response to *Aspergillus fumigatus* extract inhalation in heaves horses. *Clin Exp Allergy* 2003; 33(9): 1289–1296

77 Kulhankova K, George CL, Kline JN, Snyder JM, Darling M, Field EH et al. Early-life co-administration of cockroach allergen and endotoxin augments pulmonary and systemic responses. *Clin Exp Allergy* 2009; 39(7): 1069–1079

78 Braun-Fahrlander C. The role of the farm environment and animal contact for the development of asthma and allergies. *Clin Exp Allergy* 2001; 31(12): 1799–1803

79 Braun-Fahrlander C, Riedler J, Herz U, Eder W, Waser M, Grize L et al. Environmental

exposure to endotoxin and its relation to asthma in school-age children. *N Engl J Med* 2002; 347(12): 869–877

80 Merchant JA, Naleway AL, Svendsen ER, Kelly KM, Burmeister LF, Stromquist AM et al. Asthma and farm exposures in a cohort of rural Iowa children. *Environ Health Perspect* 2005; 113(3): 350–356

81 Portengen L, Sigsgaard T, Omland O, Hjort C, Heederik D, Doekes G. Low prevalence of atopy in young Danish farmers and farming students born and raised on a farm. *Clin Exp Allergy* 2002; 32(2): 247–253

82 Eduard W, Douwes J, Omenaas E, Heederik D. Do farming exposures cause or prevent asthma? Results from a study of adult Norwegian farmers. *Thorax* 2004; 59(5): 381–386

83 Douwes J, Travier N, Huang K, Cheng S, McKenzie J, Le GG et al. Lifelong farm exposure may strongly reduce the risk of asthma in adults. *Allergy* 2007; 62(10): 1158–1165

84 Smit LA, Heederik D, Doekes G, Blom C, van Z, I, Wouters IM. Exposure-response analysis of allergy and respiratory symptoms in endotoxin-exposed adults. *Eur Respir J* 2008; 31(6): 1241–1248

85 Castellan RM, Olenchock SA, Kinsley KB, Hankinson JL. Inhaled endotoxin and decreased spirometric values. *N Engl J Med* 1987; 317: 605–610

86 Sigsgaard T, Brandslund I, Omland O, Hjort C, Lund ED, Pedersen OF et al. S and Z alpha1–antitrypsin alleles are risk factors for bronchial hyperresponsiveness in young farmers: An example of gene/environment interaction. *Eur Respir J* 2000; 16(1): 50–55

87 Sigsgaard T, Brandslund I, Lund E, Rasmussen JB, Varming H. Low normal alpha-1–antitrypsin serum concentrations and MZ phenotype are associated with byssinosis and familial allergy in cotton mill workers. *Pharmacogenetics* 1994; 4: 135–141

88 Alexis N, Eldridge M, Reed W, Bromberg P, Peden DB. CD14-dependent airway neutrophil response to inhaled LPS: Role of atopy. *J Allergy Clin Immunol* 2001; 107(1): 31–35

89 Blaski CA, Clapp WD, Thorne PS, Quinn TJ, Watt JL, Fress KL et al. The role of atopy in grain dust-induced airway disease. *Am J Respir Crit Care Med* 1996; 154: 334–340

90 Sigsgaard T, Bonefeld-Jorgensen EC, Kjaergaard SK, Mamas S, Pedersen OF. Cytokine release from the nasal mucosa and whole blood after experimental exposures to organic dusts. *Eur Respir J* 2000; 16(1): 140–145

91 Kruger T, Sigsgaard T, Bonefeld-Jorgensen EC. Ex vivo induction of cytokines by mould components in whole blood of atopic and non-atopic volunteers. *Cytokine* 2004; 25(2): 73–84

92 Sigsgaard T, Abell A, Jensen LD, Malmros P. Lung function changes among recycling workers exposed to organic dust. *Am J Ind Med* 1994; 25: 69–72

93 Arbour NC, Lorenz E, Schutte BC, Zabner J, Kline JN, Jones M, Frees K, Watt JL, Schwartz DA. TLR4 mutations are associated with endotoxin hyporesponsiveness in humans. *Nat Genet* 2000; 25(2): 187–191

94 Raby BA, Klimecki WT, Laprise C, Renaud Y, Faith J, Lemire M et al. Polymorphisms in toll-like receptor 4 are not associated with asthma or atopy-related phenotypes. *Am J Respir Crit Care Med* 2002; 166(11): 1449–1456
95 Eder W, Klimecki W, Yu L, von ME, Riedler J, Braun-Fahrlander C et al. Toll-like receptor 2 as a major gene for asthma in children of European farmers. *J Allergy Clin Immunol* 2004; 113(3): 482–488
96 Beutler B, Hoebe K, Du X, Ulevitch RJ. How we detect microbes and respond to them: The Toll-like receptors and their transducers. *J Leukoc Biol* 2003; 74(4): 479–485
97 Lazarus R, Raby BA, Lange C, Silverman EK, Kwiatkowski DJ, Vercelli D et al. Toll-like Receptor 10 (TLR10) Genetic variation is associated with asthma in two independent samples. *Am J Respir Crit Care Med* 2004
98 Kullman GJ, Thorne PS, Waldron PF, Marx JJ, Ault B, Lewis DM et al. Organic dust exposures from work in dairy barns. *Am Ind Hyg Assoc J* 1998; 59(6): 403–413
99 Preller L, Heederik D, Kromhout H, Boleij JS, Tielen MJ. Determinants of dust and endotoxin exposure of pig farmers: Development of a control strategy using empirical modelling. *Ann Occup Hyg* 1995; 39(5): 545–557
100 Thorne PS, Ansley AC, Perry SS. Concentrations of bioaerosols, odors, and hydrogen sulfide inside and downwind from two types of swine livestock operations. *J Occup Environ Hyg* 2009; 6(4): 211–220
101 Duchaine C, Thorne PS, Meriaux A, Grimard Y, Whitten P, Cormier Y. Comparison of endotoxin exposure assessment by bioaerosol impinger and filter-sampling methods. *Appl Environ Microbiol* 2001; 67(6): 2775–2780
102 Thorne PS, Reynolds SJ, Milton DK, Bloebaum PD, Zhang X, Whitten P et al. Field evaluation of endotoxin air sampling assay methods. *Am Ind Hyg Assoc J* 1997; 58(11): 792–799
103 Smid T, Heederik D, Houba R, Quanjer PH. Dust- and endotoxin-related respiratory effects in the animal feed industry. *Am Rev Respir Dis* 1992; 146: 1474–1479
104 Schwartz DA, Thorne PS, Yagla SJ, Burmeister LF, Olenchock SA, Watt JL et al. The role of endotoxin in grain dust-induced lung disease. *Am J Respir Crit Care Med* 1995; 152(2): 603–608
105 Zock JP, Hollander A, Heederik D, Douwes J. Acute lung function changes and low endotoxin exposures in the potato processing industry. *Am J Ind Med* 1998; 33(4): 384–391
106 Roy CJ, Thorne PS. Exposure to particulates, microorganisms, beta(1–3)-glucans, and endotoxins during soybean harvesting. *AIHA J (Fairfax, VA)* 2003; 64(4): 487–495
107 Smit LA, Wouters IM, Hobo MM, Eduard W, Doekes G, Heederik D. Agricultural seed dust as a potential cause of organic dust toxic syndrome. *Occup Environ Med* 2006; 63(1): 59–67.

Allergen and irritant exposure and exposure-response relationships

Dick Heederik and Gert Doekes

Division of Environmental Epidemiology, Institute for Risk Assessment Sciences, Utrecht University, Utrecht, The Netherlands

Abstract

Exposure to allergens and irritants is a complex phenomenon. Especially the particulate nature of many natural allergens in combination with the low exposure creates remarkable phenomena. Many allergens appear to be potent sensitizers in the nanograms per cubic meter of air range. Evidence exists that workers can be sensitized even after exposure to a low number of particles. With exposure in the low nanogram range, the respiratory tract is exposed to distinct exposure quanta of a few particles, which lead to high local concentrations of allergenic molecules. With gaseous exposure, a more equal exposure over the large surface area of the respiratory organ is to be expected. These phenomena may have mechanistic and biological implications, but certainly determine exposure assessment approaches, the interpretation of exposure measurements and the evaluation of exposure-response relationships.

Introduction

Exposure-response relationships are considered important because they point towards options for prevention. Exposure is a complex phenomenon and varies considerably over time and space. Characterizing exposure for assessing relationships with asthma occurrence in epidemiological studies requires understanding of exposure phenomena. These phenomena in their turn determine the approach in the analysis to a large extent. When all this is taken in consideration, exposure-response relationships can be analyzed. Many examples exist of exposure-response relationships for low- (LMW) and high- (HMW) molecular-weight agents, mainly from industry-based studies in which the exposure has been measured in quantitative terms. Some of these examples are presented and discussed in this chapter. General population studies with less detailed exposure information are not discussed. Recent developments such as the use of exposure-response information in risk assessment is only briefly covered here.

Occupational Asthma, edited by Torben Sigsgaard and Dick Heederik

Allergens and irritants

An allergen is a non-parasitic/non-pathogenic/non-infectious antigen capable of inducing immune-mediated hypersensitivity reactions in sensitized hosts. The preceding 'sensitization' consists of allergen-specific immune responses to a previous exposure, upon which specific T cells and antibodies have been produced – as a rule, without any observable symptomatic adverse health effects. During secondary exposures of the sensitized host, the specific antibodies and/or T cells recruit and activate inflammatory cells and mechanisms that normally should protect against harmful pathogens. For normally harmless allergens like grass pollen, cat saliva or dog skin flakes, however, the costs of these inflammatory reactions – adverse health effects, and allergic symptoms – heavily outweigh the benefits of immune protection. "Atopic" or type I hypersensitivity refers to allergy based on specific IgE and so-called Th2-type sensitization. Since this is the best studied type of allergy associated with work-related respiratory disease, this chapter further focuses exclusively on type I allergens and IgE-mediated allergy.

Allergens causing type I-mediated ('atopic') immunological asthma can be both LMW and HMW sensitizers of which more than 250 have been identified. LMW sensitizers are often synthetic industrial chemicals such as isocyanates, acid anhydrides, metals and metal salts, but also natural substances such as plicatic acid from western red cedar wood. LMW sensitizers are supposed to react with and to bind covalently to human proteins in the respiratory tract mucosa, and to function as major epitopes in the thus-produced immunogenic 'hapten-carrier' complexes. The epitope specificity of the produced antibodies in the serum of the sensitized worker can be demonstrated by showing their binding in diagnostic tests with the LMW hapten (like isocyanate) coupled to a range of different carriers.

HMW sensitizers are naturally occurring water-soluble proteins in the 10–60-kDa molecular mass range that in a hydrophilic environment, like the respiratory mucosa, are readily released, e.g., from skin scales, plant fibers, pollen grains, and other tissue matrices. Some allergenic products contain only one or a few allergens. For instance, commercially graded fungal α-amylase contains the active enzyme, with a molecular mass between 51 and 54 kDa, and some other allergenic compounds of 25–27 kDa and 40 kDa, probably enzyme fragments or fungal products [1]. Wheat flour has been shown to contain more than 100 allergenic molecules, of which 40 have been identified [2]. For such complex products like wheat, latex, etc., the exposure assessment should either be based on measuring one single marker molecule, using highly specific monoclonal or polyclonal antibodies, or on characterizing and measuring the whole mixture of antigenic/allergenic proteins with a pool or mixture of polyclonal antibodies [3]. Both approaches have been used and so far have resulted in allergen assays with strongly concordant results [4, 5].

The situation may be analogous for some LMW sensitizers like isocyanates, where exposure occurs to a mixture of the monomer and monomer-derived oligomers. The most recent studies have measured several monomers and oligomer molecules, and expressed exposure in total isocyanate concentration [6–8]. This is a simplified way of combining exposure to a range of molecules with probably different allergenic potency into one metric. Theoretically it would be possible to weigh the relative contribution of an individual molecule to a mixture by its allergenic potency. However, this information is only available for a limited number of isocyanate molecules tested in experimental animal studies [9, 10] and is not possible practically.

Irritants are agents for which the effects do not depend on preceding specific sensitization. They can thus provoke acute and transient narrowing of the airways at first exposure of an individual, and may do so through a variety of non-immunological mechanisms such as mast cell mediator release, and interaction with sensory nerve endings in bronchial epithelium or receptors in smooth muscle. Irritants may have stronger effects in individuals who are bronchially hyperresponsive. A common incited acute response to irritants should be distinguished from the induction of reactive airways dysfunction syndrome (RADS). While the same chemicals that incite transient airway narrowing can also cause RADS, induction of the latter seems the result of extremely high peak exposures to chemical irritants such as chlorine compounds, ammonia, diisocyanates, etc. Irritant exposure is of interest because it may also interact with allergen exposure in the sense that the risk for developing allergy and asthma may be modified. Examples are diesel exposure and sensitization to common allergens [11] and exposure to disinfectants in farming and atopy and bronchial hyperresponsiveness [12].

Exposure and exposure routes

Exposure is defined as contact between a target, in the context of this chapter a human, and a chemical, biological or physical agent in an environmental carrier medium [13]. For occupational asthma (OA) contact between the respiratory organ, and air as a carrier containing allergens or irritant gases or particulates, is the most relevant exposure. Recent indications suggest that dermal exposure might also play a role. Uptake of an agent is determined by the concentration in the medium (concentration in the air), the uptake of the medium (ventilation, inhalation), and clearance from the lung. The dose of an agent is the amount that enters the target, in this case the respiratory mucosa and underlying tissues. The amount that enters the upper and lower airways is, therefore, not always the relevant amount, because for instance a large fraction of very small particles – in the 10–100 nm range – and inert, non-soluble gases may also be directly exhaled, thus leading to a lower effective dose. So dose should be defined as the amount that is absorbed by (in case of gases), or deposited on (in case of particulates) the respiratory mucosa. One should consider that the definition of 'dose' may depend on the mechanism of the studied health effect: whether it only requires interaction with cells and molecules in the mucosa, or also needs to migrate through the respiratory basal membrane to submucosal tissue, or even the surrounding capillaries or lymph nodes. It should be realized that most information about particle deposition is based on research with inert radiolabeled particulates. Very little is known about the role of deposition, clearance and retention of allergenic or irritant particulates. Particle deposition is size and shape dependent and differs for different regions of the respiratory organ. For near spherical particulates, behavior is well described by the aerodynamic diameter. The aerodynamic diameter is an expression of the aerodynamic behavior of a particle (for a perfect sphere with unit density, the diameter equals the aerodynamic diameter). Generally speaking, larger particulates deposit in the nasopharyngeal region (including nasopharynx, oral passages, and larynx) by sedimentation and impaction. Retention times in this region are short, usually between minutes to hours [14]. In the tracheo-bronchial tree, which includes the trachea, bronchi and bronchioli, particles are deposited by impaction in the upper part and by sedimentation in the lower part. Non-soluble particles are usually cleared within 1 day by the ciliated airways and most are swallowed. In the alveolar zone, particles deposit by sedimentation and diffusion, and are removed very slowly by cellular clearance mechanisms with clearance times from months to years. Different size fractions have been defined which can penetrate different regions of the respiratory organ [15]. For OA research, the inhalable dust fraction (50% cut-off at 10 μm) is the most important dust fraction, and is defined as those particles which can penetrate the human respiratory organ. Some literature exists that indicates that deposition in the nasal region can induce reactions distal from the nose, so larger particulates may be relevant for effects lower in the airways [16]. Traditionally, occupational hygiene studies focused on pneumoconiosis and monitoring programs commonly measured the fraction of respirable dust particles (50% cut-off at 4.25 μm) of which the majority can penetrate the alveolar region. This fraction is more relevant for toxicants for which uptake through the alveoli can take place, and for dusts which cause pneumoconiosis. These particles are smaller than most of those in the inhalable fraction. The respirable fraction underestimates the exposure to larger particulates for which deposition in both the upper and lower airways may also be of primary importance, like most of the known allergen-carrying particles. It should be further emphasized that the boundaries between the various particle fractions and the regions where these are deposited are not sharp. Thus, while the majority of allergen particles, e.g., of 10–20 μm diameter, will be deposited in the upper airways, a substantial proportions may reach the lower respiratory tract and induce not only rhinitis but also asthma symptoms.

Dermal exposure is a considerably less explored field in exposure assessment for OA. There is clear animal evidence showing that LMW sensitizers, like isocyanates, may induce sensitization after dermal exposure, with subsequent inhalation challenges resulting in asthma-like responses [17]. Several lines of evidence support a similar role for human isocyanate skin exposure, namely, that dermal exposure may contribute to the development of isocyanate asthma by inducing systemic sensitization [18]. More research is needed in this field to develop and improve dermal-exposure assessment methods for sensitizing agents [19, 20], since objective and reproducible methods are lacking and it is unclear how dermal exposure should be measured in a biologically relevant way for OA. Dermal exposure is usually measured by hand washing methods, dermal patches, or by analyzing gloves, but none of these approaches are completely satisfactory.

Variability of exposure and exposure patterns

Temporal aspects of exposure are considered important, e.g., is the exposure relatively constant and at the same level, or are there fluctuations or possibly even sharp and large increases over time (peaks)? Many allergen exposed workers are exposed to a pattern of high peaks over a working day. Measurements with continuously registering devices have shown that bakers are exposed to peaks of flour or enzymes when they empty bags, dust dough, or clean the bakery [21]. These peaks occur when flour particles become airborne because of physical forces, but since they are relatively large (aerodynamic diameter 5–15 μm and often even larger [22, 23]) they will reside in the air for only a brief period of time. As a result, even the highest peaks last for a maximum of only several minutes [21], and between these task-related high peaks the exposure will be very low. This exposure pattern is typical for many situations with exposure to HMW and non-gaseous LMW sensitizers, because relatively large particulates are involved, and peak exposures are usually the consequence of regularly performed daily tasks. Very high dust and allergen exposures, however, may also occur infrequently, e.g., due to repair or cleaning activities of damaged or neglected equipment or storage sites. Examples are environments such as laboratory animal facilities with exposure to rat and mouse urinary proteins, the farm environment with exposure to allergens and microbial agents such as endotoxins, health care settings with exposure to latex. The baker's work is typically cyclic, with a daily repeated pattern of exposure peaks, and the average exposure over the day is therefore relatively similar from day to day. Thus, within a day the exposure is highly variable because of the sequence of peaks and low background levels, but between days the differences are relatively small. Among laboratory animals workers day-to-day variation in exposure may be much larger. Typical high-exposure tasks are the handling of living animals and the cleaning of cages and removal of cage bedding. For workers routinely involved in cage cleaning there may be regular temporal patterns of high exposure, and also for animal caretakers there may be daily tasks, e.g., feeding, leading to more or less cyclic exposure patterns. Researchers performing animal experiments may, however, often have days or even weeks with practically no allergen exposure. Exposure assessment in this job category therefore strongly relies on combinations of allergen measurements and careful monitoring – using diaries or questionnaires – of performed tasks. Allergen-exposure levels in farming have hardly been studied, but may *a priori* be expected to show a very large variation. In animal farming many job tasks show daily patterns – like feeding and milking – and on many days the average daily exposure may thus be relatively constant. Other potentially high-exposure activities, however, like emptying and cleaning of stables and barns, occur regularly but with much lower frequency over the year. In crop farming the exposure to plant or microbial allergens will be strongly associated typical season-related activities, like harvesting. Although no data on allergen exposure are available, results for airborne dust and endotoxin levels in farming and various agricultural industries suggest that it indeed shows very pronounced within-day but also day-to-day and seasonal variation [24, 25]. Similar patterns may also occur for LMW sensitizers such as diisocyanates used in spray painting. In industrial spray painting, the within-day variation may be high but daily exposure patterns relatively constant, whereas in many small companies – notably car repair shops – the day-to-day variation may also be very large depending on the actual work available. Apart from that, there may be other reasons for incidental peak exposure. Spray painters usually work in highly controlled environments such as spray booths with exhaust ventilation systems. As a result, the exposure is often below the limit of detection but high exposures occur because they regularly spray outside the booth for small repairs or during formulation of paint, cleaning of equipment and because of spills [6].

Physical and chemical aspects of airborne allergen exposure

It is useful to conceptualize how exposure to allergens occurs. Large measurement series in the baking industry, as part of an exposure-response study on fungal α-amylase [26], showed that workers with a high exposure were exposed to time-weighted average levels of fungal α-amylase between 5 and as high as 100 ng/m^3. These data were obtained with full-shift (8 hour) measurements, and thus represent daily averages. Moderately exposed individuals were exposed to levels between 0.5 and 5 ng/m^3, but in this category more than 70% of the measurements were below the limit of detection [26]. Workers in the high-exposure category were mainly dough makers working with pure enzyme formulations. Workers with "moderate" exposure levels did not handle pure enzyme but batches of cereal flours to which the enzyme had been added – either elsewhere in the bakery or in the flour-supplying industry. Since amylase is added in only milligrams quantities per kilogram flour (a 1/10^6 ratio on the basis of weight), the amylase exposure at a worksite between 1 and 5 mg/m^3 flour dust exposure – common for dough makers – would be around 1–5 ng/m^3, which agrees well with the observed average amylase levels. It is, however, less easy to understand why for the majority of measurements in this exposure category the amylase levels remained under the limit of detection. A likely explanation might be the particulate nature of the amylase, which is added as solid powder to the cereal flours, with as consequence a highly heterodisperse distribution of airborne amylase. Since these allergen exposure characteristics may have important consequences for exposure-assessment strategies, and for the interpretation of exposure-sensitization relations, they are discussed below in some more detail. Both wheat and airborne amylase allergens have been mainly found in airborne particles with aerodynamic diameter between 5 and 15 μm [22, 26]. Assuming a spherical shape and density of 1–1.5 g/cm^3, one may estimate their mass to range between 0.04 and 2 ng. Thus, if amylase is added to flours as a 50–100% pure enzyme powder, each milligram of the resulting 'mixture' consists of approximately 1–10 million wheat flour, but only 1–10 amylase particles; when the mixture becomes airborne, a moderate dust exposure of 1 mg/m^3 would mean that workers will be exposed to a very limited number of amylase particles per cubic meter. Due to the random particle distribution at such low numbers, however, airborne measurements – with usually close to 1 m^3 air sampled per filter (on the basis of a sampler sampling 2–3 l/min) for personal full-shift air samples – will inevitably show a high coefficient of variation (CV) and potentially many samples with an allergen content below the detection limit. In fact, with on average only a handful of particles per air sample, there is a substantial risk of having no amylase particle at all in a sample, and this may be one of the reasons that even at moderate average levels many samples remain negative when tested for the presence of amylase.

The heterodisperse nature of some airborne allergens can be confirmed by direct staining methods, like the HALOgen procedure [27] in which allergen-specific antibodies are used to visualize the allergen molecules released from a particle trapped on a filter or adhesive tape. Application on personal inhalable dust sample from baker's work environment clearly confirmed that only very few of the many dust particles on a filter showed the presence of α-amylase (Fig. 1).

The airborne dust composition described here may be exceptional, with all allergenic (amylase) activity concentrated in a few particles per cubic meter, surrounded by ~10^6 other non-allergenic particles – or particles with other allergenic specificity like wheat proteins in this particular case. For 100% pure enzyme powder the number of allergen molecules per particle is, given a molecular mass of around 52 kDa for fungal α-amylase, extremely high and varies between 10^9 and 10^{10} per particle, depending on its exact size. So amylase exposure appears to occur in the form of a limited number of 'allergen quanta' consisting of particles with a large number of allergenic molecules per particle. For other allergens the situation might be less extreme, but the same principles may be applied, e.g., to animal dander particles, or fecal particles from house or storage mites. Although the latter contain many other molecules, it has been shown that each mite fecal particle may contain up to 2.5–5% (w/w) of the major allergen Der p1, which, assuming a particle diameter of approximately 20 μm and a molecular mass of 24 000, implicates 'allergen quanta'

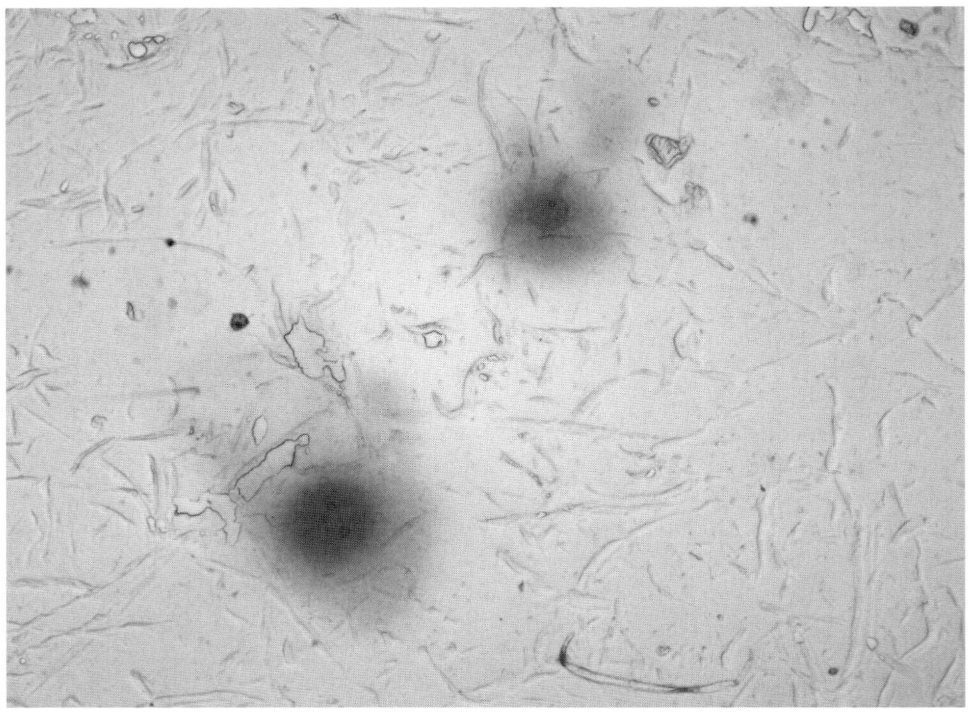

Figure 1.
HALOgen staining of α-amylase in an airborne bakery dust sample (courtesy J Bogdanovic, IRAS UU). The sample shown was taken during a 30-minute period when a bakery worker was dusting dough with enriched flour. Two amylase containing particulates are visible. The whole filter contains not more than 25 particulates, indicating that a bakery worker, handling enriched flour may be exposed to a very low number of amylase containing particulates per day.

of no less than 10^8–10^9 Der p1 molecules per particle [28]. Parallels also exist for exposure to pollen. Grass pollen exposure ranges from a few to several hundreds of pollen per cubic meter measured as long-term average concentration [29, 30]. When exposed to water, pollen grains may rupture at the single germinal aperture, releasing around 700 granules of less than 3 μm in diameter from each grain [31]. This leads to several hundreds to thousands of particulates per air samples [29, 30, 32], but still a relatively low number considering the number of allergen molecules involved.

This is in clear contrast to a spray painter working with a diisocyanate monomer or a monomer oligomer mixture of, for instance, 1,6-hexamethylene diisocyanate

(HDI). Monomer exposure will to a large extent be gaseous because of the vapor pressure of HDI. This implies that even at low exposure levels, a large number of molecules will be inhaled by, and dispersed across, the respiratory organ. Diisocyanate exposure to oligomers of HDI, however, occurs in the form of small aerosol droplets, likely with limited number of particulates containing many allergenic molecules with free isocyanate groups. There are indications from experimental animal studies that gaseous monomer exposure is more potent at eliciting respiratory responses than particulate exposure, and that differences in particle size distribution are also associated with a quantitatively different response [10, 33]. Many of these differences may be due to a different deposition pattern for different particle size distributions, leading to differences in dose in specific zones of the respiratory organ. For mixed particulate and vapor exposure, the vapor molecules may be adsorbed to the surface of the particle and penetrate deeper into the airways and lungs than in the case of gaseous exposure only. This may also contribute to a qualitatively and quantitatively different response.

It is not clear what the biological implications of localized high exposure are. It may be important to discuss the question separately for the allergic sensitization process and for the induction of symptoms in sensitized subjects. What distribution and what levels are sufficient to lead to a high sensitization risk? Results from dermal sensitization studies suggest that a few antigen-presenting dendritic cells encountering many molecules may induce a more vigorous response than many dendritic cells encountering only a few molecules [17]. Thus, the focal presentation of a very small number of allergenic molecules concentrated on a few cells may represent an exposure pattern that results in a major risk for sensitization. It therefore seems important to consider the nature of the exposure pattern in terms of aggregation phase (gaseous, particulate), particle distribution, and time pattern of exposure (peaks) [34]. Incidental (peak) exposure to a very limited number of particulates seems associated with only a mildly elevated risk for sensitization risk [26, 35]. Specific IgE titers against fungal α-amylase appeared to be low in workers with moderate exposures to fungal amylase [26]. However, workers involved in handling pure enzyme can be exposed more frequently to short exposure peaks of up to a few hundred milligram per cubic meter of pure enzyme for a few minutes [21]. Over a working day this will average out to a lower level, in the $\mu g/m^3$ range, and for longer periods – weeks to months – the average levels may be far below 1 $\mu g/m^3$. Thus, the increased sensitization risk observed at average exposure levels in the ng/m^3 range may in fact be the result of incidental 'sensitizing events' when the exposure increases suddenly but very briefly to 100–1000-fold higher levels.

The phenomena described above may also play a role in LMW sensitizer exposure. Spray painters are now more often exposed to oligomers than simply just gaseous monomers. Oligomer exposure is more likely to occur in the form of particulates. Exposure is very often below the limit of detection and is highly variable when above this limit and differs from moment to moment by more than a factor

10–1000. Spray painters often seem to face very low exposure, but during intensive spraying, or mixing of paint, brief periods of high exposure occur [6].

Exposure-response relationships

Studying exposure-response relationships for asthma is complex. The manifestation of the disease is variable and this complicates measurement of the presence of disease. The threshold concentration for elicitation of an allergic airway reaction in sensitized individuals is generally assumed to be lower than the threshold concentration to induce sensitization [17, 36]. Direct evidence for this observation is limited because elicitation levels for symptoms and other signs are poorly documented both in experimental and observational studies. It is only recently that allergen exposure data have been applied for exposure-response modeling using observational data from human populations. Some sensitizers, especially LMW ones like diisocyanates and acid anhydrides, may also have irritant properties. Irritating effects may occur in parallel at lower levels in atopic individuals who have been sensitized to common allergens, but not sensitized to the occupational allergen. Thus, although the evidence is not always very strong, different exposure-response relationships may be anticipated for different subgroups of workers. Theoretically, the slope and intercept of the exposure-response relationship might differ between individuals in the same workplace according to the mechanism of disease provocation (and therefore host factors) [36].

A clear definition of the actual health outcome studied is crucial for any statement regarding exposure-response relationships, and this is particularly true for the development of asthmatic disease. A simple model for the pathogenesis of OA induced by HMW sensitizers is usually represented as follows (Fig. 2): exposure leads to a series of events – sensitization, and development of an inflammatory response, which is accompanied by symptoms, bronchial hyperresponsiveness, airflow variability, etc. When exposure is continued, chronic changes and severe airflow impairment might occur. This process can develop rapidly and, as a result, it seems likely that workers may try to influence their exposure when they develop symptoms by migrating to jobs with lower exposure or leave the workforce (healthy worker effect). Examples of exposure-response relationships for the first step, sensitization, have been described for many allergens. For some LMW sensitizers exposure-response relationships have been observed. One prospective study included 163 previously unexposed workers with exposure to epoxy resins containing organic anhydrides: hexahydrophtalic anhydride (HHPA), methyl hexahydrophtalic anhydride (MHHPA), and methyltetrahydrophtalic anhydride (MTHPA) [38]. These workers were followed for, on average, 32 months (1–105 months). The levels of organic acid anhydrides in air and of specific IgE and IgG in serum were monitored repeatedly. The mean combined organic acid anhydride exposure was 15.4 μg/m^3

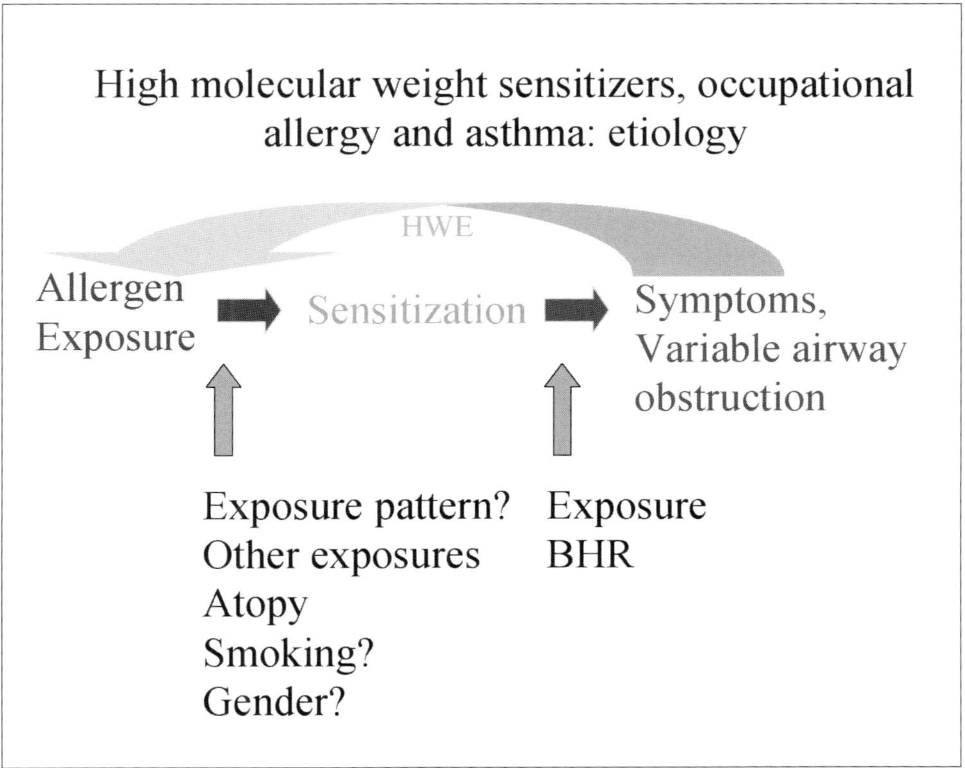

Figure 2.
Etiological model for the development of occupational asthma (after [37]).

(range < 1–189 μg/m^3). An exposure-response relationship was clearly demonstrated for the incidence of sensitization with increasing exposure. Specific IgE was demonstrated by 21 (13%) subjects with a mean induction time of 8.8 (1–35 months). The sensitization incidence was 4.1/1000 person months at risk. Atopics had a more than fivefold elevated sensitization risk compared to non-atopics.

Several other authors have also described exposure-response relationships for various organic acid anhydrides [39–41]. Similar observations have been found for some other LMW sensitizers such as platinum salts [42, 43] and isocyanates [44], although the available evidence is more limited than for organic acid anhydrides and the HMW sensitizers discussed in the following section. Early studies already gave some indications that exposure-response relationships could be observed for HMW sensitizers. Musk et al. [45] showed that bakery workers with a "high dust rank" were more often sensitized against one or more bakery allergens compared to workers with a low dust rank. The dust classification was validated with total dust measurement. More recent studies in bakers used dust sampling instead of the – from an immunological viewpoint – more valid allergen measurement [46]. These studies have probably been successful because wheat allergen levels in flour dust correlate reasonably with dust levels [26, 47]. For most other HMW allergens, however, there often is no such direct correlation between airborne dust and allergen levels, because dust and allergen levels do not always share the same sources and determinants of exposure. For these allergens, exposure-response relationships could be explored only after immunoassays became available for sensitive and specific measurement of these allergens [3]. Overviews of available exposure-response studies [17, 48, 49] show that several allergens, e.g., rat urinary proteins and fungal α-amylase, appear to be potent allergens, and are associated with increased sensitization rates at low exposure levels in the nanogram or even picogram per cubic meter range for as little as a few hours per week [26, 49]. Allergens like wheat proteins seem less potent and sensitization risk increases in the low microgram per cubic meter range [50]. A longitudinal exposure-response study in bakers has confirmed the results of the cross-sectional studies on fungal α-amylase and wheat allergen exposure [51]. Clear-cut exposure-response relationships in humans have as yet not been observed for latex proteins, since few epidemiological studies on latex sensitization have yet been conducted in which exposure was assessed with the use of latex-specific immunoassays.

Effect modification of exposure-response relationships

In most of the above-mentioned studies, modification of the exposure-response relationship by atopy has been considered. The most direct and usually optimal approach to assess effect modification by atopy is a stratified analysis, in which intercept and slope of the exposure-response relations are determined separately for atopic and non-atopic subpopulations ('strata'). In most of the studies following that approach, the slope of the exposure-response relationship is generally steeper for atopics compared to non-atopics.

One should realize that the association between exposure and sensitization is biologically specific in the sense that specific antibodies are formed against the allergen. This implies that there is only one determinant of sensitization in a strict epidemiological sense, because a confounder is required to be a determinant of the endpoint under study. Confounding cannot occur because there is only one determinant, and a confounder is by definition another determinant.

Further along the causal chain, other endpoints can also be studied. Several studies have explored the relationship between symptoms and exposure. This requires a specific strategy because the respiratory or work-related symptoms may not exclusively be caused by exposure to one specific allergen, but may also be associated with other factors in the work environment, or to non-occupational factors like smoking, exposures at home, or outdoor exposures. Thus, confounding by several other causes may occur here. If one wants to explore the association between exposure and symptoms, one needs to further stratify for specific sensitization because this is expected to be a strong modifier of risk for symptoms elicited by the specific allergen exposure. This is clearly illustrated by the example below (Tab. 1).

Table 1. Exposure-response relationship for work-related respiratory symptoms and wheat allergen exposure stratified by specific IgE sensitization to wheat (from [50]).

	Work-related symptoms	
	n/N	**%**
Sensitization to wheat		
Low exposed	1/7	14.3
Intermediated exposed	4/10	40.0
High exposed	10/19	52.6
Not sensitized to wheat		
Low exposed	17/110	15.5
Intermediate exposed	21/97	21.6
High exposed	25/103	24.3

IgE-sensitized workers had a considerably higher risk of developing symptoms at intermediate and high exposure levels than non-sensitized workers, and the exposure-response relationship in this subgroup is much steeper in the wheat-sensitized subgroup. Interestingly, additional analyses suggested that among non-wheat-sensitized workers, atopics (workers with IgE to common allergens like house dust mites and grass pollen, but not to occupational allergens) also had a somewhat higher risk than non-atopics. Atopic individuals are known to respond more often and possibly at lower exposure levels to any irritant or allergenic stimuli. The underlying mechanism is not associated with specific sensitization to a common allergen, but more likely an indirect association with bronchial hyperresponsiveness or some irritant mechanism. Similar observations are available for other allergens and from longitudinal studies [52, 53]. Some studies have shown findings indicating that sensitization does not always precede symptoms in people exposed to known allergens [54]. Mechanisms than other sensitization probably explain the occurrence of their symptoms. Thus, several exposure-response relationships exist with different underlying biological mechanisms. If one does not distinguish these different modifiers in the analysis, exposure-response relationships become diluted or may have an unexpected shape because the different associations are superimposed. This may be one of the reasons why several studies in the past have failed to find clear exposure-symptoms relationships because of the complexities and pitfalls. Several other studies explored relationships between exposure and symptoms in a straightforward way without finding a clear relationship. Exposure-symptom relationships can only be studied in a meaningful way when the analysis is stratified for modifying variables along the causal pathway, like sensitization and potentially atopy in the case of HMW sensitizers.

The most evaluated exposure-response relationships in allergic respiratory disease are exposure-sensitization and exposure-symptom relationships in cross-sectional and some longitudinal studies. However, examples in which, for instance, time to sensitization has been evaluated also exist [55]; these have shown that the time to development of disease is also dependent on exposure intensity.

Special issues in exposure-response modeling

Some studies specifically explored the existence of exposure thresholds using smoothing techniques [56–58]. There were no indications of an exposure threshold or exposure level below which the sensitization risk was not increased. Others have found levels below which sensitization did not seem to occur [40]. However, the difference between no or a few cases in the lowest exposed category and thus between observing an exposure threshold or not seems small. The power of a study, the size of the control group, the background prevalence of sensitization of the allergen, and the way sensitization has been measured may be the major driving factors for the estimated sensitization rate at the lowest exposure levels. The difference between studies that do not find exposure thresholds and those that do are to some extent relative and artificial, while the consequences for prevention and exposure standard-setting practices are obvious [59]. For some sensitizers health-based occupational exposure limits (OELs) have been defined that specify the level of exposure to an airborne substance, a threshold level below which it may reasonably be expected that there is no risk of adverse health effects. When such a threshold does not exist, an alternative approach would be to accept a low exposure, which carries a small but predefined risk in developing allergic sensitization.

For several allergens, a flattening of the exposure-response relationship at higher exposure levels has been reported [57, 58]. Some have argued that flattening off of the exposure-response relationship may be associated with specific IgG and IgG4 responses at high exposure [60, 61]. Others observed the same phenomenon in independent studies [62, 63]. However, this phenomenon was not observed in a longitudinal study looking at IgG antibody response at baseline and incidence of specific sensitization [64]. In one study it was found that the exposure-response relationship for wheat exposure with specific sensitization differed from industry to industry, possibly reflecting a differential selection bias (healthy worker effect) by industry [57]. More studies are needed to understand the underlying explanations for flattening of exposure-response relationships at high exposure levels.

Exposure-exposure interactions

Some environments with high levels of HMW allergens also appear to be associated with a strongly decreased risk of common atopy. Interactions seem to exist between exposure to microbial agents like endotoxins and sensitization. Studies among adults, some with occupational exposure data for microbial agents such as endotoxin, have shown inverse relationships between endotoxin exposure and atopic asthma [65], allergic sensitization [66], and hay fever [67, 68]. This suggests complex and interacting associations between endotoxin and allergen exposures in adult life. Similar complex interactions seem to exist with other exposures such as disinfectants [12]. Evaluation of interactions as described above will become more often the norm and not the exception. This will ask for studies with refined exposure-assessment strategies and sufficient power to be able to distinguish the effect of the different exposure variables on different phenotypes. An examples of this development will be a new generation of gene-environment studies.

References

1 Baur X, Chen Z, Sander I (1994) Isolation and denomination of an important allergen in baking additives: α-Amylase from *Aspergillus oryzae* (Asp o II). *Clin Exp Allergy* 24: 465–470

2 Sander I, Flagge A, Merget R, Halder TM, Meyer HE, Baur X (2001) Identification of wheat flour allergens by means of 2–dimensional immunoblotting. *J Allergy Clin Immunol* 107: 907–913

3 Heederik, D, Doekes G, Nieuwenhuijsen MJ (1999) Exposure assessment of high molecular weight sensitisers: Contribution to occupational epidemiology and disease prevention. *Occup Environ Med* 56: 735–741

4 Sander I, Zahradnik E, Bogdanovic J, Raulf-Heimsoth M, Wouters IM, Renström A, Harris-Roberts J, Robinson E, Rodrigo MJ, Goldscheid N, Brüning T, Doekes G (2007) Optimized methods for fungal alpha-amylase airborne exposure assessment in bakeries and mills. *Clin Exp Allergy* 37: 1229–1238

5 Bogdanovic J, Wouters IM, Sander I, Raulf-Heimsoth M, Elms J, Rodrigo MJ, Heederik DJ, Doekes G (2006) Airborne exposure to wheat allergens: Measurement by human immunoglobulin G4 and rabbit immunoglobulin G immunoassays. *Clin Exp Allergy* 36: 1168–1175

6 Pronk A, Tielemans E, Skarping G, Bobeldijk I, VAN Hemmen J, Heederik D, Preller L

(2006) Inhalation exposure to isocyanates of car body repair shop workers and industrial spray painters. *Ann Occup Hyg* 50: 1–14

7 Pronk A, Preller L, Raulf-Heimsoth M, Jonkers IC, Lammers JW, Wouters IM, Doekes G, Wisnewski AV, Heederik D (2007) Respiratory symptoms, sensitization, and exposure response relationships in spray painters exposed to isocyanates. *Am J Respir Crit Care Med* 176: 1090–1097

8 Pronk A, Preller L, Doekes G, Wouters IM, Rooijackers J, Lammers JW, Heederik D (2009) Different respiratory phenotypes are associated with isocyanate exposure in spray painters. *Eur Respir J* 33: 494–501

9 Pauluhn J (2004) Pulmonary irritant potency of polyisocyanate aerosols in rats: Comparative assessment of irritant threshold concentrations by bronchoalveolar lavage. *J Appl Toxicol* 24: 231–247

10 Pauluhn J, Eidmann P, Mohr U (2002) Respiratory hypersensitivity in guinea pigs sensitized to 1,6-hexamethylene diisocyanate (HDI): Comparison of results obtained with the monomer and homopolymers of HDI. *Toxicol* 171: 147–160

11 Diaz-Sanchez D, Proietti L, Polosa R (2003) Diesel fumes and the rising prevalence of atopy: An urban legend? *Curr Allergy Asthma Rep* 3: 146–152

12 Preller L, Doekes G, Heederik D, Vermeulen R, Vogelzang PF, Boleij JSM (1996) Disinfectant use as a risk factor for atopic sensitization and symptoms consistent with asthma: An epidemiological study. *Eur Respir J* 9: 1407–1413

13 Zartarian VG, Ott WR, Duan N (1997) A quantitative definition of exposure and related concepts. *J Expo Anal Environ Epidemiol* 7: 411–437

14 Chan TL, Lippmann M (1980) Experimental measurements and empirical modelling of the regional deposition of inhaled particles in humans. *Am Ind Hyg Assoc J* 41: 399–409

15 ISO (1992) *Air quality particle size fraction definitions for health related sampling*. ISO/CD 7708 International Standardization Organization, Geneva

16 Togias A (2003) Rhinitis and asthma: Evidence for respiratory system integration. *J Allergy Clin Immunol* 111: 1171–1183

17 Arts JH, Mommers C, de Heer C (2006) Dose-response relationships and threshold levels in skin and respiratory allergy. *Crit Rev Toxicol* 36: 219–251

18 Bello D, Herrick CA, Smith TJ, Woskie SR, Streicher RP, Cullen MR, Liu Y, Redlich CA (2007) Skin exposure to isocyanates: Reasons for concern. *Environ Health Perspect* 115: 328–335

19 Pronk A, Yu F, Vlaanderen J, Tielemans E, Preller L, Bobeldijk I, Deddens JA, Latza U, Baur X, Heederik D (2006) Dermal, inhalation, and internal exposure to 1,6-HDI and its oligomers in car body repair shop workers and industrial spray painters. *Occup Environ Med* 63: 624–631

20 Liu Y, Bello D, Sparer JA, Stowe MH, Gore RJ, Woskie SR, Cullen MR, Redlich CA (2007) Skin exposure to aliphatic polyisocyanates in the auto body repair and refinishing industry: A qualitative assessment. *Ann Occup Hyg* 51: 429–439

21 Meijster T, Tielemans E, Schinkel J, Heederik D (2008) Evaluation of peak exposures in

the dutch flour processing industry: Implications for intervention strategies. *Ann Occup Hyg* 52: 587–596
22 Houba R, van Run P, Heederik D, Doekes G (1996) Wheat allergen exposure assessment for epidemiologic studies in bakeries using personal dust sampling and inhibition ELISA. *Clin Exp Allergy* 26: 154–163
23 Sandiford CP, Nieuwenhuijsen MJ, Tee RD, Taylor AJ (1994) Determination of the size of airborne flour particles. *Allergy* 49: 891–893
24 Spaan S, Wouters IM, Oosting I, Doekes G, Heederik D (2006) Exposure to inhalable dust and endotoxins in agricultural industries. *J Environ Monit* 8: 63–72
25 Eduard W, Douwes J, Mehl R, Heederik D, Melbostad E (2001) Short term exposure to airborne microbial agents during farm work: Exposure-response relations with eye and respiratory symptoms. *Occup Environ Med* 58: 113–118
26 Houba R, Heederik D, Doekes G, van Run P (1996) Exposure-sensitization relationship for α-amylase allergens in the baking industry. *Am J Respir Crit Care Med* 154: 130–136
27 Tovey E, Lucca SD, Poulos L, O'Meara T (2008) The Halogen assay – A new technique for measuring airborne allergen. *Methods Mol Med* 138: 227–46
28 Tovey ER, Chapman MD, Platts-Mills TA (1981) Mite faeces are a major source of house dust allergens. *Nature* 289: 592–593
29 Holmquist L, Vesterberg O (1999) Luminescence immunoassay of pollen allergens on air sampling polytetrafluoroethylene filters. *J Biochem Biophys Methods* 41: 49–60
30 Holmquist L, Vesterberg O (2000) Miniaturized direct on air sampling filter quantification of pollen allergens. *J Biochem Biophys Methods* 42: 111–114
31 Suphioglu C, Singh MB, Taylor P, Bellomo R, Holmes P, Puy R, Knox RB (1992) Mechanism of grass-pollen-induced asthma. *Lancet* 339: 569–572
32 Holmquist L, Vesterberg O (2003) Immunochromatographic direct on sampling filter test for aeroallergens. *J Biochem Biophys Methods* 57: 183–190
33 Pauluhn J, Thiel A, Emura M, Mohr U (200l) Respiratory sensitization to diphenylmethane-4,4'-diisocyanate (MDI) in guinea pigs: Impact of particle size on induction and elicitation of response. *Toxicol Sci* 56: 105–113
34 Nieuwenhuijsen MJ, Sandiford CP, Lowson D, Tee RD, Venables KM, Newman Taylor AJ (1995) Peak exposure concentrations of dust and flour aeroallergen in flour mills and bakeries. *Ann Occup Hyg* 39: 193–201
35 Nieuwenhuijsen MJ, Heederik D, Doekes G, Venables KM, Newman Taylor AJ (1999) Exposure-response relationships for α-amylase sensitization in British bakeries and flour mills. *Occup Environ Med* 56: 197–201
36 Becklake M (2006). Epidemiological approaches in occupational asthma. In: Bernstein IL, Chan-Yeung M, Malo J-L, Bernstein DI (eds): *Asthma in the Workplace*, 3rd and revised edition, Marcel Dekker, New York
37 Chan-Yeung, M, Malo J-L (1999) Natural history of occupational asthma. In: Bernstein IL, Chan-Yeung M, Malo J-L, Bernstein DI (eds) *Asthma in the Workplace*, 2nd edition, Marcel Dekker, New-York

38 Welinder H, Nielsen J, Rylander L, Ståhlbom B (2001). A prospective study of the relationship between exposure and specific antibodies in workers exposed to organic acid anhydrides. *Allergy* 56: 506–511
39 Zeiss CR, Mitchell JH, Van Peenen PF, Kavich D, Collins MJ, Grammer L, Shaughnessy M, Levitz D, Henderson J, Patterson RA (1992) Clinical and immunologic study of employees in a facility manufacturing trimellitic anhydride. *Allergy Proc* 13: 193–198
40 Grammer LC, Shaughnessy MA, Kenamore BD, Yarnold PR (1999) A clinical and immunologic study to assess risk of TMA-induced lung disease as related to exposure. *J Occup Environ Med* 41: 1048–1051
41 Nielsen J, Welinder H, Jönsson B, Axmon A, Rylander L, Skerfving S (2001) Exposure to hexahydrophthalic and methylhexahydrophthalic anhydrides – Dose-response for sensitization and airway effects. *Scand J Work Environ Health* 27: 327–334
42 Calverley AE, Rees D, Dowdeswell RJ, Linnett PJ, Kielkowski D (1995) Platinum salt sensitivity in refinery workers: Incidence and effects of smoking and exposure. *Occup Environ Med* 52: 661–666
43 Merget R, Kulzer R, Dierkes-Globisch A, Breitstadt R, Gebler A, Kniffka A, Artelt S, Koenig HP, Alt F, Vormberg R, Baur X, Schultze-Werninghaus G (2000) Exposure-effect relationship of platinum salt allergy in a catalyst production plant: Conclusions from a 5-year prospective cohort study. *J Allergy Clin Immunol* 105: 364–370
44 Karol, MH (1981) Survey of industrial workers for antibodies to toluene diisocyanate. *J Occup Med* 23: 741–747
45 Musk AW, Venables KM, Crook B, Nunn AJ, Hawkins R, Crook GD, Graneek BJ, Tee RD, Farrer N, Johnson DA, Gordon DJ, Darbyshire JH, Newman Taylor AJ (1989) Respiratory symptoms, lung function, and sensitisation to flour in a British bakery. *Br J Ind Med* 46: 636–642
46 Brisman J, Jarvholm B, Lillienberg L (2000) Exposure-response relations for self-reported asthma and rhinitis in bakers. *Occup Environ Med* 57: 335–340
47 Nieuwenhuijsen MJ, Lowson D, Venables KM, Newman Taylor AJ (1995) Correlation between different measures of exposure in a cohort of bakery workers and flour millers. *Ann Occup Hyg* 39: 291–298
48 Baur X, Chen Z, Liebers V (1998) Exposure-response relationships of occupational inhalative allergens. *Clin Exp Allergy* 28: 537–544
49 Heederik D, Venables K, Malmberg P, Hollander A, Karlsson A-S, Renström A, Doekes G, Nieuwenhuijsen M (1999) Exposure-response relationships for occupational respiratory sensitization in workers exposed to rat urinary allergens: Results from an European study in laboratory animal workers. *J Allergy Clin Immunol* 103: 678–684
50 Houba R, Heederik D, Doekes G (1998) Wheat sensitization and work related symptoms in the baking industry are preventable: An epidemiological study. *Am J Respir Crit Care Med* 158: 1499–1503
51 Cullinan P, Cook A, Nieuwenhuijsen MJ, Sandiford C, Tee RD, Venables KM, McDonald JC, Newman Taylor AJ (2001) Allergen and dust exposure as determinants of work-

related symptoms and sensitization in a cohort of flour-exposed workers; a case-control analysis. *Ann Occup Hyg* 45: 85–87

52 Nieuwenhuijsen MJ, Putcha V, Gordon S, Heederik D, Venables KM, Cullinan P, Newman-Taylor AJ (2004) Exposure response relationships among laboratory animal workers exposed to rats. *Occup Environ Med* 61: 551–553

53 De Zotti R, Bovenzi M (2000) Prospective study of work related respiratory symptoms in trainee bakers. *Occup Environ Med* 57: 58–61

54 Skjold T, Dahl R, Juhl B, Sigsgaard T (2008) The incidence of respiratory symptoms and sensitisation in baker apprentices. *Eur Respir J* 32: 452–459

55 Kruize H, Post W, Heederik D, Martens B, Hollander A, van der Beek E (1997). Respiratory allergy in laboratory animal workers: A retrospective cohort study using pre-employment screening data. *Occup Environ Med* 11: 830–835

56 Heederik D (2003) Allergen exposure and occupational respiratory allergy and asthma. In: MJ Nieuwenhuijsen (ed): *Exposure Assessment in Occupational and Environmental Epidemiology*. Oxford University Press, Oxford, UK

57 Peretz C, de Pater N, de Monchy J, Oostenbrink J, Heederik D (2005) Assessment of exposure to wheat flour and the shape of its relationship with specific sensitization. *Scand J Work Environ Health* 31: 65–74

58 Jacobs JH, Meijster T, Meijer E, Suarthana E, Heederik D (2008) Wheat allergen exposure and the prevalence of work-related sensitization and allergy in bakery workers. *Allergy* 63: 1597–1604

59 Rijnkels JM, Smid T, Van den Aker EC, Burdorf A, van Wijk RG, Heederik DJ, Houben GF, Van Loveren H, Pal TM, Van Rooy FG, Van der Zee JS; Health Council of the Netherlands (2008) Prevention of work-related airway allergies; summary of the advice from the Health Council of the Netherlands. *Allergy* 63: 1593–1596

60 Platts-Mills T, Vaughan J, Squillace S, Woodfolk J, Sporik R (2001) Sensitisation, asthma, and a modified Th2 response in children exposed to cat allergen: A population-based cross-sectional study. *Lancet* 357; 752–756

61 Platts-Mills TA, Vaughan JW, Blumenthal K, Pollart Squillace S, Sporik RB (2001) Serum IgG and IgG4 antibodies to Fel d 1 among children exposed to 20 microg Fel d 1 at home: Relevance of a nonallergic modified Th2 response. *Int Arch Allergy Immunol* 124: 126–129

62 Matsui EC, Krop EJ, Diette GB, Aalberse RC, Smith AL, Eggleston PA (2004) Mouse allergen exposure and immunologic responses: IgE-mediated mouse sensitization and mouse specific IgG and IgG4 levels. *Ann Allergy Asthma Immunol* 93: 171–8

63 Matsui EC, Diette GB, Krop EJ, Aalberse RC, Smith AL, Curtin-Brosnan J, Eggleston PA (2005) Mouse allergen-specific immunoglobulin G and immunoglobulin G4 and allergic symptoms in immunoglobulin E-sensitized laboratory animal workers. *Clin Exp Allergy* 35: 1347–1353

64 Portengen L, de Meer G, Doekes G, Heederik D (2004) Immunoglobulin G4 antibodies to rat urinary allergens, sensitization and symptomatic allergy in laboratory animal workers. *Clin Exp Allergy* 34: 1243–1250

65 Eduard W, Douwes J, Omenaas E, Heederik D (2004) Do farming exposures cause or prevent asthma? Results from a study of adult Norwegian farmers. *Thorax* 59: 381–386

66 Portengen L, Preller L, Tielen M, Doekes G, Heederik D (2005) Endotoxin exposure and atopic sensitization in adult pig farmers. *J Allergy Clin Immunol* 115: 797–802

67 Smit LA, Zuurbier M, Doekes G, Wouters IM, Heederik D, Douwes J (2007) Hay fever and asthma symptoms in conventional and organic farmers in The Netherlands. *Occup Environ Med* 64: 101–107

68 Smit L, Heederik D, Doekes G, Lammers J-W, Wouters I (2010) Occupational endotoxin exposure reduces the risk of atopic sensitization but increases the risk of bronchial hyperresponsiveness. *Int Arch Allergy Immunol* 152: 151–158

Gene-environment interactions in occupational asthma

Francine Kauffmann[1,2], *Francesc Castro-Giner*[3,4,5], *Lidwien A. M. Smit*[1,2], *Rachel Nadif*[1,2] *and Manolis Kogevinas*[3,4,5,6]

[1]Inserm, U780 – Epidemiology and Biostatistics, Villejuif, France
[2]Université Paris Sud, IFR69, Villejuif, France
[3]Center for Research in Environmental Epidemiology (CREAL), Barcelona, Spain
[4]Municipal Institute of Medical Research, Barcelona, Spain
[5]CIBER Epidemiologia y Salud Publica (CIBERESP), Spain
[6]Medical School, University of Crete, Heraklion, Greece

Abstract

This chapter reviews the existing knowledge regarding gene-environment interactions in occupational asthma. So far, studies have been conducted on relatively small samples, considering workers exposed to specific hazards such as isocyanates or red cedar. HLA class II, genes in the antioxidant defense, and more recently genes in the innate immunity pathway have been studied. As yet, few interactions have been demonstrated; however, the development of large-scale genetic studies of asthma will likely change the situation. Two types of approach can be developed based on testing hypotheses (candidate interactions) or in searching interactions with genes of yet-unknown function that may be evidenced through genome-wide associations. Current challenges concern the improvement of phenotypic and environmental characterization and setting up interdisciplinary research to understand the determinants of asthma. Building large international consortia on asthma with data on occupational exposure is warranted.

Introduction

It is only recently that active search for both environmental and genetic determinants of common diseases, such as asthma has been undertaken [1, 2]. For classical occupational diseases such as coal workers' pneumoconiosis, associations of exposure with disease could be very strong. For such disease, exposure was a necessary cause. On the other hand, not all those exposed develop the disease, leading to the idea of individual susceptibility. However, there was some reluctance to search genetic determinants because of concerns about the potential use of the results. Moreover, the technology available for studying genetic factors was limited. In one word, there was moderate interest for genetics by (traditional) epidemiologists. What were then called "genetic diseases" were in fact monogenic diseases and without the deleterious variant, the disease did not exist. Finding the relevant gene

Occupational Asthma, edited by Torben Sigsgaard and Dick Heederik

was done through familial studies on affected subjects by positional cloning. The association of the identified deleterious variants with disease was usually very high. Geneticists talked of penetrance to explain why not all individuals with the variant get the disease. The heterogeneity of phenotypic expression was searched in relation to different variants of the gene, and possible gene-gene interactions, such as modifier genes in cystic fibrosis. In other words, geneticists had little interest in the environment at that time. It is now widely accepted that for complex diseases, such as asthma, a more balanced view regarding the role of environmental and genetic determinants is warranted.

Occupational asthma: A complex disease

Addressing the heterogeneity of asthma both at the phenotypic and etiological level is a priority of research [3]. In that context, occupational asthma represents one particular category of the disease among the persistent adult asthmas. Perhaps more than in other complex diseases that occur only in adulthood, time is a crucial element in asthma, a disease that can occur over the whole lifespan. Figure 1 shows

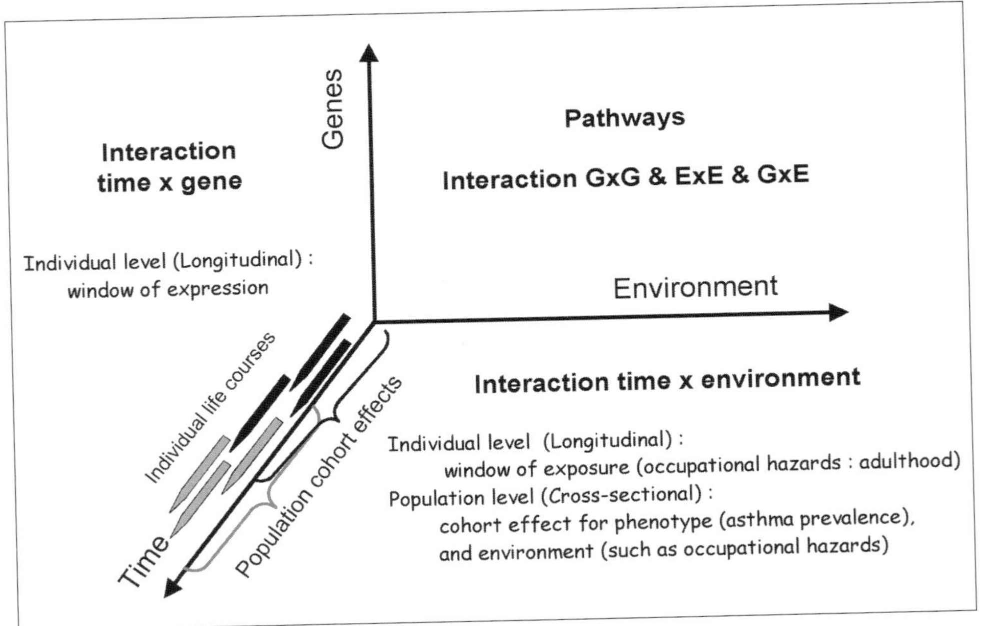

Figure 1.
Environment, genes, and time.

that time plays a role both through cohort effects and during the lifespan of individuals of the same cohort. For example, the prevalence of asthma has increased two- or threefold during the last few decades, and occupational exposures in the industrial and tertiary workforce have changed both qualitatively and quantitatively. During the life of an individual, it is critical to consider the window of environmental exposure, i.e., when a specific exposure occurs, and the window of genetic expression, i.e., when a given gene will play a role. Although time invariant, genotypes do not play the same role over the lifespan. For example, some genes can play a specific role in childhood growth or in the occurrence of adult onset asthma. Early infancy appears to be a critical period for the development of allergy and asthma. According to the so-called hygiene hypothesis, early contact with microbial agents, for instance through contact with livestock may protect from allergy by influencing immune system development. This hypothesis is consistent with immunological and epidemiological observations, but it is still lacking direct proof [4]. Adolescence with the occurrence of puberty, changing lifestyle and the beginning of occupational exposures during training is a sensitive period. In occupational asthma, interactions of genes with occupational exposures will occur in individuals who already have a history regarding exposure to allergy and asthma risk factors since birth. This is less the case for other work-related diseases, which do not share as many features with non-occupational diseases. Interactions between various genes, various environmental factors and between genes and environmental factors act through specific pathways, and it is important to note that pathways are "ignorant" of the source of the exposures. In other words, the underlying mechanisms explaining occupational asthma are general pathways that depend on numerous non-occupational factors.

Whereas occupational factors are not always adequately considered in general reviews regarding the etiology of asthma, occupational asthma may provide a model to study asthma in general through a semi-experimental situation, inasmuch as the start of exposure may be determined. Thus, understanding gene-environment interactions in the context of occupational asthma may provide clues to key pathways. As detailed elsewhere in the book, occupational asthma is now considered the main respiratory occupational disease in developed countries, and has been related to exposure to many different substances (more than 300 have been described), with a recent interest in irritants as a potential additional cause [5]. Most of the studies have been conducted in occupational cohorts, a very efficient method for assessing exposure, but one that is subject to the healthy worker effect bias. The other approach, by looking at the general population, is less subject to the healthy worker effect, but faces the problem of assessing exposure. Methods have been developed to assess exposure in these instances, such as asthma-specific job-exposure matrices, as described in other chapters. It is worth noting that there has not as yet been a single published study on gene-environment interaction regarding occupational asthma in general populations. Most studies with occupational characterization have not included data on genetic factors and most genetic studies on asthma have not included data on occupational exposures.

The limited evidence regarding gene-environment studies suggests questioning the pertinence of the issue: 'Why do we need to study genetics in occupational asthma?' 'What will we gain from knowledge of genetics in the occupational setting?' As mentioned before, reluctance to conduct these studies may relate to anxiety regarding the potential use of findings on gene-environment interactions in the context of occupational exposures. It should be stated clearly that such knowledge is needed to improve the understanding of asthma and not to propose the selection of workers based on genetic factors. It is the work that should be adapted to the most vulnerable. Legal protection regarding potential discrimination in relation to genetic tests has been addressed both in Europe, and more recently in United States [6, 7]. While remaining vigilant about the implications of research, occupational epidemiologists should do more studies on the combined effects of genes and environment to improve the understanding of such complex diseases, to ultimately improve primary and secondary prevention [8, 9].

This chapter reviews the existing knowledge and discusses strategies in the changing context of genetic research. A glossary of genetic terms is given to help the reader (Tab. 1). The candidate interactions strategy, based on *a priori* hypotheses or knowledge is discussed. Finally, new challenges regarding the search of gene-environment interactions for occupational asthma are discussed in the context of genome-wide associations.

Table 1. Glossary of genetics terminology

Genetic term	Definition
Gene	The fundamental unit of heredity, made up of a sequence of DNA that can be transcribed into messenger RNA and translated into protein.
Chromosome	An organized gene-carrying structure composed primarily of DNA and protein.
Genome	The whole set of DNA of an organism or a species.
Phenotype	Observable traits or characteristics of an individual.
Gene expression	The process by which inheritable information from a gene is made into a functional gene product such as messenger RNA and protein. Gene expression may be modulated as a response to different developmental and environmental factors.
Common disease or Complex disease	A disease or trait that is the result of multiple genetic and environmental factors and the interaction between them. Asthma is regarded as a complex disease.

Monogenic disease or Mendelian disease	Relatively rare disease caused by a modification in a single gene.
Penetrance	The probability that a genetic variant will be expressed on a phenotypic level. For example, if the penetrance is 100% (completely penetrant), then all individuals with the genetic variant will express the phenotype.
Locus	A position on a chromosome of a gene or other chromosome marker.
Allele	Alternative form of a genetic locus; a single allele for each locus is inherited from each parent. The term allele is also used to refer to DNA sequence variants.
Genotype	The genetic constitution of an organism; genotype can refer to the entire genetic makeup, or the alleles at a specific locus.
Single Nucleotide Polymorphism (SNP)	DNA sequence variation in a single nucleotide.
Functional SNP	SNP that influences a trait in a measurable way by altering the activity of the protein or the gene expression.
Haplotype	Combination of genetic markers at different sites present on neighboring, closely linked loci on the same chromosome.
Linkage disequilibrium	Describes the situation in which alleles occur together more often than can be accounted for by chance.
Haplotype tagging SNPs	A relatively small subset of representative SNPs that are needed to uniquely identify a complete haplotype.
Positional cloning	Method to identify a gene for a specific disease or trait based on its chromosomal location.
Candidate gene	A known gene which is suspected to be associated with the disease or trait under study on the basis of the biological function of its protein.
Genome-wide Association Study (GWAS)	Association study with a large set of genetic markers (up to 1 000 000) which captures a large proportion of common variation in the human genome sequence. The objective is to identify susceptibility genes associated with a disease or trait.
Multiple Comparisons	Refers to the problem that arises when multiple hypotheses are tested, and some significant results are expected even if the null hypothesis is true.
False Discovery Rate (FDR) control	An approach to correct for multiple comparisons. FDR is the expected ratio of erroneous rejections of null hypotheses to the total number of rejected hypotheses.

Literature review

Gene-environment interactions have been reported for only some of the agents known to cause occupational asthma. In general, studies were based on small sample sizes and not always comparable phenotypes. Most studies investigated workers exposed to isocyanates, which is to date the most evaluated occupational exposure with at least 13 studies (Tab. 2). The genes evaluated reflect the two main pathogenetic mechanisms suggested for isocyanates: immunological and oxidative stress. Interaction with the gene for human leukocyte antigen-II (*HLAII*) has been evaluated in 6 studies [10–15], leading to contradictory results but suggesting a critical role of the *HLAII DQB1* locus. Three studies evaluating polymorphisms in glutathione S-transferases (*GSTs*), which are enzymes involved in antioxidant defense, have shown the importance of this mechanism in the protection against isocyanate damage [16–18]. Other genes that have been associated with isocyanate-induced asthma are involved in the metabolism of these compounds (*N*-acetyltransferases *NAT1* and *NAT2*), and in the inflammatory response [interleukin *(IL)-4* receptor α chain, *IL-13*, *CD14*, and neurokinin 2 receptor] [18–20]. More recently, in the first genome-wide association study (GWAS) performed on occupational asthma, Kim and co-workers [21] identified the catenin alpha 3, alpha-T catenin gene (*CTNNA3*) as a new candidate for susceptibility to isocyanate-induced asthma.

Studies investigating other occupational exposures, including low-molecular-weight sensitizers (acid anhydrides, platinum, plicatic acid), aluminum emissions, and laboratory animal allergens are summarized in Table 3 and some illustrative examples are presented in Tables 4 and 5. Most studies are underpowered, with only two studies including at least 100 cases [22, 23]. In addition, there is almost a complete lack of replication of results from these studies. Polymorphisms of the *HLA* system have been associated with occupational asthma and/or sensitization related to acid anhydrides [24–26], platinum [27], western red cedar wood [28], and laboratory animal allergens [22, 29]. Two studies evaluating asthma among aluminum smelter workers did not find significant associations for the genes assessed [30, 31]. A study among young farmers (16–26 years) did not find associations between genes of the innate immunity pathway (*CD14*, *TLR2*, or *TLR4*) and new-onset asthma [23]. However, a statistically significant effect of *CD14/-260* and *CD14/-651* on atopy was reported, and effects of both *CD14* single nucleotide polymorphisms (SNPs) appeared to be stronger among farmers who were born and raised on a farm.

Table 2. Gene-environment interactions in asthma. Exposure to isocyanates.

Place (ref)	Type of study	Phenotype	Genes, genotype	Exposure	Cases/ controls	Main results
France and Italy [12]	Case-control	Occupational asthma	*HLAII-DQA1* *HLAII-DQB1* *HLAII-DPB1* *HLAII-DR*	TDI	28/16	Risk alleles: *DQB1*0503* and *DQB1*0201/0301* Protective alleles: *DQB1*0501*, *DQA1*0101*, and *DQA1*0101-DQB1*0501-DR1* haplotype
Italy [10]	Case-control	Occupational asthma	*HLAII-DQA1* *HLAII-DQB1*	TDI	30/12 and 126 non-exposed	Frequency in cases vs controls *DQB1*0503*: 30% vs 0%; pc=NS *DQB1*0501*: 0% vs 25%; pc=0.04, RR=0.044 Frequency in cases vs non-exposed *DQB1*0503*: 30% vs 13%; pc=0.05, RR=2.95
USA [11]	Case-control	Occupational asthma	*HLAII-DRB1* *HLAII-DQB1*	MDI, TDI, HDI	10/15	Non-significant results
Central Europe [15]	Case-control	Occupational asthma Total and specific IgE	*HLAII-DRB1* *HLAII-DQB1* *HLAII-DQA1*	MDI, TDI, HDI	32/23 and 90 non-exposed	Non-significant results
Italy [14]	Case-control	Occupational asthma	*HLAII-DQA1* *HLAII-DQB1* *HLAII-DRB1*	TDI	67/27	Frequency in cases vs controls *DQA1*0104*: 24% vs 0%; $p=0.005$ *DQB1*0503*: 21% vs 0%; $p=0.005$ *DQA1*0101*: 10% vs 37%; $p=0.004$ *DQB1*0501*: 13% vs 37%; $p=0.01$
Italy [48]	Case-control	Occupational asthma	*HLAI A, B,* *CTNF-α*: A308G	TDI	*HLA-I*: 16/41 *TNF-α*: 142/45	Non-significant results

Table 2. (continued)

Place (ref)	Type of study	Phenotype	Genes, genotype	Exposure	Cases/ controls	Main results
Korea [13]	Case-control	Occupational asthma	*HLAI A, B, C* *HLAII-DRB1* *HLAII-DQB1* *HLAII-DPB1*	TDI	55/47 and 95 non-exposed	Frequency in cases vs controls *DRB1*15–DPB1*05*: 11% vs 0%; $p=0.001$ Frequency in cases vs non-exposed controls *DRB1*15–DPB1*05*: 11% vs 2.5%; $p=0.003$
Finland [17]	Case-control	Occupational asthma IgE levels Specific bronchial provocation	*GSTM1*: null(–) *GSTM3*: A, B *GSTP1*: Val105/ Ile105 *GSTT1*: null(–)	MDI, HDI, TDI	109/73	*GSTM1(–)*: OR=1.89 (1.01–3.52) asthma, OR=0.18 (0.05–0.61) specific IgE *GSTM3* AA: OR=3.75(1.26–11) late reaction *GSTP1*Val/Val: OR=5.46 (1.15–26) specific IgE *GSTM1(–)* + *GSTM3* AA: OR=0.09 (0.01–0.73) specific IgE, OR=11.0 (2.19–55) late reaction
Italy [16]	Case-control	Occupational asthma BHR	*GSTP1:* Val105Ile	TDI	92/39	*GSTP1* Val/Val vs Ile/Ile: OR=0.23(0.05–1.13) Protective effect is greater at a longer duration of exposure
Finland [18]	Case-control	Occupational asthma	*NAT1* and *NAT2*: slow acetylation genotypes *GSTM1*: null(–) *GSTM3*: A, B *GSTP1*: Val105/ Ile105 GSTT1: null(–)	MDI, TDI, HDI	109/73	*NAT1*sa: OR=2.54 (1.32–4.91) diisocyanate *NAT1*sa: OR=7.77 (1.18–52) TDI *NAT1*sa+*GSTM1*null: OR=4.20 (1.51–12) *NAT2*sa+*NAT1*sa: OR=3.12 (1.11–8.78) *NAT2*sa+*GSTM1*null: OR=4.53 (1.76–12)
Korea [20]	Case-control	Occupational asthma BHR IgE and IgG VEGF	*NK2R*: G7853A, G11424A	TDI	59/93	Non-significant results for case-control study 7853 GG: increased VEGF levels in exposed; $p=0.04$

Canada [19]	Case-control	Occupational asthma	*IL4RA* *IL13* *CD14*	MDI, TDI, HDI	62/75	Significant results only for HDI: *IL4RA* 50Ile/Ile: OR=3.29 (1.33–8.14) *IL4RA* 50Ile/Ile + IL13 110Arg/Arg: OR=4.13 (1.35–13) *IL4RA* 50Ile/Ile + *CD14/*–159CT: OR=5.20 (1.82–15) *IL4RA* 50Ile/Ile + *IL-13* 110Arg/Arg + *CD14/*–159CT: OR=6.40 (1.57–26)
Korea [21]	Case-control	Occupational asthma	GWAS	TDI	84/263	*CTNNA3* rs10762058: OR=1.68 (1.15–2.47) rs7088181: OR=1.80 (1.24–2.61) rs4378283: OR=1.68 (1.15–2.47)

Modified from [49].

BHR, bronchial hyperresponsiveness; *CTNNA3*, catenin alpha 3, alpha-T catenin; *GST*, glutathione S-transferase; GWAS, genome-wide association study; HDI, hexamethylene diisocyanate; *HLA*, human leukocyte antigen; *IL4RA*, interleukin 4 receptor α chain; *IL-13*, interleukin 13; MDI, methylene diisocyanate; *NAT*: N-acetyltransferase; *NK2R*, neurokinin 2 receptor; TDI, toluene diisocyanate; *TNF*-α, tumor necrosis factor alpha; VEGF, vascular endothelial growth factor

Table 3. Gene-environment interactions in asthma - Exposure to other occupational exposures.

Place (ref)	Type of study	Phenotype	Genes, genotype	Exposure	Cases/ controls	Main results
Australia [31]	Case-control	Occupational asthma and atopy	Alpha 1-antitrypsin: *M*, *MM*, *MS*, *MZ* *HLA* Ig: GM, KM allotypes	Aluminum emissions	33/127	Non-significant results
USA [30]	Case-control	Occupational asthma and atopy	*ADRB2*: Gly 16, Gln 27 High affinity-receptor of IgE: Gly237Glu *TNF*-α: A308G	Aluminum emissions	13/39	Non-significant results
UK [26]	Case-control	Sensitization to trimellitic anhydride	*HLA*	Acid anhydride	30/28	*DR3*: OR=6; $p=0.05$
Sweden [25]	Case-control	Sensitization to acid anhydride	*HLAI A, B, C* *HLAII-DR* *HLAII-DQ*	Acid anhydride	53/47	Frequency cases vs controls *A25*: 0% vs 9%; $p<0.05$ *A32*: 0% vs 13%; $p<0.01$
Sweden [24]	Case-control	Sensitization to acid anhydride	*HLAII-DQB1* *HLAII-DRB1*	Acid anhydride	52/73	*DQ5*: OR=4.3 (1.7–11) *DR1*: OR=3.0 (1.2–7.3) *DQB1*0501*: OR=3.0 (1.2–7.4)
South Africa [27]	Case-control	Skin prick test positive to ACP	*HLAII-DRB* *HLAII-DPB* *HLAII-DQA* *HLAII-DQB*	Platinum (Ammonium hexachloro-platinate ACP)	44/57	*D3*: OR=2.3 (1.0-5.6) *D6*: OR=0.4 (0.2-0.8) Associations are stronger in lower exposed subjects
Canada [28]	Case–control	Occupational asthma	*HLAII-DRB1* *HLAII-DQB1*	Western Red Cedar (plicatic acid)	56/63	*DQB1*0603*: OR=2.9; $p=0.05$ *DQB1*0302*: OR=4.9; $p=0.02$ *DQB1*0501*: OR=0.3; $p=0.02$ *DRB1*0401-DQB1*0302*: OR=10.3; $p=0.01$ *DRB1*0101-DQB1*0501*: OR=0.27; $p=0.04$

Sweden [29]	Case–control	Occupational allergy	*HLAI A, B, C* *HLAII-DR*	Laboratory animals	92/27	Frequency cases vs controls *B16*: 0% vs 30%; $p<0.05$
UK [22]	Case-control	Sensitization to rat lipocalin	*HLAII-DQB1* *HLAII-DRB1*	Laboratory rats (lipocalin allergens)	109/397	*DR7*: OR = 1.82 (1.12-2.97) sensitization *DR7*: OR=2.96 (1.64-5.37) work-related chest symptoms *DR7*: OR = 3.81 (1.90-7.65) sensitization and work-related chest symptoms *DR3*: OR = 0.55 (0.31-0.97) sensitization
US [50]	Case-control	Sensitization to lab animal allergens	*TLR4*: Asp299Gly, Thr399Ile	Laboratory animals, endotoxin	69/266	*TLR4* 299Gly: OR = 2.5 (1.5-5.5)
Denmark [23]	Nested case-control	New-onset asthma Atopy: skin prick test	*CD14*: C-651T, C-260T, C+1342A *TLR4*: Asp299Gly, Thr399Ile *TLR2*: A-16934T, Pro631His, Arg753Gln	Farm environment, endotoxin	100/88	*CD14*/-260T: OR = 0.39(0.21-0.72) atopy *CD14*/-651T: OR = 2.53(1.33-4.88) atopy

Modified from [49].
ADRB2, adrenergic receptor beta-2; *HLA*, human leukocyte antigen; *TNF-α*, tumor necrosis factor alpha; *TLR*, toll like receptor

Table 4. Example 1– Distribution of DRB1 *and* DQB1 HLA *class II alleles in occupational asthma due to western red cedar [28].*

	Cases (56)	**Controls (63)**	**OR [95%CI]**
*DRB1*0101*	7.1	23.4	0.25 [0.08-0.79]
*DQB1*0501*	10.7	28.1	0.30 [0.11-0.82]
*DQB1*0603*	23.2	9.4	2.90 [1.01-8.17]
*DQB1*0302*	19.6	4.7	4.90 [1.28-18.6]

For the case control comparison, 37 other alleles were tested (17 with at least 5% in controls).
Lowest p value = 0.0201 ; $-\log(p) = 1.7$ [28].

Table 5. Example 2 – Occupational sensitization to rat lipocalin allergens and specific symptoms [22].

A				
	Sensitized employees (*n*=109)	**Non sensitized employees (*n*=397)**	**UK blood donors (603)**	**OR [95% CI]**
*DRB1*03*	18.4	28.7	26.1	0.56 [0.33–0.95]
*DRB1*07*	39.5	28.5	26.7	1.64 [1.05–2.55]

B		
Logistic regression (including age, sex, exposure)	**Sensitization**	**Sensitization and work-related chest symptoms**
*DRB1*07*	1.8 [1.1–3.0]	3.8 [1.9–7.7]
Atopy	4.8 [2.9–3.6]	5.0 [2.41–10.5]
Daily work in animal housing facility	3.8 [1.9–7.4]	5.5 [1.8–16.5]

Candidate interactions

In the 'old' days, that is in the 1970s, researchers were studying ad hoc genes known at that time, such as *ABO* and *HLA*. Subsequently, there has been a move to the study of 'candidate genes', i.e., genes for which what was known on their physiological function appears relevant to explain the disease and a reasonable hypothesis for the interaction. By qualification of a gene as a candidate, geneticists mean that the gene is studied because of a hypothesis, as opposed to genome-wide approaches. This latter approach has been characterized by some as being agnostic (etymologically: without knowledge) research [32]. By analogy, gene-environment interactions defined by using previous knowledge can be named candidate interactions [33] (Tab. 6).

Knowledge may derive from preliminary findings regarding environment or genes. In the context of occupational asthma, environment-gene interaction research is primarily conducted using information on the potential mode of action of putative or established occupational asthmagens. As shown by the literature review above, interactions studied so far were based on a hypothesis-driven approach with genes implicated on allergen recognition, second line antioxidant defense, and inflammatory response. Starting from the environment calls for pathways rather than single genes, and until now it was more the excess rather than the lack of hypotheses regarding potential genes that was a limitation. Hypotheses can be formulated based on physiology, including animal models [34]. Because of the potential oxidative role of numerous occupational asthmagens, it may be relevant to study all genes in the antioxidant pathway, as well as all genes related to innate immunity when considering farming. However, very few studies have actually considered more than one gene from the same pathway in a given study.

Numerous new candidate interactions could be studied such as interactions of irritant exposures with genes from the transient receptor potential (*TRP*) family [35]. There is increasing concern that exposures to irritants less extreme than those observed in reactive airway syndrome occurring after inhalation accidents could lead to asthma. Thus, genes from the *TRP* family, which includes the channel receptor for capsaicin and in particular *TRPV1* (also named vanilloid receptor, *VR1*) are good candidates. Capsaicin is a strong irritant, inducing a cough, and is an occupational hazard in chili pepper workers [36]. As women usually exhibit a more nocturnal cough, and cough at a lower level of exposure to capsaicin, it could be hypothesized that, in such an example, it is not asthma in general that should be studied but the subphenotype in which nocturnal cough is present and taking gender into account.

Studying all genes in the genome-wide association era?

Since 2007, numerous genome-wide associations have led to discoveries of new genes for a variety of disorders. A current format is to genotype for 100 000–1 000 000 SNPs per individual in series of at least 1000 cases and 1000 controls. In the Wellcome trust case-control study for example, 14 000 cases of seven common diseases (not asthma) were studied *versus* 3000 shared controls. It allows most established loci for these diseases to be replicated – an important proof of concept of the method – and to determine new pathways [37].

Table 6. Gene-environment interactions – From the simplest to the most complex strategy of analysis in the GWAS era.

Strategy	Rationale	Examples	Comments
I - Candidate interaction	(Known) pathway approach		
G known × E known	Precise hypothesis	*HLA* with TDI	+ Biological plausibility and easy interpretation More robust result – Subject to *a priori* knowledge
G known × E not very precise		*HLA*, *GST* with any asthmagen	+ Relevant in general population studies
II - No candidate interaction	Possibly find new pathway		– Need for replication in another population. – Possibly lack of biological plausibility Need for further experimental studies to determine the underlying biological process
E known for asthma × G known for asthma	Hypothesis driven: additive effect expected, test for synergy, possibly new pathway	TDI × *IL-13* Plicatic acid × *ADAM33*	+ Data will be available, low cost + Easy statistically – Lack of biological plausibility if function of both G and E are known but pertain to different pathways – Possibility of chance finding
Marginal effects first G asthma and E asthma	Most G × E interactions are weak	Studies on exposures without considering genetics Studies on genotypes without considering environment	+ Good power + Fits with GWAS strategy – Loss of G × E evidence

G × E for all genes	Focus on the question of interaction	Search of interactions of all genes with TDI (done by [21])	+ Not loosing the evidence of interaction – Dimensional problem not solved – Exposures usually basic, or sample size problem
Subphenotypes first (independent of exposure)	Relevance for occupational exposure (adult onset, immunological or non immunological, etc.)	GWAS on IgE-dependent occupational asthma, studies on asthma with irritant cough	+ Increase strength of association, address phenotypic heterogeneity – Small samples – Need of collaboration
All G with all E	No *a priori* hypothesis of any sort	Consider hundreds of occupational asthmagens or all putative environmental determinants of asthma with all genes	Huge problem of multiple comparison, E not well measured

G, gene; E, environment
+ Advantage of the strategy
– Limitation of the strategy
ADAM33, a disintegrin and metalloprotease 33; *GST*, glutathione S-transferase; GWAS, genome-wide association study; *HLA*, human leukocyte antigen; *IL-13*, interleukin 13; TDI, toluene diisocyanate

A genome-wide association study (GWAS) for asthma was performed in the Gabriel European consortium among children [38]. Potential associations of asthma (yes/no, simply defined) with approximately 300 000 SNPs across the genome were searched. The analysis took into account multiple comparisons using the false discovery rate statistic. The results evidenced the role of *ORMDL3* on chromosome 17q21, with the first replication sample from the International Study of Asthma and Allergies in Childhood (ISAAC) [38]. An important aspect to consider is that, similar to GWAS in other diseases, the effect size was small, with an odds ratio for *ORMDL3* of only 1.5. Hence, the new genes that are currently being discovered may correspond to weak associations with the phenotype under study. Analyses conducted in the French epidemiological study on the genetics and environment of asthma (EGEA) have confirmed the association of 17q21 variants with asthma and showed that, in this population including both children and adults, the association was restricted to early-onset asthma [39], and therefore not a candidate for occupational asthma. In the future, industrial samples will also be included in such GWAS, and it is anticipated that genes common to asthma in general and specific to the exposures will be found. In addition, it would be interesting to study genes in relation to intermediate phenotypes or subphenotypes in contrasted groups of exposure. However, very large numbers are needed to allow interactions with specific exposures, and the necessary pooling and replication raise questions regarding population ascertainment, comparability of phenotypes, the heterogeneity of exposure, and geographical/ethnic differences regarding allele frequencies.

Although starting from hypotheses related to occupational asthmagens was the primary rationale in the past, the situation may evolve with the evaluation of results from GWAS. An example of this is the search of exposure by gene interactions that is using previous knowledge on exposure to choose the genes to study. Using the increasing knowledge on new genes (e.g., the association with age at onset or a precise knowledge of its function) should help to focus the search of genes involved in occupational hazard exposure interactions. To discover gene-environment interactions, strategies without hypotheses are also possible, but these face major problems of sample size. Although too underpowered to be really conclusive, the first GWAS conducted for toluene diisocyanate (TDI)-induced asthma suggested the involvement of a gene not previously hypothesized to play a role (*CTNNA3*) [21]. However, as there is no specific hypothesis for interaction with TDI, the primary replication to be performed may be with asthma in general, and not specifically with TDI-induced occupational asthma. On the other hand, it could point to a gene specific for the subphenotype of TDI-induced occupational asthma. In that case, replication with appropriate confidence would need a much larger sample size.

If GWAS show genes with an already known function, the strategy that should be followed is that of candidate interactions, i.e., using the existing knowledge. In the case of discoveries of genes with unknown function, other strategies may be implemented. Table 6 illustrates that numerous strategies are possible to assess environment by gene interactions from the most hypothesis-driven to the most agnostic ones. Some are common; some may seem unfeasible for now. Unless the interaction is hypothesized to be massive, it can also be argued that it is more appropriate to look first at marginal effects instead of looking at every environment in potential interaction with every genetic marker.

Challenges on the genetic, phenotypic, and environmental aspects

Multiple comparisons

Multiple comparisons are not a new issue. In the example presented in Table 4, the odds ratio of 4.9 for *DQB1*302* in relation to exposure to red cedar asthma has to be put in the context of the study in which 37 different alleles were tested [28]. The association is not statistically significant if the number of comparisons is taken into account. To illustrate the issue of multiple comparisons, a p value of 5×10^{-6}, i.e., $-\log(p)$ around 6, is needed in the context of GWAS done with 300 000 SNPs, such as in Gabriel [38] based on a 5% false discovery rate, i.e., a classical p value for a simple comparison. If one considers now an MHC-wide test for only 1270 SNPs, $-\log(p)$ needs to be around 4.4, based on Bonferroni correction [40]. However, if the significance of only 183 *HLA* class II SNPs were examined in that array, $-\log(p)$ would decrease to 3.6 [41]. Finally, if looking only at 3 SNPs in the *CTNNA3* gene for example, the requested p value for significance will remain in the area of classical studies.

Extracting the relevant information from large tables, such as those of GWAS is difficult

Informatic tools are currently being developed to reduce extremely large data sets to study either gene-gene or gene-environment interactions [42, 43]. Other methods, hypothesis-driven, can be considered, e.g., Bayesian combination of candidate genes, using the accumulation of knowledge on the first genes to go further either by studying genes in a given pathway (such as a gene controlling the production of a protein and the gene controlling the receptor of that protein) or not (such as by taking into consideration prior evidence – possibly belief – regarding the role of genetic determinants). Relaxing the level of significance when studying associations with selected exposures may be considered, i.e., balancing the cost benefit of lack of power and false discovery. Note that in searching for an association with genes, we are in a situation different from that in a clinical trial: a wrong conclusion will not kill any patient to whom the inappropriate treatment is given, we just loose time by pursuing on wrong hypotheses that will not be replicated.

A difficulty in the current period when studying candidate genes is the mode of choice of SNPs in large series of genotyping. If they are chosen based only on known function, the possibility of discovering new genes is limited. If they are chosen based only on haplotype blocks, the possibility of testing functional SNPs is limited. Furthermore, it is current practice not to genotype low frequency alleles due to power issues, whereas these may be the functional ones. It is well possible that the common disease-common variant model will not be sufficient to understand complex diseases such as asthma, and that rare alleles of major effect may explain the observed heterogeneity [44]. To address this question, the relevance of sequencing DNA in the context of specific studies is currently discussed. Such a strategy puts emphasis on improving the genetic characterization. Clearly, the appropriate balance in the improvement of phenotypic, environmental and genetic characterization is a challenge.

Looking at the appropriate phenotype is a challenge

What needs to be done after finding some new genes associated with asthma? Since GWAS in asthma and other diseases tend to evaluate a single phenotype that can be easily measured in different studies, the next step should probably be to look back at that same question but with improved phenotyping. One proposal is that the second step should be to consider a few of the SNPs (e.g., less than 10) evidenced for the "new" gene and to search associations with numerous phenotypes, i.e., the phenome. The order of magnitude may then be of the order of 1000 comparisons, representing a problem much easier to handle statistically than comparisons on 300 000 SNPs. This analysis on subphenotypes may suggest clues regarding the function of the gene. Subphenotypes may relate to age of onset, allergic characteristics, but more generally to a variety of subphenotypes. Asthma starting in adulthood is a pertinent subphenotype regarding the role of occupational determinants, whereas the subphenotype of asthma active in adulthood is pertinent regarding the role of occupational factors implicated in work-aggravated asthma as well as (new-onset) occupational asthma. Obviously other means to understand gene function exist (including expression studies, animal models, etc.). The difficulty with the above phenome strategy will come from the absolute need for replication. Therefore, either such studies should be planned when relatively similar phenotypic characterization exists in various data sets, or when it is easy to improve phenotypic characterization very quickly. Large consortia with standardized detailed phenotyping are necessary and such consortia are currently being built.

There is a need of refining phenotypic characterization in complex diseases such as asthma. Improved phenotyping concerns clinical phenotypes with the development of more international standards. Further, ordinal or quantitative scores instead of dichotomous (diagnosis) definitions seem of great interest. That particular aspect is similar to issues regarding classification of occupational exposures using probability and intensity in job exposure matrices, instead of yes/no criteria. Another aspect is to study intermediate phenotypes, sometimes called endophenotypes. This may vary from total IgE, to gene expression data obtained from RNA, or to proteomics, which is likely to represent a source of major improvement in phenotypic characterization in the next few years. Such data are often quantitative. However, it is not always obvious whether they are true intermediate phenotypes (i.e., between the gene and the disease) or only associated traits (i.e., possibly a consequence of the disease). In fact, the pertinent item is not an SNP, or a gene, but rather biological pathways. Improving phenotypic characterization towards more biological-oriented approaches should be an efficient means to decrease the multiple comparison issue, using for example Bayesian approaches.

After that step, potential interactions with the environment may remain totally obscure or not. A genetic variant only associated with childhood onset asthma will not be a good candidate for interaction with occupational exposure; a genetic variant only associated with asthma with nocturnal cough might be candidate for an interaction with exposure to irritants, etc. If a candidate interaction approach cannot be taken after step 2, a step 3 approach could be implemented that searches all the potential interactions of the few SNPs (less than 5) with very few subphenotypes (less than 5), considering now all the environmental characteristics (termed the envirome or exposome). Here again, the number of variables will remain much lower than for the genetic variants, probably the same order of magnitude as for the phenome phase, i.e., 1000 variables. Again, without a replication sample, such a strategy cannot be set up.

Improving environmental characterization is a challenge

There is a general need for standardization in an interdisciplinary context. Measurement bias is known for genotypes by geneticists, for phenotypes by epidemiologists and clinicians, for exposures by environmental epidemiologists and toxicologists. Interdisciplinary teams should address those comprehensively [45]. The insufficiency of the precision regarding exposure is a key aspect, and as plied by Wild [46], it is necessary to complement the genome by an "exposome" with good precision. Beyond the disease phenotype, new "omics" such as proteomics and metabolomics should improve the assessment of exposure.

Conclusion

Research on gene-environment interactions in occupational asthma has been limited and findings have not been adequately replicated. Research regarding genetics in common diseases is rapidly evolving, and it is likely that in the next few years several new genes, possibly of yet-unknown function, will be suggested as potential determinants of asthma following GWAS. These genes with relatively common variants will probably have relatively weak effects but some of these genes may be relevant to study further and and help us understand the development and evolution of occupational asthma. Other studies will be needed to find potentially new genes with rare variants but larger effects, which may also explain the occurrence of occupational asthma. Based on hypotheses (candidate interactions) or directly using "omics" approaches on interactions by strategies not yet determined, new studies may help to find other genetic variants that interact with occupational asthmagens. The study of gene-environment interactions focused on occupational asthmagens will increase our understanding of the disease in general. It is important to remind that association does not mean prediction [47], and that risks need to be very high to predict disease in a given individual. Identification of gene-environment interactions, at least in the short term, will probably not help improve primary and secondary prevention of asthma or the management of the disease. Improvement of the evaluation of environmental/occupational exposures is needed for studies, irrespective of whether they consider or not the role of potential interactions with genetic determinants. Gene-environment interaction studies should not slow the study focused on the search for the associations of occupational exposures with asthma and prevention of such workplace exposures.

Acknowledgments

This review was supported by the Ga2len project (Global Allergy and Asthma European Network) EU-FOOD-CT-2004-506378 (working packages 2.9 and 2.4). F Castro-Giner was partly supported by a grant from the MaratoTV3, Catalonia, Spain. LAM Smit was supported by an European Academy of Allergy and Clinical Immunology (EAACI) – Ga^{2}len exchange fellowship.

References

1 Cookson W (1999) The alliance of genes and environment in asthma and allergy. *Nature* 402: B5–11

2 Ober C, Thompson EE (2005) Rethinking genetic models of asthma: The role of environmental modifiers. *Curr Opin Immunol* 17: 670–678

3 Wenzel SE (2006) Asthma: Defining of the persistent adult phenotypes. *Lancet* 368: 804–813

4 Strachan DP (2000) Family size, infection and atopy: The first decade of the "hygiene hypothesis". *Thorax* 55 (Suppl 1): S2–10

5 Zock JP, Plana E, Jarvis D, Anto JM, Kromhout H, Kennedy SM, Kunzli N, Villani S, Olivieri M, Toren K et al (2007) The use of household cleaning sprays and adult asthma: An international longitudinal study. *Am J Respir Crit Care Med* 176: 735–741

6 Hudson KL, Holohan MK, Collins FS (2008) Keeping pace with the times – The Genetic Information Nondiscrimination Act of 2008. *N Engl J Med* 358: 2661–2663

7 Van Hoyweghen I, Horstman K (2008) European practices of genetic information and insurance: Lessons for the Genetic Information Nondiscrimination Act. *JAMA* 300: 326–327

8 Khoury MJ, Gwinn M, Yoon PW, Dowling N, Moore CA, Bradley L (2007) The continuum of translation research in genomic medicine: How can we accelerate the appropriate integration of human genome discoveries into health care and disease prevention? *Genet Med* 9: 665–674

9 Schulte PA, Lomax GP, Ward EM, Colligan MJ (1999) Ethical issues in the use of genetic markers in occupational epidemiologic research. *J Occup Environ Med* 41: 639–646

10 Balboni A, Baricordi OR, Fabbri LM, Gandini E, Ciaccia A, Mapp CE (1996) Association between toluene diisocyanate-induced asthma and DQB1 markers: A possible role for aspartic acid at position 57. *Eur Respir J* 9: 207–210

11 Bernstein JA, Munson J, Lummus ZL, Balakrishnan K, Leikauf G (1997) T-cell receptor V beta gene segment expression in diisocyanate-induced occupational asthma. *J Allergy Clin Immunol* 99: 245–250

12 Bignon JS, Aron Y, Ju LY, Kopferschmitt MC, Garnier R, Mapp C, Fabbri LM, Pauli G, Lockhart A, Charron D et al (1994) HLA class II alleles in isocyanate-induced asthma. *Am J Respir Crit Care Med* 149: 71–75

13 Kim SH, Oh HB, Lee KW, Shin ES, Kim CW, Hong CS, Nahm DH, Park HS (2006) HLA DRB1*15–DPB1*05 haplotype: A susceptible gene marker for isocyanate-induced occupational asthma? *Allergy* 61: 891–894

14 Mapp CE, Beghe B, Balboni A, Zamorani G, Padoan M, Jovine L, Baricordi OR, Fabbri LM (2000) Association between HLA genes and susceptibility to toluene diisocyanate-induced asthma. *Clin Exp Allergy* 30: 651–656

15 Rihs HP, Barbalho-Krolls T, Huber H, Baur X (1997) No evidence for the influence of HLA class II in alleles in isocyanate-induced asthma. *Am J Ind Med* 32: 522–527

16 Mapp CE, Fryer AA, De Marzo N, Pozzato V, Padoan M, Boschetto P, Strange RC, Hemmingsen A, Spiteri MA (2002) Glutathione S-transferase GSTP1 is a susceptibility gene for occupational asthma induced by isocyanates. *J Allergy Clin Immunol* 109: 867–872

17 Piirila P, Wikman H, Luukkonen R, Kaaria K, Rosenberg C, Nordman H, Norppa H, Vainio H, Hirvonen A (2001) Glutathione S-transferase genotypes and allergic responses to diisocyanate exposure. *Pharmacogenetics* 11: 437–445

18 Wikman H, Piirila P, Rosenberg C, Luukkonen R, Kaaria K, Nordman H, Norppa H, Vainio H, Hirvonen A (2002) N-Acetyltransferase genotypes as modifiers of diisocyanate exposure-associated asthma risk. *Pharmacogenetics* 12: 227–233

19 Bernstein DI, Wang N, Campo P, Chakraborty R, Smith A, Cartier A, Boulet LP, Malo

JL, Yucesoy B, Luster M et al (2006) Diisocyanate asthma and gene-environment interactions with IL4RA, CD-14, and IL-13 genes. *Ann Allergy Asthma Immunol* 97: 800–806

20 Ye YM, Kang YM, Kim SH, Kim CW, Kim HR, Hong CS, Park CS, Kim HM, Nahm DH, Park HS (2006) Relationship between neurokinin 2 receptor gene polymorphisms and serum vascular endothelial growth factor levels in patients with toluene diisocyanate-induced asthma. *Clin Exp Allergy* 36: 1153–1160

21 Kim SH, Cho BY, Park CS, Shin ES, Cho EY, Yang EM, Kim CW, Hong CS, Lee JE, Park HS (2008) Alpha-T-catenin (CTNNA3) gene was identified as a risk variant for toluene diisocyanate-induced asthma by genome-wide association analysis. *Clin Exp Allergy* 39: 203–12

22 Jeal H, Draper A, Jones M, Harris J, Welsh K, Taylor AN, Cullinan P (2003) HLA associations with occupational sensitization to rat lipocalin allergens: A model for other animal allergies? *J Allergy Clin Immunol* 111: 795–799

23 Smit LA, Bongers SI, Ruven HJ, Rijkers GT, Wouters IM, Heederik D, Omland O, Sigsgaard T (2007) Atopy and new-onset asthma in young Danish farmers and CD14, TLR2, and TLR4 genetic polymorphisms: A nested case-control study. *Clin Exp Allergy* 37: 1602–1608

24 Jones MG, Nielsen J, Welch J, Harris J, Welinder H, Bensryd I, Skerfving S, Welsh K, Venables KM, Taylor AN (2004) Association of HLA-DQ5 and HLA-DR1 with sensitization to organic acid anhydrides. *Clin Exp Allergy* 34: 812–816

25 Nielsen J, Johnson U, Welinder H, Bensryd I, Rylander L, Skerfving S (1996) HLA and immune nonresponsiveness in workers exposed to organic acid anhydrides. *J Occup Environ Med* 38: 1087–1090

26 Young RP, Barker RD, Pile KD, Cookson WO, Taylor AJ (1995) The association of HLA-DR3 with specific IgE to inhaled acid anhydrides. *Am J Respir Crit Care Med* 151: 219–221

27 Newman Taylor AJ, Cullinan P, Lympany PA, Harris JM, Dowdeswell RJ, du Bois RM (1999) Interaction of HLA phenotype and exposure intensity in sensitization to complex platinum salts. *Am J Respir Crit Care Med* 160: 435–438

28 Horne C, Quintana PJ, Keown PA, Dimich-Ward H, Chan-Yeung M (2000) Distribution of DRB1 and DQB1 HLA class II alleles in occupational asthma due to western red cedar. *Eur Respir J* 15: 911–914

29 Sjostedt L, Willers S, Orbaek P (1996) Human leukocyte antigens in occupational allergy: A possible protective effect of HLA-B16 in laboratory animal allergy. *Am J Ind Med* 30: 415–420

30 Arnaiz NO, Kaufman JD, Daroowalla FM, Quigley S, Farin F, Checkoway H (2003) Genetic factors and asthma in aluminum smelter workers. *Arch Environ Health* 58: 197–200

31 Mackay IR, Oliphant RC, Laby B, Smith MM, Fisher JN, Mitchell RJ, Propert DN, Tait BD (1990) An immunologic and genetic study of asthma in workers in an aluminum smelter. *J Occup Med* 32: 1022–1026

32 Hoover RN (2007) The evolution of epidemiologic research: From cottage industry to "big" science. *Epidemiology* 18: 13–17
33 Kauffmann F, Nadif R (2007) Candidate interactions. *Eur Respir J* 30: 3–4
34 Willis-Owen SA, Valdar W (2009). Deciphering gene-environment interactions through mouse models of allergic asthma. *J Allergy Clin Immunol* 123: 14–23
35 Brooks SM (2008) Irritant-induced chronic cough: Irritant-induced TRPpathy. *Lung* 186 (Suppl 1): S88–93
36 Blanc P, Liu D, Juarez C, Boushey HA (1991) Cough in hot pepper workers. *Chest* 99: 27–32
37 Wellcome Trust Case Control Consortium (2007) Genome-wide association study of 14 000 cases of seven common diseases and 3,000 shared controls. *Nature* 447: 661–678
38 Moffatt MF, Kabesch M, Liang L, Dixon AL, Strachan D, Heath S, Depner M, von Berg A, Bufe A, Rietschel E et al (2007) Genetic variants regulating ORMDL3 expression contribute to the risk of childhood asthma. *Nature* 448: 470–473
39 Bouzigon E, Corda E, Aschard H, Dizier MH, Boland A, Bousquet J, Chateigner N, Gormand F, Just J, Le Moual N et al (2008) Effect of 17q21 variants and smoking exposure in early-onset asthma. *N Engl J Med* 359: 1985–1994
40 Tharrault H, Le Moual N, Aschard H, Bouzigon E, Vervloet D, Siroux V, Dizier MH, Oryszczyn MP, Nadif R, Pin I et al (2008) Associations of asthma with 1270 SNPs from the MHC region and potential interactions with occupational asthmagens in adults from the EGEA study. *Am J Respir Crit Care Med* 177: A335
41 Horton R, Wilming L, Rand V, Lovering RC, Bruford EA, Khodiyar VK, Lush MJ, Povey S, Talbot CC Jr, Wright MW et al (2004) Gene map of the extended human MHC. *Nat Rev Genet* 5: 889–899
42 Bush WS, Dudek SM, Ritchie MD (2006) Parallel multifactor dimensionality reduction: A tool for the large-scale analysis of gene-gene interactions. *Bioinformatics* 22: 2173–2174
43 Motsinger-Reif AA, Dudek SM, Hahn LW, Ritchie MD (2008) Comparison of approaches for machine-learning optimization of neural networks for detecting gene-gene interactions in genetic epidemiology. *Genet Epidemiol* 32: 325–340
44 Gibson G (2009). Decanalization and the origin of complex disease. *Nat Rev Genet* 10: 134–140
45 Wong MY, Day NE, Luan JA, Chan KP, Wareham NJ (2003) The detection of gene-environment interaction for continuous traits: Should we deal with measurement error by bigger studies or better measurement? *Int J Epidemiol* 32: 51–57
46 Wild CP (2005) Complementing the genome with an "exposome": The outstanding challenge of environmental exposure measurement in molecular epidemiology. *Cancer Epidemiol Biomarkers Prev* 14: 1847–1850
47 Pepe MS, Janes H, Longton G, Leisenring W, Newcomb P (2004) Limitations of the odds ratio in gauging the performance of a diagnostic, prognostic, or screening marker. *Am J Epidemiol* 159: 882–890

48 Beghe B, Padoan M, Moss CT, Barton SJ, Holloway JW, Holgate ST, Howell WM, Mapp CE (2004) Lack of association of HLA class I genes and TNF alpha-308 polymorphism in toluene diisocyanate-induced asthma. *Allergy* 59: 61–64

49 Castro-Giner F, Kauffmann F, de Cid R, Kogevinas M (2006) Gene-environment interactions in asthma. *Occup Environ Med* 63: 776–786, 761

50 Pacheco K, Maier L, Silveira L, Goelz K, Noteware K, Luna B, du Bois R, Murphy J, Rose C (2008) Association of Toll-like receptor 4 alleles with symptoms and sensitization to laboratory animals. *J Allergy Clin Immunol* 122: 896–902 e894

Asthma in apprentice workers
The birth cohort parallel: Using apprentices as a powerful cohort design for studying occupational asthma

Denyse Gautrin and Jean-Luc Malo

Axe de recherche en santé respiratoire, Hôpital du Sacré-Coeur de Montréal, 5400 Gouin Blvd West, Montreal, Canada

Abstract

This chapter presents a review of longitudinal studies of apprentices in trades and professions entailing substantial risks for the development of occupational asthma (OA). Prospective studies of OA enable the assessment of host characteristics before apprentices/workers enter a particular workforce, thus before being exposed to a suspected etiological agent, as well as the early detection of sensitization to a specific work-related antigen and the evaluation of bronchial responsiveness before onset of symptoms of asthma. Since 1973, several cohort studies have been conducted in Europe and Canada among apprentices exposed to high- and low-molecular-weight agents. The investigated outcomes were, apart from OA, work-aggravated asthma, bronchial hyperresponsiveness, work-related symptoms and specific sensitization. The rate of onset of the relevant outcomes was high even after 1 year of training; the implications for setting timing of surveillance programs would be to screen for sensitization and symptoms in the first 2–3 years of apprenticeship. Several host factors assessed at baseline were identified as risk factors for the incidence of work-related outcomes. However, more investigations are needed to explore the extent to which the risk of work-related allergy and asthma increases with exposure characteristics during apprenticeship. Directions for research in the existing cohorts and in future ones are suggested.

Introduction

This chapter reviews studies of apprentices in trades and professions entailing substantial risks for the development of occupational asthma (OA). Most of the apprentice studies were designed with the objective of gaining a better understanding of the natural history of work-related asthma and identifying the host risk factors; a few of these aimed at a better characterization of the causal exposure.

Occupational Asthma, edited by Torben Sigsgaard and Dick Heederik

Concept of the model of occupational asthma

It was suggested by Becklake [1] that studying OA could provide useful information on the relationship between some environmental risk factors and the development of asthma since, with OA, etiological agents can be identified and measured. In the early nineties Malo and Chan-Yeung [2–4] proposed that the natural history of OA be used as an 'experimental' model in studying the development of asthma. This model enables the assessment of host characteristics before workers enter a particular workforce, thus before being exposed to a suspected etiological agent, as well as the early detection of sensitization to a specific work-related antigen [in the case of exposure to a high-molecular-weight (HMW) agent] and the evaluation of bronchial responsiveness before any possible onset of symptoms of asthma. Furthermore, the prognosis for asthmatics as well as the reversal of bronchial hyperresponsiveness (BHR) can be studied after workers are removed from exposure (Fig. 1).

To document the natural history of work-related asthma, the most suitable populations to study would be newly hired individuals, apprentices, or students in workplaces or vocational schools where there are high risk exposures. Since these groups are mostly naïve in terms of contact with work-specific allergens, the

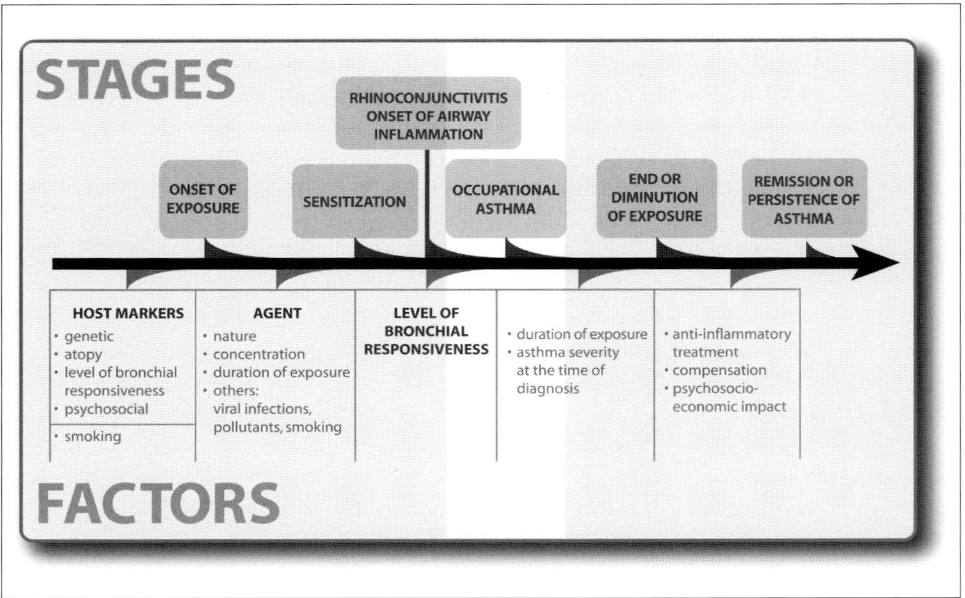

Figure 1.
Natural history of occupational asthma; stages of the natural history; factors influencing the onset and prognosis.

approach of choice would be to set up epidemiological prospective cohorts of these specific populations.

In prospective studies, subjects are selected on the basis that they are exposed to the factor under investigation, but in whom the disease has not yet manifested itself. The investigator must conduct a follow-up of the cohort members for an appropriate period to ascertain the disease's status; for example, the outcome(s) of interest. The most appropriate approach is to assemble the cohort prior to exposure, or upon their initial employment, thus allowing for the comparisons to be made internally; for example, between cases and non-cases to determine the effect of exposure and other potential determinants [5]. When the cause of the disease is known, prospective cohort studies may be undertaken to meticulously assess exposure to quantify exposure-response relationships. There are examples of recent longitudinal studies in workers exposed to laboratory animals or baker's allergens to explore exposure-response relationships with the long-term objective of reducing the incidence of allergic sensitization and respiratory symptoms through a better control of exposure [6].

From a different perspective, the natural history of asthma has been assessed in birth cohorts such as the well known Dunedin (New Zealand) study, initiated in 1972–1973, to study the development of a broad spectrum of diseases [7]. There have been European birth cohorts on asthma, allergic rhinitis and atopic diseases that were initiated in the 1990s in eight countries [8].

However, birth cohorts and apprentice cohorts on asthma present some similarities. They are both designed to assess periodically selected outcome measures for atopy, allergic sensitization to specific agents, rhinitis (allergic or not) and asthma. The cohort members are enrolled at birth or upon starting their apprenticeship while they are still naïve with respect to exposure(s) that is specific to their new environment; in particular to allergens. At that time point, the so-called baseline host characteristics and other potential risk factors, e.g., smoking (maternal/personal), are documented. Birth cohorts are usually assembled to represent the general population in a determined geographic area over 1 or more calendar years; whereas apprentice cohorts are restricted to individuals at risk of developing work-related asthma and related conditions, the latter possibly being more limited in terms of size since the expected rate of outcomes is greater than in birth cohorts. A major difference arises in the identification of the causal agent(s) with one or several ubiquitous allergens of various types (pets, pollens, mites, molds, etc.) in birth cohorts, as opposed to a limited number of agents specific to the environment of a particular training program such as, flour and α-amylase in baking apprenticeship.

The application of the model of occupational asthma

The profile of individuals prior to being exposed at work/during apprenticeship can be assessed through a number of tools. Questionnaires, in particular those developed for the European Respiratory Health Survey [9], are administered to determine the history of allergic diseases, symptoms suggestive of asthma, allergic symptoms, other respiratory symptoms, as well as smoking habits and exposure to pets. Other standardized questionnaires have just started being used in prospective studies of OA to assess mental health, in particular depression and anxiety status. Skin-prick tests [10] and serological tests are used to determine the immunological status to common allergens and also to the specific work-related allergen(s) under investigation. Finally, methacholine/histamine/adenosine-5'-monophosphate challenge tests are used to assess bronchial responsiveness [11–13]. All these tests can be and have been administered within the confines of the teaching institutions by trained research nurses and medical technologists. A modified protocol for bronchial challenge tests was developed and the safety of the test has been confirmed [14].

The design of these studies enables the prospective assessment of exposure to the agent(s) under investigation as well as of the potential confounding factors such as exposure to other contaminants in the workplace (e.g., to irritant products), viral infections, and continuous or discontinuous smoking.

The repeated assessments of health outcomes from the beginning of the apprenticeship onwards provide the opportunity of observing the trend in the incidence of relevant signs and symptoms of occupational allergy in the population studied as well as following the sequence of individual outcomes over time.

A pitfall in all prospective studies is the loss to follow-up and the effects this may have on the interpretation of the results. In occupational studies, the 'healthy worker' effect is known to occur when workers who experienced work-related health conditions have left the workplace. In the proposed apprentice model, both the assessment of the baseline host characteristics and the on-going evaluations of new sensitizations and work-related symptoms provide information to characterize those who quit the apprenticeship and assess the likelihood of selection biases [15]. The selected study population can theoretically be workers newly hired in an industry or apprentices starting a training program in a vocational school; indeed both populations are recruited when they have no earlier exposure to the agent. However, it is more efficient to select a cohort of apprentices since groups of individuals start exposure at the same point in time (study year) rather than spread over time such as for new workers.

A possible limitation worth considering for some apprentices studies (e.g., those involving laboratory animal workers and agricultural workers), is that they may have had exposure to the relevant allergens earlier. Lab animal workers sometimes had a past in agriculture like farmer apprentices and so they are not truly naïve with regard to the exposure. However, interestingly, in a study of 769 apprentices in four different sectors: lab animal technology, veterinary medicine, pastry-making and dental hygiene technology, the prevalence of allergic sensitization to laboratory animals at entry into the apprenticeship was the same (6.8–7.4%) in each group [11].

Studied apprentice populations

Cohorts of apprentices in trades that entail exposures to various respiratory sensitizers and irritants, who are thus at risk of developing OA, have been studied in several countries. Published by Herxheimer in 1973 [16], the first long-term examination was completed in Germany in a large group of 880 apprentice bakers, a small number ($n = 37$) of them were followed for 5 years. The percentage of skin sensitization increased gradually over the years until the third year when it reached 19% (54/290); at that time, complaints suggestive of an allergic disease occurred in 7% of apprentices, half of them were skin positive to either flour or other allergens. Since then, a number of prospective studies in trainee bakers and pastry makers have been conducted in Sweden [17], Italy [18], The Netherlands [13], Canada [19], Poland [12] and Denmark [20]; details of most of these studies, and main findings are summarized in Table 1. In Canada, inception cohort studies of apprentices exposed to different types of HMW agents derived from laboratory animals and latex were conducted among animal-health technicians [11, 21, 22] and dental hygienists [23]. Other populations of apprentices followed prospectively were mainly exposed to low-molecular-weight (LMW) agents; they included a Canadian cohort of apprentice machinists exposed to metalworking fluids [24], another Canadian cohort of apprentice welders exposed to welding fumes [25], a group of hairdressing apprentices in France [26], and apprentice car-painters in Canada [27]. Furthermore, an Italian group of investigators conducted a longitudinal study of apprentices from different trades exposed to various airway occupational sensitizers and irritants [28].

Investigated outcomes (events)

The central and long-term outcomes considered in the published cohorts of apprentices are OA and more recently its variants such as work-aggravated asthma [20]. OA was only confirmed objectively using specific inhalation challenge tests in the Polish cohort study [12]. The nearest outcome to OA was a combination of: (1) a significant increase in bronchial responsiveness defined as a 3.2-fold (or 2-fold) decrease in PC_{20} in a methacholine challenge test; and (2) sensitization to apprenticeship-specific allergens when the causal agent is an HMW allergen [22] or incident work-related asthma-like symptoms in the case of LMW agents when an immunological mechanism has not been confirmed [24, 25]; the term 'probable OA' has been used for these groupings of outcomes. Several other endpoints related to OA or considered as intermediate conditions have been evaluated. These include occupational rhinitis, confirmed through nasal specific inhalation tests as performed in symptomatic persons within the Polish cohort of apprentice bakers [12], or defined as the incidence of both specific sensitization to an occupational allergen and work-related symptoms of rhinitis [19].

Table 1. Summary from prospective cohort studies of apprentices in high-risk industrial sectors with exposure to agents causing occupational asthma.

Apprentice population, agent(s)	No. recruited; no. followed	Duration (years)	Outcomes of interest	Incidence	Factors			First author, year, country	Ref.
					Baseline host	During follow-up	Exposure		
Bakers, flour	880; 290, (37)	3, (5)	Skin sensitization to flour	19%	Skin sensitization to pollen	Skin sensitization to pollen	ND	Herxheimer, 1973, Germany	[16]
Bakers, flour, α-amylase	125	2.5	Skin sensitization to occupational allergens	10.1%	ND	ND	ND	De Zotti, 2000, Italy	[18]
			Work-related respiratory symptoms	9%	History of allergic disease	Skin sensitization to wheat, flour/α-amylase	ND		
Pastry makers, flour	230; 188	1.4	Skin sensitization to flour	4.2 per 100 PY	Hay fever; skin reactivity to grass-pollen; father with asthma	ND	ns	Gautrin, 2002, Canada	[29]
			Work-related symptoms of RC	13.1 per 100 PY	Skin sensitization to wheat flour; persistent rhinitis	ND	ND		
			Skin sensitization to flour + work-related RC symptoms	1.3 per 100 PY	–	–	–		

Bakers, flour	461; 287	2	Hypersensitivity to occupational allergens	8.2%	Atopy; history of skin symptoms	ND		Walusiak, 2004, Poland	[12]
			Work-related chest symptoms	8.6%		ND			
			Occupational rhinitis†	12.5%	Atopy	ND			
			Occupational asthma‡/chronic cough	8.7%	Atopy; skin sensitization to occupational allergens				
Bakers, flour, α-amylase, moulds, mites	187; 114	2	Work-related rhinitis	22.1 per 100 PY				Skjold, 2008, Denmark	[20]
			Asthma-like symptoms	10.0 per 100 PY	Atopy; female	BHR			
			Occupational sensitization	6.1%					
Animal-health technicians, laboratory animals	417; 387	1.6–3.6	Skin sensitization to lab animals	8.9 per 100 PY	Atopy; respiratory symptoms in the pollen season	ND	Duration of exposure	Gautrin, 2000, Canada	[21]
			Skin sensitization to lab animals + Increase in BR (3.2-fold decrease in PC_{20})	2.7 per 100 PY	Skin sensitization to pets; BR	ND		Gautrin, 2001, Canada	[22]
			Work-related RC symptoms	24%	Skin sensitization to grass pollen; rhinorrhea on contact with dust; chest tightness; cough	ND	ns	Rodier, 2003, Canada	[19]
			Skin sensitization to lab animals + work-related RC symptoms	9.6%	Skin sensitization to cats; BR	ND	ns		

Table 1. (continued)

Apprentice population, agent(s)	No. recruited; no. followed	Duration (years)	Outcomes of interest	Incidence	Factors			First author, year, country	Ref.
					Baseline host	During follow-up	Exposure		
Dental hygienists, latex	122; 110	1.5–2.5	Skin sensitization to latex	2.5 per 100 PY	Atopy; history of asthma	ND	ND	Archambault, 2001, Canada	[23]
			Skin sensitization to latex + increase in BR (3.2-fold decrease in PC_{20})	1.8 per 100 PY	ND	ND	ND		
Hairdressers, sensitizing materials with irritant exposure	297; 191 (referents: 248; 189)	2–3	Respiratory symptoms (wheezing)	10.0% vs 11.5%	Atopy	ND	ND	Iwatsubo, 2003, France	[26]
			Change in FEV_1 (% predicted)	Mean (SD) –2.5 (8.4) vs 0 (7.4)	ns	ND	No specific hair-dressing activity; no working conditions		
Machinists, metalworking fluids (MWF)	95; 82 (referents: 202; 157)	2	Increase in BR (2-fold decrease in PC_{20}) 13% vs 7%				Duration of exposure to synthetic MWF	Kennedy, 1999, Canada	[24]
			BHR + asthma-like symptoms	7% vs 2%					
Welders, welding fumes	286; 194	1.25–1.5	Increase in BR (3.2-fold decrease in PC_{20})	11.9%	ND	ND	ND	El-Zein, 2003, Canada	[25]
			Increase in BR + work-related chest symptoms	3.1%					

Welders, welding fumes	286; 232	1.25–1.5	Welding-related chest symptoms	13.8%	none	Possible MFF		El-Zein, 2005, Canada	[37]
Car-painters, diisocyanates (HDI)	385; 298	1.5	HDI-specific IgE and IgG				Duration of exposure during training	Dragos, 2008, Canada	[27]
			Work-related nasal symptoms	6.4%	Inversely related to IgG4 levels				
			Work-related chest symptoms	4.4%	Inversely related to IgE levels; physician-diagnosed asthma; BHR				

†: Based on questionnaire data and positive reaction to a specific inhalation challenge (SIC);
‡: work-related chest symptoms and positive SIC;
MWF: metalworking fluids; PC_{20}: provocative concentration of nonspecific agent causing a 20% decrease in FEV_1; FEV_1: forced expiratory volume in 1 second; BHR: bronchial hyperresponsiveness; BR: bronchial responsiveness; RC: rhinoconjunctivitis; PY: person-years; ND: not assessed; ns: non significant; MFF: metal fume fever.

The aforementioned outcomes – sensitization to allergens specific to the apprenticeship (specific IgE or skin-prick test reactivity), work-related nasal, ocular and chest symptoms, and increase in bronchial reactivity – have also been considered separately to determine their incidence and/or determinants (see Tab. 1).

Major findings

Incidence

OA can develop during a 2-year apprenticeship in a bakery. In the Polish cohort the proportion of cases was 8.7% after 2 years of training, with symptoms of wheezing occurring after a mean (± SD) latency period of 15.1 ± 5.1 months [12]. In the Canadian cohort of apprentice bakers, no cases of probable OA were observed. However, incident cases of probable OA were detected in the cohort of apprentices in animal health with a rate of 2.7 per 100 person-years (PY) [22]. Among apprentice machinists exposed to metalworking fluids, 7% developed new bronchial responsiveness with asthma-like symptoms [24], while the incidence was 3.1% in apprentice welders [25]; both these Canadian cohorts were followed over 2 years.

Occupational rhinitis was also detected and confirmed in 12.5% of Polish apprentice bakers, a slightly higher proportion than for OA [12]; the incidence of probable occupational rhinitis among Canadian pastry-making apprentices was low (1.3 per 100 PY) compared to that of work-related symptoms of rhinoconjunctivitis with no specific sensitization to flour (13.1 per 100 PY) [29].

Specific (skin) sensitization to the relevant work-related allergen(s) was assessed in all cohorts of apprentices exposed to HMW agents. The findings are reported in Table 1 and suggest that the incidence is greater among individuals exposed to laboratory animals than to baker's allergens. The proportions of apprentices showing a twofold dose decrease or more in PC_{20} was 13% and 11.9% in apprentice machinists and welders, respectively. Interestingly, although an increase in bronchial responsiveness may be believed to be nonspecific, the increase was significantly greater in machinists than in apprentices in various other construction trades [24].

A proportion of individuals without prior exposure to an occupational allergen may be sensitized to such allergens before enrolling into a vocational program [11, 12]. Sensitization to flour or α-amylase present when starting training in pastry-making or bakery is a risk factor for the future development of work-related respiratory symptoms [12, 18, 29].

Time course of 'events' (stages)

The time course of relevant outcomes during an apprenticeship was described through repeated assessments [12, 30]. The rate of new work-related rhinoconjunctivitis symptoms and sensitization to training-specific allergens assessed yearly among apprentice animal-health technicians was greater than 10% after 1 year of training and remained high after 2 and 3 years; the rate of new work-related chest symptoms was highest only after 2 and 3 years [30]. On the other hand, in a cohort of apprentice bakers, the incidence of all respiratory symptoms was higher in the second year of training; the incidence of skin reactivity to occupational allergens also increased from 4.6% to 8.2% between the first and second year in training [12]. Differences in the time course of occurrence of these outcomes for these different populations of apprentices are difficult to interpret; they may be attributable to differences in duration and intensity of exposure to the causative agent(s), or to the varying pathogenicity of the allergens. Nevertheless, the implications for setting the timing of surveillance programs are the same, and would be to screen for sensitization and symptoms in the first 2–3 years of apprenticeship.

The 'allergic march'

It is generally believed that rhinitis precedes asthma [31]. There is some evidence that rhinitis of occupational origin progresses into asthma [32, 33]. Cohorts of apprentices can offer a powerful approach to verify the assumption of an allergic march. However, the published data from apprentice studies have not yet provided clear evidence to confirm this hypothesis. Indeed, results from the prospective study of apprentice bakers conducted by Walusiak [12] showed that the latency period for new nose and chest symptoms was almost the same; the diagnosis of occupational rhinitis (36/287) and of OA (25/287) by specific inhalation challenges were concurrent in 25/36 individuals. For only 5/25 apprentices with confirmed OA was it shown, during the clinical examination, that OA was preceded by allergic rhinitis, which was not necessarily work-related, but present prior to entering the apprenticeship [12]. From a different perspective, in a prospective study among apprentice animal-health technicians, the predictive values of work-related rhinitis symptoms for the development of respiratory symptoms and of probable OA were estimated at 9.0% and 11.4%, respectively; these rather low values failed to provide evidence for the 'allergic march' [30]. Nonetheless, the length of follow-up of most studies published since 1999 has been limited to the duration of the apprenticeship, which does not exceed 3 or 4 years (see Tab. 1).

Factors associated with asthma

The factors associated with asthma that are consistently reported in the cohorts of apprentices are host factors assessed at baseline; some studies have evaluated the role of 'intermediate' outcomes, such as skin sensitization for the development of work-related symptoms. Exposure parameters have not been considered as much.

Factors at inception

The prospective cohorts of apprentices document host factors at baseline, which are essential from different perspectives: first, for detecting the incidence of 'endpoints' that may already be prevalent before starting an apprenticeship (e.g., sensitization to training-specific allergens and BHR), and second, for identifying determinants of OA and associated features with knowledge of the sequence of events. In the following section, 'Factors' are regarded as 'determinants' or risk factors.

Atopy

Atopy evaluated by skin tests to common allergens is a determinant of skin sensitization to training-specific HMW allergens. Where ubiquitous allergens were individually considered, the effect of individual allergens was shown; for example, grass pollen for sensitization to flour [16, 29] and pets in the case of sensitization to laboratory animals [21]. As shown in Table 1, atopy is an important determinant for the other endpoints studied in apprentice cohorts exposed to HMW agents and also in hairdressing apprentices [26]. However, investigators have mostly uncovered a predominant role of individual aeroallergens.

Although in a smaller proportion, non-atopic subjects also develop work-related sensitization and symptoms when exposed to HMW occupational agents. Interestingly, the factors associated with various endpoints vary according to the atopic status; for example, rhinitis symptoms on contact with pets and skin sensitization to pets were associated with work-related rhinoconjunctivitis symptoms in atopic apprentices exposed to laboratory animals, while perennial rhinitis and having a $PC_{20} \leq 32$ mg/ml were found in non-atopics [34]. In apprentice pastry makers, atopic at inception, no other factor was associated with the incidence of work-related rhinoconjunctivitis symptoms, whereas in non atopics symptoms of rhinitis on contact with pets was the factor most strongly related [34].

Skin sensitization to the training-specific allergen(s)

In cohorts of apprentices, the prospective design offers the possibility of assessing sensitization to training-specific agents at inception. A proportion showed signs of immunological sensitization to laboratory animals [11] or flour [16] on early exposure during the apprenticeship; this may result from immunological cross-reactivity with ubiquitous allergens derived from animal or plant species. Prior specific sensitization to baker's allergens was related to incidence of work-related rhinoconjunctivitis symptoms in apprentice pastry makers [29] and of OA in apprentice bakers [12].

History of symptoms of allergy

Similar to studies in workers, a history of nasal, skin and chest allergic symptoms were associated with work-related sensitization and symptoms. The summary results of the cohorts of apprentices presented in Table 1 show that chest and rhinoconjunctivitis symptoms, on contact with pets or pollen or in any nonspecific circumstances, are the main determinants of several endpoints, mainly work-related symptoms of rhinoconjunctivitis, or are of similar importance as skin-prick atopy. However, being highly correlated with atopy, they do not add as significant determinants in multivariate analyses.

History of allergic disease

Physician-diagnosed asthma (reported by the participants) was an important determinant of sensitization to latex in dental hygiene apprentices [23] and of work-related respiratory symptoms in apprentice car painters [35].

Bronchial responsiveness

BR has only rarely been assessed at recruitment into apprentice cohorts. A PC_{20} equal to, or less than 32 mg/ml (measurable bronchial responsiveness) was associated with probable OA and probable occupational rhinitis [19, 20, 22].

Smoking and other host factors

Smoking status has been documented, but has not yet shown any association with the development of the endpoints. Genetic studies are in progress to investigate the link between selected polymorphisms and the development of sensitization to training-related allergens and other hallmarks of OA.

Intermediate outcomes assessed throughout an apprenticeship

In cohorts of apprentice bakers, skin sensitization to pollens developed during the apprenticeship was related to the development of sensitization to flour [16] and to the onset of OA [12]. On the other hand, new sensitization to baker's allergens was associated with work-related respiratory symptoms [18]. The role of intermediate outcomes in the development of a work-related disease has now been explored further in a long-term follow-up of cohorts of apprentices exposed to HMW agents [36] and the main findings are summarized below.

Exposure

Although the period of apprenticeship spans only a few years, Kennedy and colleagues found an association between the duration of exposure to metalworking fluids and the development of the combination of BHR and asthma-like symptoms. Similarly, in apprentice animal-health technicians, the number of hours in contact with rodents in the laboratory was an independent determinant of a new sensitization to laboratory animals, after accounting for an allergic diathesis [21].

Previous epidemiological and exposure assessment studies considering either currently employed or retired welders were unable to account for a critical window of first-time exposure, which usually occurs during the apprenticeship. The prospective study by El-Zein and colleagues [25] considered this early window and found that being exposed to welding fumes and gases during apprenticeship, over an average period of 15 months, was associated with pulmonary function changes and the development of welding-related systemic and respiratory symptoms. The concentrations of metal fumes present in the breathing zone of apprentice welders were quantified for four common welding processes (shielded metal arc welding, tungsten inert gas welding, metal inert gas welding, and flux cored arc welding). Throughout the duration of the apprenticeship, 247 samples were gathered. The findings suggested the presence of rather low concentrations of metals; iron seemed to be the best marker. The low concentrations prohibited further analysis with the outcome variables assessed in the epidemiological study [25, 37]. The low concentrations found could be explained in part by the short sampling time, depending on the actual time the students performed welding operations on a given sampling day. Another explanatory factor could be the presence of a probably well-functioning general ventilation system (personal communication by El-Zein, PhD).

Apprentices probably experience a different exposure compared to the fully trained workers because of disparities in training, experience and products used. We know very little about exposure of apprentices and this really needs further exploration. We will then need to investigate the extent to which the risk of work-related allergy and asthma increases with parameters of exposure during apprenticeship. So far, evidence of exposure-response relationship between exposure and work-related allergies in cohorts of individual at risk is scarce, even among workers. The first long-term longitudinal study to address this question in workers showed an increased risk of laboratory animal allergy (LAA) related to duration of exposure to animals and work in animal-related tasks [38].

Assessment of selection bias

No apparent self selection into the apprenticeship due to prior sensitization to the relevant allergen(s) was observed in three populations of apprentices (animal health technology, pastry making and dental hygiene); i.e., the proportion of subjects sensitized to laboratory animals at inception did not differ between career programs [11]. However, a healthy worker effect was suspected in hairdressing apprentices, who showed fewer respiratory symptoms and higher lung function values in comparison with office apprentices upon starting their training [26]. In general, participation in prospective studies has raised satisfactory interest among apprentices. However, the characteristics of non-participants and reasons for declining to participate are worth investigating in order to assess the presence and/or the magnitude of a potential selection bias. When non-participant baker apprentices to a Danish cohort study were asked why they refused, reasons were fear of blood sampling and the time commitment to the follow-up study [39]. Attrition or selection out of the cohort may also, in some circumstances, introduce a bias. Factors associated with quitting an apprenticeship may be associated with the health status before entering and during the training. These factors were investigated in a cohort of apprentices exposed to HMW agents; a history of hay fever before entering the apprenticeship was a mild, but significant determinant. Among apprentices in animal health, quitting was associated with baseline sensitization to laboratory animals and symptoms of asthma during apprenticeship, but not with work-related respiratory symptoms [40]. Interestingly, in the same cohort of apprentices, acquiring sensitization, symptoms or BHR during training did not significantly influence the decision of pursuing a career in the same field. Indeed, around 80% of the individuals chose a job related to their training, but those who complained of work-related rhinoconjunctivitis symptoms during apprenticeship tended not to have a job with a risk of exposure to sensitizers during the 8-year post-apprenticeship span [36]. Radon and co-workers reported similar findings in a prospective cohort study of nearly 5000 people, showing no association between an atopic diathesis at baseline and subsequent choice of a job [41].

Long-term follow-up

A follow-up study of the Canadian cohort of apprentices exposed to HMW agents, 8 years after ending an apprenticeship in animal-health technology, pastry making and dental hygiene was carried out between 2002 and 2006. This was the first prospective study of an inception cohort of apprentices after they entered a workforce, regardless of whether or not their job was related to their training [36]. Of note, this cohort is one of those where apprentices (also named students) attend specialized vocational training schools; they seek employment into a workforce only after their 2–3-year training. The incidences of work-related skin sensitization, rhinoconjunctivitis, chest symptoms, and BHR were, respectively, 1.3, 1.7, 0.7 and 2.0 per 100 PY in individuals who had, at anytime during the follow-up period, held a job related to their training (78%). These incidence figures were lower than those found during the apprenticeship; i.e., 7.3, 12.9, 1.7 and 5.8 per 100 PY for the respective endpoints. We hypothesize that the most vulnerable individuals acquire these features early after starting exposure to specific sensitizers. This is in agreement with results from studies with a short-duration follow-up; however, these findings need to be confirmed in other long-term follow-up studies. Of interest, a high proportion of apprentices who had developed these outcomes during training were in remission at the follow-up assessment, even if they were still working in the same field (i.e., 67%, 65%, 71% and 53% for work-specific skin sensitization, rhinoconjunctivitis symptoms, chest symptoms and BHR, respectively); and more so in participants with a work history not related to their apprenticeship (i.e., 80%, 76%, 75% and 86%). Several clinical, immunological and functional characteristics present at inception of the cohort or developed during the apprenticeship were found to be significantly associated with incidence (post-apprenticeship) of the endpoints listed above or with remission of those acquired while training. Clinical determinants acquired during the apprenticeship included non-work-related respiratory symptoms for later incidence of work-related chest symptoms and BHR, as well as nasal or conjunctival symptoms at work for a later incidence of BHR. In this cohort, new cases of probable OA (defined in '*Investigated outcomes*' above) were identified: 28 among animal-health technicians and 2 among dental hygienists during their training. Of the 23 evaluated at the 8-year follow-up, two had left the field and no longer showed the features of probable OA, while 7/21 had persistent probable OA. Among 201 individuals at risk and still working in the same domain, 3 developed probable OA.

Other long-term follow-up studies have been conducted in settings where the apprenticeship was undertaken in the workplace. A retrospective cohort study of laboratory animal workers used pre-employment screening data to assess the incidence of LAA symptoms in "naïve" individuals at the time they were accepted for a job at a Dutch research institute [42]. It was shown that the risk of developing LAA was still present after 3 years or more of exposure in contrast to an earlier notion.

A long-term longitudinal study in a large dynamic cohort of workers exposed to laboratory animals (from a pharmaceutical company in North Carolina, USA), although not an inception cohort in apprentices, has further described the natural history of asthma and confirmed that laboratory animal allergy is a major risk factor for the development of asthma [43].

Conclusions

Cohorts of apprentices provide an excellent experimental model to follow the natural history of OA, as the stages preceding the first manifestations of asthma can be assessed prospectively in addition to the prognosis of the disease itself or associated features or pre-clinical manifestations after interruption or diminution of exposure. Extensive assessment of baseline clinical, immunological, functional and psychosocial status, before exposure to the causal occupational sensitizers begins, is possible. Exposure to known causal agents can be well characterized, both qualitatively and quantitatively, and very importantly, its variation in intensity and duration over time.

Studies of prospective cohorts of apprentices initiated before starting apprenticeship offer the possibility of following its members for long periods of time, as for birth cohort studies.

Directions of future research

Long-term follow-up of cohorts of apprentices initiated in the early 1990s should be encouraged and supported.

Research on on-going and especially new cohorts should encompass an improved identification of the stages of the disease and of its determinants such as:

- Better evaluations of environmental factors and exposures that may influence, potentiate, or attenuate the effect of occupational sensitizers on the development of asthma, e.g., the general urban *versus* rural environment, concomitant exposure to endotoxins, ozone, SO_2, solvents, or any relevant contaminant.
- Use of available tools to sample induced sputum to measure markers of disease.
- Measurements of exhaled NO.
- Better and more refined biological markers including: genetic polymorphisms, markers of inflammation including inflammatory cells, chemotactic factors and mediators of activation for these cells, and markers of remodeling such as matrix metalloproteinases.
- New genetic investigations to gain a better understanding of possible changes in genetic markers or their expression as a result of a specific environmental exposure.
- Psychosocial determinants.

Although apprentice cohort studies were primarily designed to study the natural history of OA, the data now available can be used to develop prognostic models for sensitization to occupational allergens and other markers of asthma during the apprenticeship. The models would be based upon host characteristics at baseline, outcomes assessed prospectively and characteristics of exposure as predictors. By determining the individual probabilities of developing asthma and related endpoints, such models may serve to advise young people in their career orientation and support surveillance programs targeted towards individuals at high risk.

References

1 Becklake MR. Epidemiology: Prevalence and Determinants. In: Bernstein IL, Chan-Yeung M, Malo J, Bernstein DI (eds): *Asthma in the Workplace*. Marcel Dekker, New York 1993, p. 29–59

2 Malo JL. Occupational Asthma: A Model for Environmental Asthma. In: Godard P, Bousquet J (eds): *Advances in Allergology and Clinical Immunology*. Parthenon Publishing Group, Carnforth 1992, p. 391–400

3 Chan-Yeung M, Malo JL. Natural History of Occupational Asthma. In: Bernstein IL, Chan-Yeung M, Malo JL, Bernstein DI (eds): *Asthma in the Workplace*. Marcel Dekker, New York 1993. p. 299–322

4 Chan-Yeung M, Malo JL. Occupational asthma. *N Engl J Med* 1995 Jul 13; 333(2): 107–12

5 McDonald JC. Study design. In: Corbett McDonald (ed.): *Epidemiology of work-related diseases*. BMJ Publishing Group, London 1995, p. 325–51

6 Nieuwenhuijsen MJ, Putcha V, Gordon S, Heederik D, Venables KM, Cullinan P, et al. Exposure-response relations among laboratory animal workers exposed to rats. *Occup Environ Med* 2003 Feb; 60(2): 104–8

7 Silva PA, Stanton WR. *From child to adult: The Dunedin Multidisciplinary Health and Development Study*. Oxford University Press, Auckland 1996

8 Keil T, Kulig M, Simpson A, Custovic A, Wickman M, Kull I, et al. European birth cohort studies on asthma and atopic diseases: I. Comparison of study designs – A GALEN initiative. *Allergy* 2006 Feb; 61(2): 221–8

9 Burney PG, Luczynska C, Chinn S, Jarvis D. The European Community Respiratory Health Survey. *Eur Respir J* 1994 May; 7(5): 954–60

10 Pepys J. Types of allergic reaction. *Clin Allergy* 1973 Dec; 3 Suppl: 491–509

11 Gautrin D, Infante-Rivard C, Dao TV, Magnan-Larose M, Desjardins D, Malo JL. Specific IgE-dependent sensitization, atopy, and bronchial hyperresponsiveness in apprentices starting exposure to protein-derived agents. *Am J Respir Crit Care Med* 1997 Jun; 155(6): 1841–7

12 Walusiak J, Hanke W, Gorski P, Palczynski C. Respiratory allergy in apprentice bakers: Do occupational allergies follow the allergic march? *Allergy* 2004 Apr; 59(4): 442–50

13 De Meer G, Postma DS, Heederik D. Bronchial responsiveness to adenosine-5'-monophosphate and methacholine as predictors for nasal symptoms due to newly introduced allergens. A follow-up study among laboratory animal workers and bakery apprentices. *Clin Exp Allergy* 2003 Jun; 33(6): 789–94

14 Troyanov S, Malo JL, Cartier A, Gautrin D. Frequency and determinants of exaggerated bronchoconstriction during shortened methacholine challenge tests in epidemiological and clinical set-ups. *Eur Respir J* 2000 Jul; 16(1): 9–14

15 Monso E, Malo JL, Infante-Rivard C, Ghezzo H, Magnan M, L'Archeveque J, et al. Individual characteristics and quitting in apprentices exposed to high-molecular-weight agents. *Am J Respir Crit Care Med* 2000 May; 161(5): 1508–12

16 Herxheimer H. The skin sensitivity to flour of bakers' apprentices. *Acta Allergol* 1973; 28: 42–9

17 Brisman SJ, Jarvholm BG. Occurrence of self-reported asthma among Swedish bakers. *Scand J Work Environ Health* 1995 Dec; 21(6): 487–93

18 De Zotti R, Bovenzi M. Prospective study of work related respiratory symptoms in trainee bakers. *Occup Environ Med* 2000 Jan; 57(1): 58–61

19 Rodier F, Gautrin D, Ghezzo H, Malo JL. Incidence of occupational rhinoconjunctivitis and risk factors in animal-health apprentices. *J Allergy Clin Immunol* 2003 Dec; 112(6): 1105–11

20 Skjold T, Dahl R, Juhl B, Sigsgaard T. The incidence of respiratory symptoms and sensitisation in baker apprentices. *Eur Respir J* 2008 Aug; 32(2): 452–9

21 Gautrin D, Ghezzo H, Infante-Rivard C, Malo JL. Incidence and determinants of IgE-mediated sensitization in apprentices. A prospective study. *Am J Respir Crit Care Med* 2000 Oct; 162(4 Pt 1): 1222–8

22 Gautrin D, Infante-Rivard C, Ghezzo H, Malo JL. Incidence and host determinants of probable occupational asthma in apprentices exposed to laboratory animals. *Am J Respir Crit Care Med* 2001 Mar; 163(4): 899–904

23 Archambault S, Malo JL, Infante-Rivard C, Ghezzo H, Gautrin D. Incidence of sensitization, symptoms, and probable occupational rhinoconjunctivitis and asthma in apprentices starting exposure to latex. *J Allergy Clin Immunol* 2001 May; 107(5): 921–3

24 Kennedy SM, Chan-Yeung M, Teschke K, Karlen B. Change in airway responsiveness among apprentices exposed to metalworking fluids. *Am J Respir Crit Care Med* 1999 Jan; 159(1): 87–93

25 El-Zein M, Malo JL, Infante-Rivard C, Gautrin D. Incidence of probable occupational asthma and changes in airway calibre and responsiveness in apprentice welders. *Eur Respir J* 2003 Sep; 22(3): 513–8

26 Iwatsubo Y, Matrat M, Brochard P, Ameille J, Choudat D, Conso F, et al. Healthy worker effect and changes in respiratory symptoms and lung function in hairdressing apprentices. *Occup Environ Med* 2003 Nov; 60(11): 831–40

27 Dragos M, Jones M, Malo J-L, Ghezzo H, Gautrin D, Specific antibodies to diisocyanate and work-related respiratory symptoms in apprentice car-painters. *Occup Environ Med* 2009; 66: 227–234

28 Talini D, Monteverdi A, Lastrucci L, Buonocore C, Carrara M, Di PF, et al. One-year longitudinal study of young apprentices exposed to airway occupational sensitizers. *Int Arch Occup Environ Health* 2006 Mar; 79(3): 237–43

29 Gautrin D, Ghezzo H, Infante-Rivard C, Malo JL. Incidence and host determinants of work-related rhinoconjunctivitis in apprentice pastry-makers. *Allergy* 2002 Oct; 57(10): 913–8

30 Gautrin D, Ghezzo H, Infante-Rivard C, Malo JL. Natural history of sensitization, symptoms and occupational diseases in apprentices exposed to laboratory animals. *Eur Respir J* 2001 May; 17(5): 904–8

31 Bousquet J, Vignola AM, Demoly P. Links between rhinitis and asthma. *Allergy* 2003 Aug; 58(8): 691–706
32 Piirila P, Estlander T, Hytonen M, Keskinen H, Tupasela O, Tuppurainen M. Rhinitis caused by ninhydrin develops into occupational asthma. *Eur Respir J* 1997 Aug; 10(8): 1918–21
33 Karjalainen A, Martikainen R, Klaukka T, Saarinen K, Uitti J. Risk of asthma among Finnish patients with occupational rhinitis. *Chest* 2003 Jan; 123(1): 283–8
34 Gautrin D, Ghezzo H, Infante-Rivard C, Malo JL. Host determinants for the development of allergy in apprentices exposed to laboratory animals. *Eur Respir J* 2002 Jan; 19(1): 96–103
35 Dragos MC, Malo JL, Gautrin D. Specific IgG and IgE to hexamethyl diisocyanate (HDI) among car-painting apprentices at risk of developing occupational asthma (OA). *Am J Respir Crit Care Med* 2004 169(7), A647
36 Gautrin D, Ghezzo H, Infante-Rivard C, Magnan M, L'Archeveque J, Suarthana E, et al. Long-term outcomes in a prospective cohort of apprentices exposed to high-molecular-weight agents. *Am J Respir Crit Care Med* 2008 Apr 15; 177(8): 871–9
37 El-Zein M, Infante-Rivard C, Malo JL, Gautrin D. Is metal fume fever a determinant of welding related respiratory symptoms and/or increased bronchial responsiveness? A longitudinal study. *Occup Environ Med* 2005 Oct; 62(10): 688–94
38 Elliott L, Heederik D, Marshall S, Peden D, Loomis D. Incidence of allergy and allergy symptoms among workers exposed to laboratory animals. *Occup Environ Med* 2005 Nov; 62(11): 766–71
39 Skjold T, Nielsen SC, Adolf K, Hoffmann HJ, Dahl R, Sigsgaard T. Allergy in bakers' apprentices and factors associated to non-participation in a cohort study of allergic sensitization. *Int Arch Occup Environ Health* 2007 Apr; 80(5): 458–64
40 Monso E, Magarolas R, Radon K, Danuser B, Iversen M, Weber C, et al. Respiratory symptoms of obstructive lung disease in European crop farmers. *Am J Respir Crit Care Med* 2000 Oct; 162(4 Pt 1): 1246–50
41 Radon K, Huemmer S, Dressel H, Windstetter D, Weinmayr G, Weiland S, et al. Do respiratory symptoms predict job choices in teenagers? *Eur Respir J* 2006 Apr; 27(4): 774–8
42 Kruize H, Post W, Heederik D, Martens B, Hollander A, van der BE. Respiratory allergy in laboratory animal workers: A retrospective cohort study using pre-employment screening data. *Occup Environ Med* 1997 Nov; 54(11): 830–5
43 Elliott L, Heederik D, Marshall S, Peden D, Loomis D. Progression of self-reported symptoms in laboratory animal allergy. *J Allergy Clin Immunol* 2005 Jul; 116(1): 127–32

Management of an individual worker with occupational asthma

Sherwood Burge

Heart of England NHS Foundation Trust, Birmingham Heartlands Hospital, Bordesley Green East, Birmingham B9 5SS, UK

Abstract

The aim of management of an individual with occupational asthma is to preserve their health and wealth, preferably to leave their employer in business, and to prevent other workers from developing occupational asthma. To do this a confident diagnosis must be made. Occupational asthma should be suspected when asthma symptoms improve on days away from work or on holiday. As these questions have many false-positive answers, the diagnosis needs objective confirmation. The most appropriate first test is to carry out good quality peak flow measurements every 2 hours for about 3 weeks during periods of usual work exposure. Specific IgE is helpful for most high-molecular-weight allergens, and can be used to monitor allergen avoidance. Specific bronchial challenge testing is required in new or difficult situations. Non-specific bronchial hyperresponsiveness is not sufficiently sensitive to use as a screening test for those requiring further investigation. Once a diagnosis has been made workers should be separated into those in whom further (usual level) exposure is unlikely to cause further deterioration in their asthma (mostly those with acute irritant-induced asthma) and those who are sensitised to a workplace agent in whom further usual level exposure commonly leads to deteriorating asthma. There is a hierarchy of control methods when exposure must be eliminated or substantially reduced, going from substitution, source exposure control and individual protection. Examples of each strategy are given. The availability and scope of compensation schemes also affect management; some facilitate re-training and ensuring income preservation much better than others. Successful management nearly always involves cooperation between the affected worker, their employer and their compensation scheme. An accurate clinical diagnosis is a requirement for all of these.

Introduction

The aim of management of an individual with occupational asthma (OA) is to preserve their health and wealth, preferably to leave their employer in business, and to prevent other workers from developing OA. There is good evidence that, in general, removal from exposure within the first year of work-related symptoms leads to a better prognosis than that of those who remain exposed [1–7]. Also, those who have reduced exposure generally do worse than those with no exposure at all [4, 8–12]. Within this generalisation, however, are individual workers who remain exposed

Occupational Asthma, edited by Torben Sigsgaard and Dick Heederik

and symptomatic, but in whom the severity of the disease does not progress (similar to a person with non-OA who remains exposed to mites or animals to which they are sensitised). The management of the individual worker depends crucially on the context in which you are working (as the treating Physician or the Occupational Physician) and the compensation system within which you work.

As the treating Physician your responsibility is to the individual worker. Not all workers will allow you to contact their workplace, for which they need to give consent. In my practice, about one third of all new patients with OA refuse consent to contact their workplace, at least in the initial part of their management. They are often worried that they will loose their job, which at least in the UK is common. Under these circumstances, all you can do is give advice to the individual worker about diagnosis, the likely poorer medical outcome if exposure continues and offer follow-up.

For the majority, satisfactory resolution of OA requires cooperation with the workplace, preferably *via* an Occupational Physician. As an Occupational Physician, you may be in an even more difficult position as again you have a duty of confidentiality but also a duty to protect individuals from harm in the workplace.

The choices available to eliminate or reduce exposure, in descending order of preference, are:

- Remove the causative agent from the workplace (substitution); solves the problem for the index case and prevents further cases.
- Relocate the index case to an area without exposure to the causative agent; leaves others exposed and needs careful monitoring to make sure relocation is successful. Re-exposure when getting to the new workplace, toilets, meal breaks, etc., is common. The causative agent needs enclosure to one part of the workplace. Relocation often involves a less satisfactory job (e.g. to a labouring job in an outside yard).
- Substantial reduction of exposure to the causative agent; this is a good solution to reduce further sensitisation but has usually to be done very efficiently to reduce exposure sufficiently in the index case to prevent symptoms. Enclosure of the source with extraction to the outside would be an example. Extraction through a filter to the workplace is often less satisfactory and requires careful maintenance of the filters.
- Respiratory protective equipment (RPE); regarded as a last resort, often satisfactory for short intermittent exposures. If needed for the whole work shift it has to be organised and maintained to prevent exposure. This involves donning and removing outside the work area, maintenance by someone else wearing their own RPE, and correct use and replacement of filters. All of this is more difficult to achieve than it may seem.
- Terminating employment; this should achieve removal from exposure, at least temporarily. This could be a good option if there is a compensation scheme

with a large re-training element, it would then appear much higher up the list of options. Without access to good re-training, the affected worker is often left with the option of unemployment, or getting a similar job to the one causing OA. This may involve concealing the original diagnosis and re-exposure to the original cause; often, however, in a better maintained workplace with lower exposures than before.

I illustrate the options using data needed for diagnosis and management. A fuller account of the tests illustrated here appears in the chapter by A. Cartier.

Evidence-based guidelines

There are many guidelines for the management of OA, but only two so far are based on a critical evidence-based review. The British Occupational Health Research Foundation (BOHRF) is a charitable body; it commissioned the first review concerning the occupational health aspects of the prevention, identification and management of OA. After identification of specific questions, there was a systematic search of all published, methodologically sound and original scientific studies, with each publication rated for the strength of the evidence plus a narrative overview by agreement between two experienced and independently minded reviewers. Where reviewers disagreed about the score of the paper or its relevance to this research, they discussed it to reach resolution. Where resolution was not achieved, a third reviewer was involved. Evidence tables were made for each pre-defined question and formed the basis to formulate evidence statements and recommendations. The evidence statements related to the management of an individual are as follows:

- What is the prognosis of OA?

Generally, OA is reported to have a poor prognosis and to be likely to persist and deteriorate unless identified early and managed effectively. The symptoms and functional impairment of OA caused by various agents may persist for many years after avoidance of further exposure to the causative agent.

- Which factors increase the probability of a favourable prognosis after a diagnosis of OA?

Complete avoidance of exposure may or may not improve symptoms and bronchial hyperresponsiveness. Both the duration of continued exposure following the onset of symptoms and the severity of asthma at diagnosis may be important determinants of outcome. Early diagnosis and early avoidance of further exposure, either by relocation of the worker or substitution of the hazard offer the best chance of complete recovery. Workers who remain in the same job and continue to be exposed to the same causative agent after diagnosis are unlikely to improve and symptoms may worsen. The likelihood of improvement or resolution of symptoms or of preventing deterioration is greater in workers who have no further exposure to the causative agent. The likelihood of improvement or resolution of symptoms or of preventing deterioration is greater in workers who have relatively normal lung function at the time of diagnosis, who have shorter duration time between first exposure and first symptom, or a shorter duration of symptoms prior to avoidance of exposure.

- What evidence is there for benefit of redeployment within the same workplace?

Ideally, complete and permanent avoidance of exposure is the mainstay of management. In practice, workers may reject this advice for social or financial reasons. If it is possible to relocate the worker to low or occasional exposure work areas, he or she should remain under increased medical surveillance. Where present, specific IgE can be monitored, although this has not been shown to affect outcome. Redeployment to a low-exposure area may lead to improvement or resolution of symptoms or prevent deterioration in some workers, but is not always effective.

- What evidence is there for the benefit of the enhanced use of respiratory protective equipment?

Once sensitised, a worker's symptoms may be incited by exposure to extremely low concentrations of a respiratory sensitiser. Respiratory protective equipment is effective only insofar as it is worn when appropriate, that there is a good fit on the face and proper procedures are followed for removal, storage and maintenance. The few studies that investigate the effectiveness of respiratory protective equipment are limited to small studies in provocation chambers or limited case reports. There are no large studies of long-term outcome. Air-fed helmet respirators may improve or prevent symptoms in some but not all workers who continue to be exposed to the causative agent.

- What is the impact of OA on employment?

There is consistent evidence derived from clinical and workforce case series in a limited number of countries that about one third of workers with OA are unemployed after diagnosis. The risk may or may not be higher than among other adult asthmatics, although this has been examined in only three studies. The risk of unemployment may fall with increasing time after diagnosis. There is consistent evidence that loss of employment following a diagnosis of OA is associated with loss of income. In comparison with other adult asthmatics those whose disease is related to work may find employment more difficult. Approximately one third of workers with OA are unemployed up to 6 years after diagnosis. Workers with OA suffer financially.

- What is the effectiveness of compensation being directed towards rehabilitation?

There are no studies that have made direct comparisons between different systems of rehabilitation either under different jurisdictions or within the same jurisdiction at different times. Systems that incorporate re-training may be more effective than those that do not.

- What is the effect of inhaled corticosteroids on recovery from OA?

A single small randomised-controlled trial has examined the effect of inhaled corticosteroids on the recovery from OA after cessation of exposure. Small but statistically significant improvements in some symptoms, peak expiratory flow (PEF) and quality of life were reported.

These guidelines can be accessed interactively, allowing you to add further evidence or comment on the existing evidence, at www.occupationalasthma.com/bohrf.aspx. They are currently being updated. The Canadian evidence-based guidelines were only concerned with the diagnosis of OA, and used statistical methods to calculate the sensitivity and specificity of individual tests. They used specific inhalation testing as the reference standard following a systematic review of literature regarding the diagnosis of OA in which specific inhalation challenge testing was compared with alternative tests [13]. The results complement the BOHRF non-statistical approach and provide confidence limits for the BOHRF statements. The following conclusions were reached:

- What are the sensitivity and the specificity of a normal measurement of non-specific reactivity, while at work, in the diagnosis of OA?

Non-specific hyperresponsiveness had a sensitivity of 79.3% [95% confidence interval (CI) 68–88%] for high-molecular-weight (HMW) agents and 66.7% (95% CI 58–74%) for low-molecular-weight (LMW) agents. Specificity was 51.3% (95% CI 35–67) for HMW and 63.9% (56–71%) for LMW agents.

- What are the sensitivity and the specificity of specific IgE testing in the diagnosis of validated cases of OA?

Specific IgE had a sensitivity of 73.3% (95% CI 64–81%) for HMW agents and 31.2% (95% CI 23–41%) for LMW agents for which tests were available. Specificity was 79.0% (95% CI 50–93%) for HMW agents and 88.9% (95% CI 77–92%) for LMW agents.

The highest sensitivity among LMW asthmagens occurred with combined non-specific reactivity and skin prick tests (100%; 95% CI 74.1–100%). Specific IgE and skin prick tests had similar specificities (88.9%; 95% CI 84.7–92.1%; and 86.2%; 95% CI 77.4–91.9%, respectively). For HMW agents, high specificity was demonstrated for positive non-specific reactivity tests and skin prick tests alone

(82.5%; 95% CI 54.0–95.0%) or when combined with specific IgE (74.3%; 95% CI 45.0–91.0%). Sensitivity was somewhat lower (60.6% and 65.2%, respectively). While positive results of a single non-specific reactivity test, specific skin prick tests, or serum-specific IgE testing would increase the likelihood of OA, a negative result could not exclude OA.

Confidence in the diagnosis

The degree of confidence that you require for diagnosis depends on the consequences for the worker. For instance, if an individual may lose his or her employment because of a diagnosis of OA, then a much greater degree of certainty is required than if relocation is easy to a non-exposed job without loss of income or status. Table 1 gives the sensitivity and specificity of the various diagnostic tests available. Testing for specific IgE has been omitted as it is very variable from antigen to antigen, but in some situations (e.g. prick tests to ammonium hexachlorplatinate) can be both sensitive and specific for OA [14, 15]. Specific IgE measurements can be very useful for finding a specific cause for HMW agents once OA has been confirmed by other means.

There is one study of workers with a good history of OA and negative specific challenges, who subsequently had workplace challenges and serial PEF measurements [16]. OA was confirmed in 29%, and asthma or rhinitis (of any sort) excluded in 34%.

Table 1. Sensitivity and specificity of different diagnostic tests for occupational asthma; averages from the BOHRF evidence-based review. Specific challenge tests were usually taken as the gold standard [7].

	Sensitivity %	Specificity %
History and examination	95	55
PEF before and after day shift (Δ >5 l/min)	50	95
Non-specific reactivity away from work (Δ 3.2 times)	48	64
Serial PEF <4/day or <3 weeks (Oasys score >2.5)	64	83
Serial PEF ≥4/day and ≥3 weeks (Oasys score >2.5)	78	92
Serial PEF ≥4/day and ≥4 work and rest days (mean PEF rest days – workdays >16 l/min)	67	100
Serial PEF ABC (area between curves) ≥15 l/min/hour	62–71	92
Workplace challenge	No comparative data	
Specific challenge	Unknown but <100%	

Use of Oasys plotter of serial PEF measurements in diagnosis and management of workers with OA

If occupational exposure causes or exacerbates asthma, this must be measurable with serial measurements of PEF or FEV1. The problems arise because the effects of occupational exposure may be delayed, may increase with successive exposures, and recovery may be delayed. The effects of work exposure needs separating from those due to diurnal variation, treatment, non-specific exposures such as exercise, infection and other allergen exposures. The Oasys plotter is a validated tool for plotting and analysing serial measurements of PEF. Recording should be made at approximately 2-hour intervals. For day shifts measurements on waking, arriving at work, during each work break, leaving work, mid evening and bedtime, with most importantly readings similarly spaced on days away from work. Each "days" plot starts with the first reading at work, and continues until the last recording before work on the next day, with special adjustments during shift changes (the day interpreter).

There are three validated methods of analysis of Oasys plotted records, with different minimum data quantity requirements. The original Oasys score was based on a discriminant analysis comparing a period of days at work with the preceding and following periods away from work (a rest-work-rest complex) and its counterpart a work-rest-work complex. Complexes were scored from 1 (no evidence of a work effect) to 4 (definite work effect). The complexes were summed with double weighting for scores of 1 and 4; a mean of >2.5 was found to be highly specific for independently diagnosed OA. This analysis is tolerant of missing or mistimed readings; its published specificity includes any prefabricated readings in the self-recorded records. The minimum data quantity for optimal sensitivity and specificity is ≥5 complexes (about 3 weeks), ≥3 consecutive days at work, ≥4 readings/day, no changes in treatment, with no respiratory infections and with typical exposures during the record (see Figs 3 and 4 for examples).

The area between curves (ABC) score compares the mean value for each 2-hourly segment between days at work and days away from work. Plotting hours from waking allows different shift patterns to be compared; the plot also separates days with different work exposures. Accurate timing of the readings is more important for this analysis; minimum data quantity is ≥8 readings/day with ≥8 workdays and ≥3 days away from work. The specificity was 92% and sensitivity 62–71% with the ABC score ≥15 l/min/hour for day-shift work (see Fig. 1 for example).

The final method compares the mean PEF on days away from work with those on workdays, after day interpretation. The upper 95% CI for asthmatics without OA, and asymptomatic workers exposed to high levels of irritants (grain dust) is 16 l/min. Values over this have a sensitivity of 70% for OA. The minimum data quantity for this analysis has not yet been assessed. Oasys analyses are supported by the website www.occupationalasthma.com.

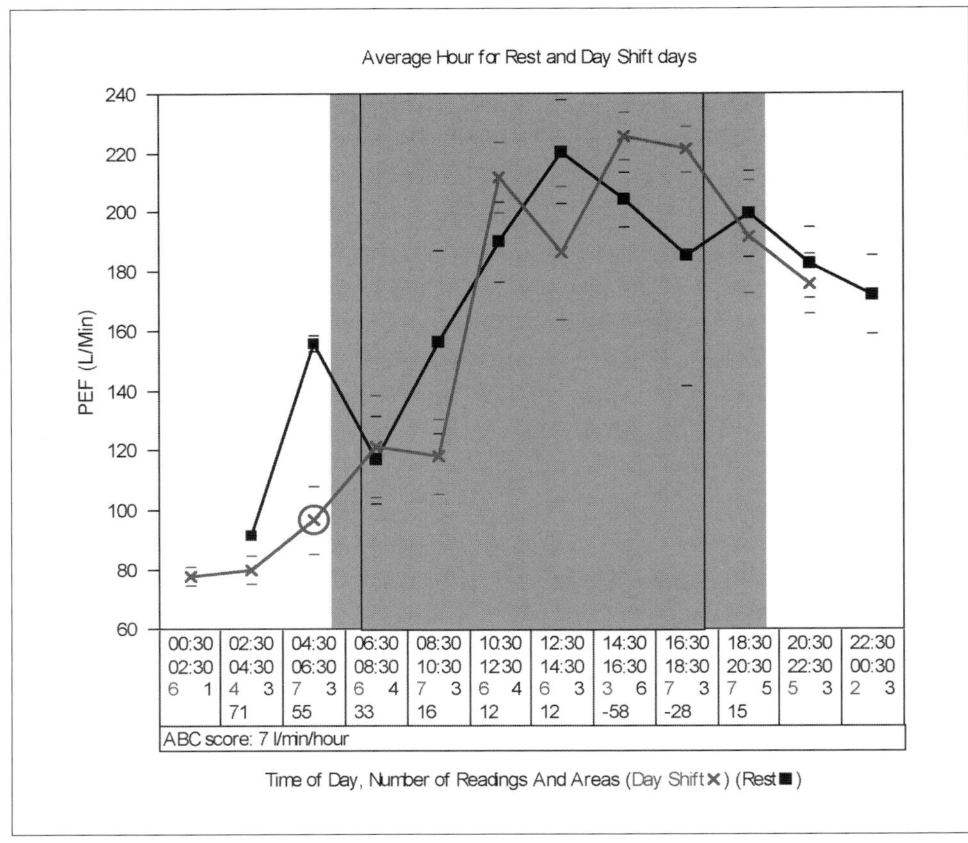

Figure 1.
Mean 2-hourly value of PEF on 7 workdays and 6 days away from work. The period at work is shaded (centre section always at work, end panels sometimes at work). Taken from an Oasys Utilities plot; the bottom panel shows the time in 2-hour blocks, the number of readings on workdays (left) and rest days (right) and the difference between work and rest days. The graph is only plotted when there are at least three measurements at each data point. The area between the curves (ABC) score is 7 l/min/hour. A score >15 is required to show a significant work effect.

Is the current work exposure causing temporary or permanent damage to the lungs?

Workers with acute irritant-induced asthma (toxic asthma) have asthma induced by a single large exposure but have not become sensitised to the agent and should be able to tolerate low levels of exposure to the same agent without problems. Although they are now asthmatic, most will be able to remain in their original jobs. Heightened surveillance would then be required.

Workers with work-aggravated asthma who have regular deterioration with work exposures and improvement away from work, or workers with OA from any mechanism will need careful assessment before continuing exposure is recommended. Evidence shows that the majority (but not all) of these will have deteriorating lung function and the longer the symptomatic exposure continues, the worse the long-term prognosis. There are, however, individuals who have regular asthma in relation to work exposures who show no identifiable long-term consequences. At the moment we do not know how to identify those with a good prognosis from those with a poor prognosis at the time of diagnosis and it is only after prolonged follow-up that the situation becomes clear. There does not seem to be a relationship between the type of agent, the magnitude of reaction to the occupational agent, atopy, smoking or treatment between those with good and poor prognoses. Those with a low lung function at presentation are amongst those with a poorer prognosis but these compose the minority of all those with OA.

A security guard with acute exposure to diesel fumes

A previously well 46-year-old security guard was locked in the back of a 16-ton security van that was stuck in a traffic jam on a busy intercity road on a foggy November morning for 90 minutes, while the diesel exhaust was escaping into his compartment through a ruptured exhaust pipe. His eyes started to smart and run, he felt tired, he had difficulty breathing, wheeze and a hoarse voice. On being released he vomited, and was taken to the Accident and Emergency department where he was found to be wheezy and breathless. He was awake during the next 2 nights with wheeze and breathlessness, and returned to work on the third day. Six days later he saw his General Practitioner who found him wheezy and breathless, PEF was 275 l/min. He was given prednisolone and salbutamol and had non-specific reactivity to histamine within the asthmatic range. For the next year he woke twice each night breathless, was wheezy for 2.5 hours each morning, and missed much time from work. He found it difficult to carry much money upstairs. He continued to smoke 35 g pipe tobacco/week. His employer wondered whether his current job was detrimental to his health. He kept serial measurements of PEF, the mean value for each 2-hour period for work and rest days are shown in Figure 1.

The plot shows that he wakes with a low PEF, which improves similarly whether at work or not. He has developed acute irritant-induced asthma, but continuing work is not associated with worse PEF. The problems he is having at work are likely to be due to his underlying asthma, provoked by exercise. Increased asthma treatment to help him cope with the exercise and carrying is likely to be the best way forward.

Removal from exposure or reduction of exposure?

There are some individuals where reducing exposure is sufficient to abolish work-related asthma and some where complete removal from exposure is required. For those with the most extreme sensitivity, contact with workers with antigen on their clothes outside the workplace may be sufficient to provoke asthma. Cases of this sort have been shown in laboratory animal workers, isocyanates and complex salts of platinum amongst others. Antigen may be taken home on the hair and clothes of the worker and contaminate the home environment as well (shown with laboratory animal workers) [17].

Substitution

The best solution is to remove the offending agent completely from the workplace so that the individual sensitised worker can continue with employment and others at work no longer run the risk of sensitisation. There are a number of good examples of this, including the removal of isocyanates from an undercoat in a steel-coating works [18]; the substitution of glutaraldehyde with non-aldehyde sterilising agents for endoscopes and its removal from x-ray developer; the substitution of latex examination gloves for vinyl or nitrile gloves and the substitution of charged platinum salts with tetraamine platinum dichloride in the manufacture of catalytic car exhausts [15]. Sometimes technological changes may remove the need for particular exposures, for instance moving to cell cultures from live animal work, or moving to digital radiology from developed x-ray films. However, sometimes an agent causing OA is replaced by another for which there is no information, which subsequently turns out to be a sensitising agent. This for instance has occurred particularly with isocyanates, where originally methylene diphenyl 4,4'-diisocyanate (MDI) was proposed as a safer substitute for toluene diisocyanate (TDI); subsequently MDI has been shown to be a major sensitising agent. The replacement of diisocyanates with pre-polymers and partially reacted isocyanate products has also not solved the problem. Recently, hydroxylamine used to replace glutaraldehyde for paper de-inking has caused OA [19].

Two workers coating steel sheet with PVC

Two workers in a factory coating steel sheet with a PVC coating presented to their occupational physician with symptoms suggestive of OA, subsequently confirmed with serial measurements of PEF. Both worked on the paint line where a continuous steel strip was passed through rollers; first an undercoat and then the PVC topcoat were applied, passing through ovens after each application.

The undercoat was known to contain epoxy resins, acrylics, phenol formaldehyde and chromates, all possible causes of OA. A survey of the 241 workforce identified symptoms suggestive of OA in 9.5%, a further 28.5% had less specific work-related respiratory symptoms. Workers on any part of the paint line were at increased risk compared with workers in other parts of the factory. Unknown to the factory, TDI had been added to the undercoat 8 years previously. The two index cases had positive specific challenge testing to TDI. (Fig. 2) The isocyanate was removed from the undercoat and the workforce restudied 1 year later. No new cases of OA had occurred, and nocturnal waking from asthma was reduced in both those with symptoms originally suggestive of OA (from 55% to 18%), but also in those with less specific symptoms (from 40% to 16%). This outbreak shows the need to make a specific aetiological diagnosis with a challenge test, and the value of removing the causative agent, extending beyond those originally thought to have OA [18].

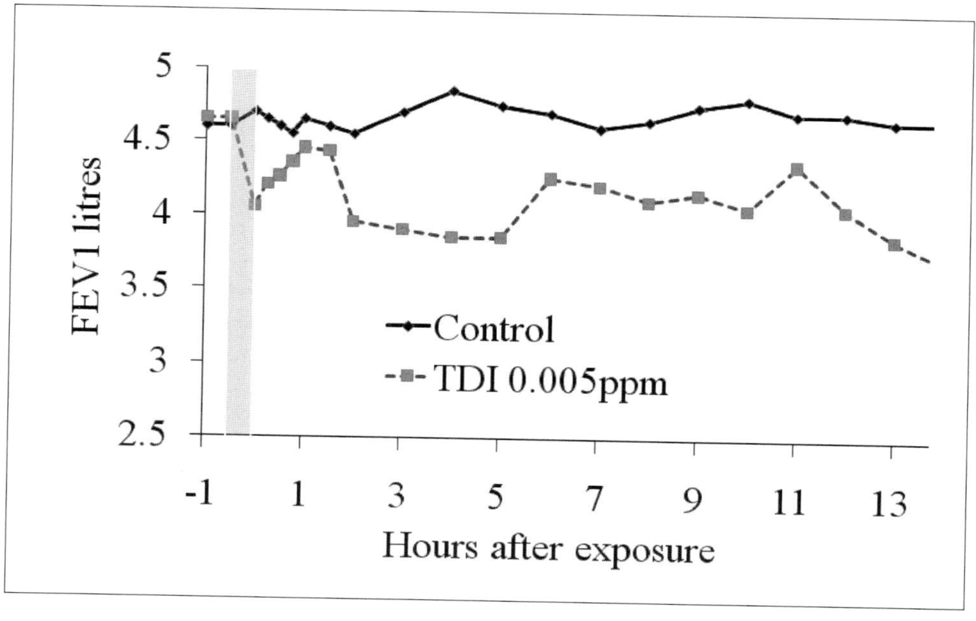

Figure 2.
Specific challenge tests to toluene diisocyanate (TDI) in an index worker in a factory coating steel sheet, showing a late asthmatic reaction to TDI. As there were several other possible causes of occupational asthma (OA) in the workplace, the specific challenge allowed the precise cause of the outbreak to be identified and the correct remedial action to take place.

Reducing exposure

There is reasonable evidence that higher levels of exposure lead to greater levels of sensitisation for most agents. Reducing inhalable exposure to an occupational allergen should be a primary aim of control. This is best done by engineering methods and there are good examples of this in the literature. For instance, biological detergents were a major cause of OA. Inhalable levels of the detergent enzymes have been reduced by reformatting the powder into a pelletised version, which is less dusty, enclosing the process particularly in the packing areas and by local exhaust ventilation [20]. Lapses in this control process particularly related to compression into tablets have resulted in a recent outbreak of OA in a biological detergent factory [21]. Detergent enzyme sensitisation can be measured with skin prick tests or specific IgE assays, which can be used for surveillance. There are more detergent workers with sensitisation than with OA, but controlling sensitisation should control disease.

Respiratory protective equipment

This is regarded as the last method for exposure control and requires substantial attention to detail to make it effective. Unpowered masks are difficult to breathe through as the work of drawing the air through the filter needs to be done by the worker and few are acceptable for day-long use. Powered units either with an external air supply or air drawn through a filtering system give more acceptable protection but are unsuitable for workers who have to get into difficult places, for instance maintaining machinery, and requires changing outside the work area and the cleaning and maintenance of RPE and air filters by somebody else wearing RPE.

Two workers manufacturing car engines

Figure 3 shows the Oasys PEF plot of a car engine manufacturer exposed to metalworking fluid aerosols. The first panel shows deterioration in 3/3 work periods and improvement in 3/3 periods away from work in 2003. The Oasys score was 4.0; as there were only two readings a day the sensitivity of this record is 64% and specificity 83% (the improvement from week to week invalidates interpretation of the rest–workday score). He was then relocated to an area of reduced exposure in 2004, although improved, he continued to deteriorate on workdays and improve on days off work; the Oasys score is now 4.0 and rest–workday difference 42 l/min (although there are now six to eight reading/day the record is too short for optimal sensitivity/specificity). In 2005 he was wearing RPE in the same job, the record was probably normal; however, there are only two readings on rest days which are inadequate for computer scoring. Visual inspection of the whole record in this situation is preferable.

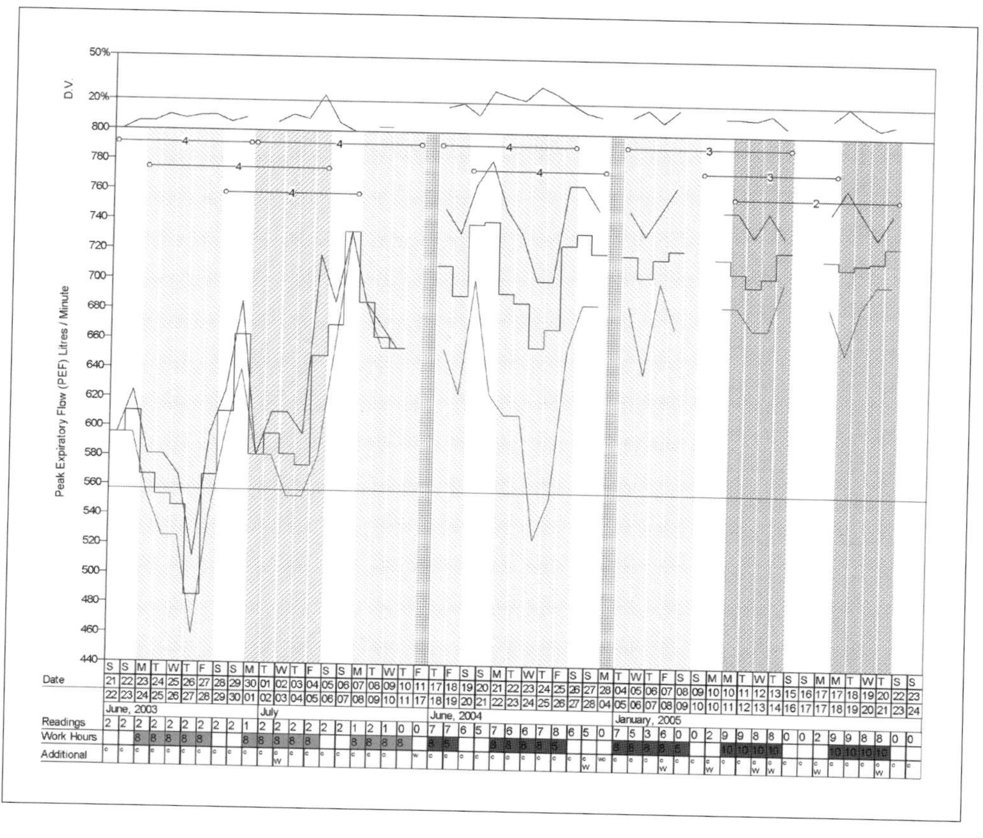

Figure 3.
Oasys plot of serial PEF of an car engine manufacturer exposed to metal-working fluid aerosols. The top panel shows daily PEF diurnal variation. The centre panel shows the daily maximum (upper dotted line), mean (middle horizontal bars) and minimum (lower dotted line). Days away from work have a clear background, days at work a shaded background (back hatching morning shift, forward hatching afternoon shift, cross hatching night shift). The predicted PEF is the horizontal line at 559 l/min. The bottom panel shows the date, the number of readings per day, the number of hours worked and comments. An explanation of the findings is given in the text.

Figure 4 shows another worker from the same engine manufacturing shop who kept serial PEF measurements before the metal working fluid was replaced. The left panel shows an Oasys score of 3.91 and a rest–work difference of 45 l/min; this fulfils all the criteria for an optimal record with Oasys score sensitivity 78% and specificity 92%. After cleaning (centre panel) there is improvement, but the Oasys

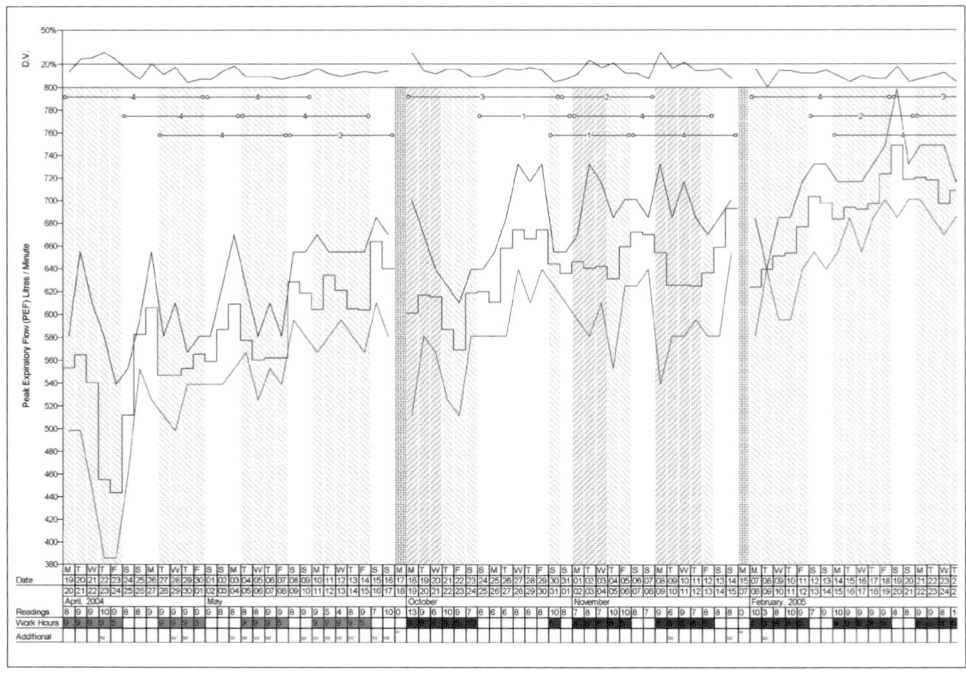

Figure 4.
Oasys plot of serial PEF in another worker exposed to the same metal-working fluid aerosols as the worker in Figure 3. The first 4 weeks are before remedial action, the middle 4 weeks after a complete clean and replacement of the metal-working fluid, and the right 4 weeks while wearing full air-fed RPE. An explanation is given in the text.

score remains positive at 2.5 and the rest–workday difference 35 l/min. While wearing full air-fed RPE (right panel) the PEF has improved but still shows an Oasys score of 3.56 and a rest–work difference of 32 l/min. Each change was associated with an improvement in PEF, but even while wearing RPE he still deteriorated on workdays and improved away from work showing that relocation away from exposure was required.

The role of compensation

The primary assessment of a worker with OA should separate workers who are unlikely to be able to work again because of the severity of their disease or their nearness to a normal retirement age and those who could work productively again, provided that they are not exposed to the agent to which they are sensitised. Those who are unlikely to work again are best handled by some sort of compensation to make up for their loss of earnings.

Those who may work again often need re-training and have income preserved during this period of re-training. There are only a few schemes in the world where compensation includes a major resource for re-training and, even in these, only a minority have substantial re-training. Good examples come for Quebec and Finland.

If re-training or preservation of income is assured through a compensation scheme, it is much easier to remove somebody from exposure than for a similarly affected worker who is not eligible for compensation in a particular country. For instance, in some countries, OA is only recognised to a limited list of agents and if a worker has the same disease from an unrecognised agent, removal from exposure may lead to unemployment and no extra income at all.

Heightened surveillance for relocated workers

Any worker who continues in the workplace with possible exposure to the agent to which they are sensitised needs heightened surveillance, which should at least include a questionnaire and spirometry. If the OA is *via* an IgE mechanism, measuring the IgE serially should allow continued exposure to be monitored as specific IgE has a relatively short half life and reduces with cessation of exposure. The interpretation of longitudinal data, particularly spirometry, is difficult, as measurement error and spontaneous variability (95% CIs for FEV1 measured on two occasions around 160 ml in good hands) is far higher than the expected decline of 25–30 ml/year due to aging. A minimum of 5 years readings is usually required. The following show examples of IgE and FEV_1 used in surveillance of relocated workers.

A laboratory scientist

A laboratory scientist developed urticaria, rhinitis and asthma that improved on days away from work. Her job was mainly administrative but she did do some hands on work for which she used latex gloves. She had a positive skin prick test and specific IgE to latex, making latex the most likely cause of her symptoms. She stopped wearing latex gloves herself but had little change in her asthma, or her specific IgE, suggesting continuing exposure. Latex gloves were then replaced with nitrile gloves in the whole laboratory, with improvement in her symptoms and a reduction in her specific IgE to latex as shown in Figure 5.

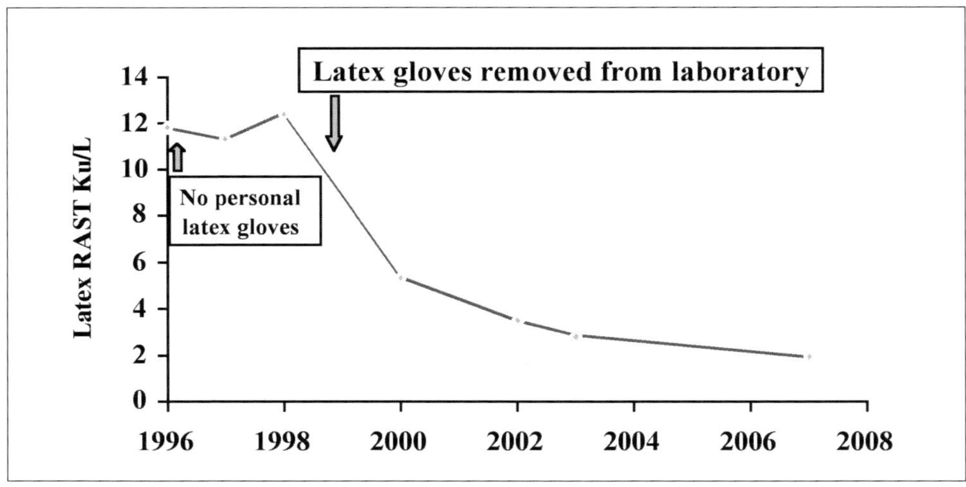

Figure 5.
Serial measurements of specific IgE to latex in a laboratory scientist with OA, rhinitis and urticaria. It shows no reduction when she stopped using latex gloves personally, but an exponential fall when latex gloves were removed from the whole laboratory, confirming satisfactory avoidance of exposure.

A university professor with OA from rats

This professor developed severe asthma 8 years after starting work with rats and mice. He was the only member of the department with an animal licence and was responsible for bleeding mice occasionally. Following diagnosis in 1994 he stopped working with animals, which were now transported in filter-top cages to reduce exposure during movement. The results of trivial exposure to the rats when his lecturer left and was not replaced is shown in Figure 6.

Taking action on serial measurements of lung function carried out during medical surveillance is even more difficult as the measurement error and biological variations are substantial in relation to suspected annual declines. SPIROLA is a useful program for analysing serial measurements of FEV_1 to detect abnormal FEV_1 declines [22] (see examples in Figs 7 and 8).

SPIROLA

This program is available free of charge from National Institute for Occupational Safety and Health (NIOSH). It helps interpret longitudinal changes in FEV_1

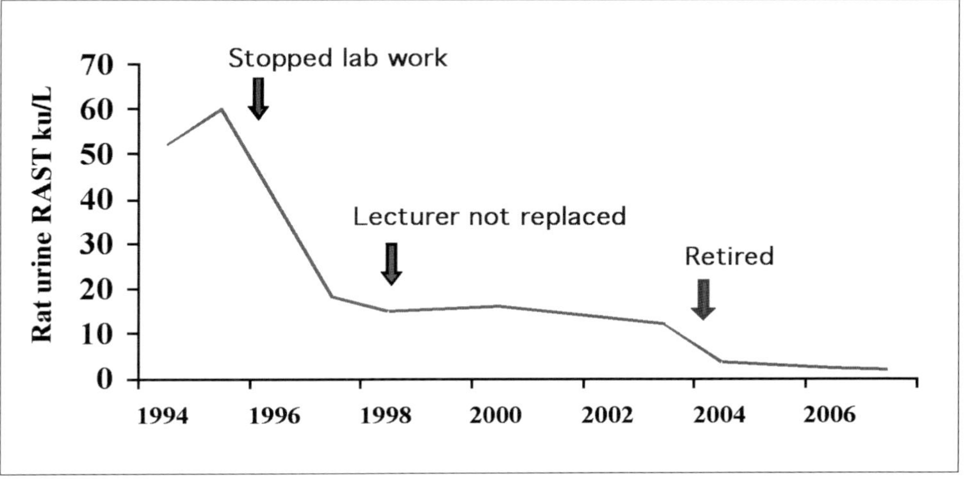

Figure 6.
Serial measurements of specific IgE to a rat urinary antigen in a university professor whose research used with rats and mice. There was initially a satisfactory fall in specific IgE until his lecturer left and was not replaced, leaving the professor to do very occasional teaching sessions with rat exposure (30 minutes twice a year). His rat IgE stopped falling indicating continuing exposure, levels fell again after retirement.

in individual workers, and detects excess decline when statistically significant. It requires measurements over several years unless the FEV_1 decline is very rapid, for instance a decline of 400 ml in 1 year may be within the 95% CI for an individual. The interpretation of a result for an individual depends on the precision of measurement for the group (and operators) from which the worker comes. This is calculated by measuring the change in FEV_1 percent predicted from two measurements within 18 months, and calculating the standard deviation of this change for the group. The 95% CI for this change is then calculated, which reduces the longer the series of measurements for an individual proceeds. Over the first 8 years of an individual's follow-up, SPIROLA uses the limit of longitudinal decline (LLD) to determine whether or not the individual's decline in FEV_1 may be excessive. After 8 years of follow-up, the age at which the individual may be expected to develop moderate-severe lung function impairment is taken into consideration in the evaluation, which also shows how the last measurement has increased or decreased the estimate of FEV_1 decline. When the regression line of FEV_1 for an individual crosses the 95% limit of longitudinal decline, accelerated decline for that individual can be confirmed with confidence. The program

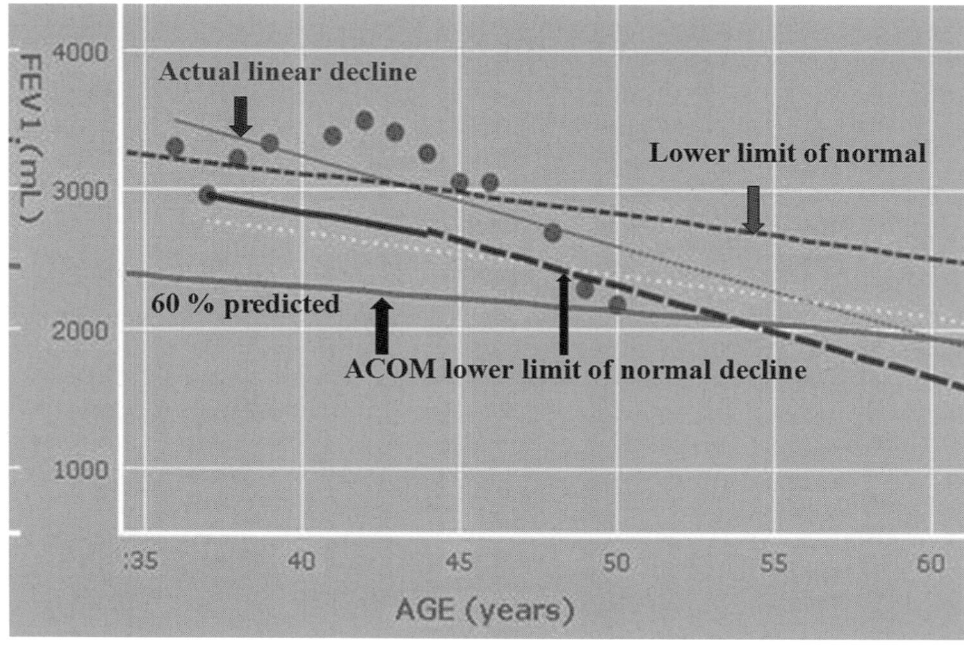

Figure 7.
The SPIROLA plot of a cereal manufacturer. The round dots are the actual FEV_1 measurements; the upper small dashed line the lower limit of normal; the upper solid line the estimated annual decline using linear regression; the lower heavy solid line the value for 60% predicted at each age and the pale dotted line the lower 95% CI for the rate of FEV_1 decline using the centres precision estimate.

is supported by the website http://www.cdc.gov/niosh/topics/spirometry/spirola.html.

The plot includes the actual FEV_1 measurements, the lower limit of normal from predicted equations, the estimated annual decline for the individual using linear regression, the value for FEV_1 that is 60% of that predicted at each data point, and the lower 95% CI for the rate of FEV_1 decline for the individual using the centres precision estimate (Fig. 7). After 5 years of measurements, SPIROLA also plots the effect of the last measurement on the calculated FEV_1 slope, and FEV_1 decline calculated on the last 8 years measurements only, allowing the detection of a change in slope, for instance after the development of sensitisation to a workplace agent (Fig. 8).

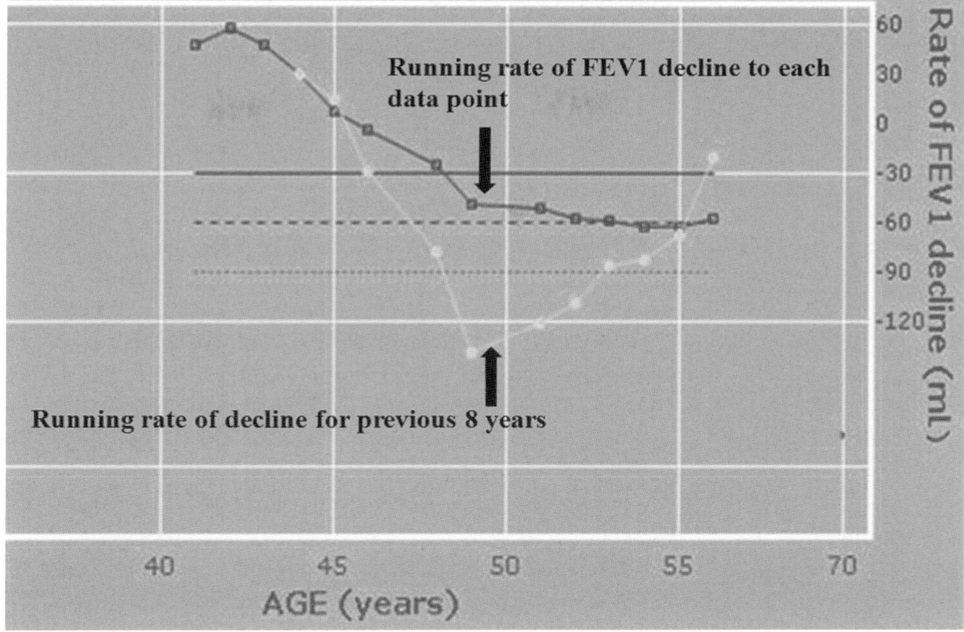

Figure 8.
SPIROLA plot of the same worker extended for 6 years after relocation away from thiamine exposure, while working as a fork-lift truck driver in the stores. The upper panel shows whether the last measurement has altered the calculated FEV_1 slope (upper line), and FEV_1 decline calculated on the last 8 years measurements only (lower line). There is a clear improvement on relocation away from thiamine exposure.

A manufacturer of breakfast cereals

A 45-year-old non-smoking manufacturer of breakfast cereals developed rhinitis shortly followed by asthma that improved away from work but was only worse on some workweeks. He was under regular medical surveillance because of his exposure to wheat and maize, which are recognised respiratory sensitisers. He was removed from exposure to wheat and maize and continued to have annual spirometry. His FEV_1 continued to fall. His annual FEV_1 was plotted with SPIROLA and is shown in Figure 7.

His estimated FEV_1 decline crosses the 95% CI at the age of 49. It was now clear that relocation had failed and that the standard of proof for the diagnosis of wheat asthma based on history and PEF readings was insufficient. Interestingly, IgE to wheat had been negative initially, but wheat asthma sometimes occurs with a

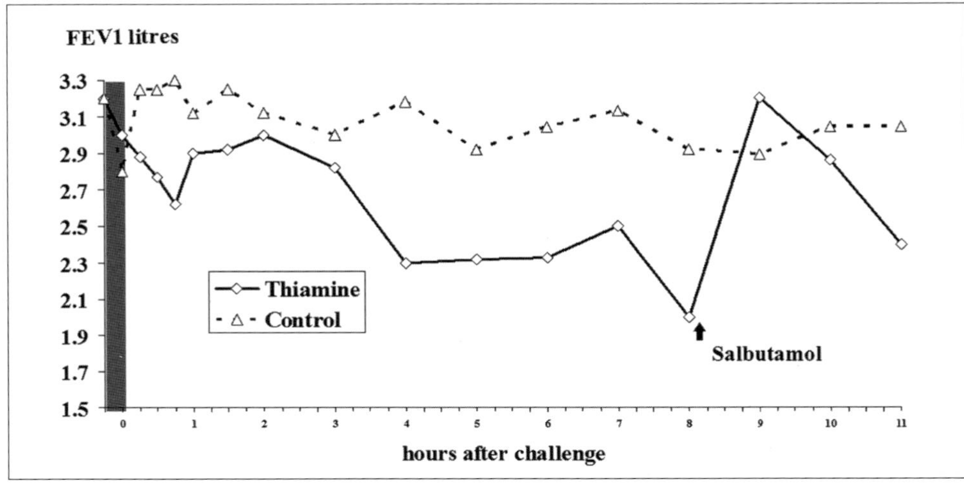

Figure 9.
The results of specific bronchial challenge testing to nebulised thiamine showing a dual asthmatic reaction.

negative IgE. At this point he was investigated with specific challenge tests, which showed no reaction to wheat but a dual asthmatic reaction to thiamine, sprayed onto the cereals for added nutritional value (Fig. 9). He was then removed from thiamine exposure aged 50 and continued with annual spirometry while working as a fork-lift truck driver in the stores. The updated SPIROLA plot is shown in Figure 8.

Treatment

Treatment should be of benefit to those with OA in the same way as in non-OA. There is pressure to treat rather than investigate when the patient first presents. Treatment rarely if ever fully controls OA; it is much better to validate the diagnosis of OA or non-OA first before starting (or increasing) treatment as the diagnostic tests are less sensitive when more treatment is being taken [23]. If a worker elects to remain exposed to the causative agent usual asthma treatments should be used. The proportion of non-eosinophilic asthma is probably greater in OA caused by LMW molecules than in non-OA [24], but as yet there are no studies which have investigated the benefits of inhaled corticosteroids in occupational asthmatics separated into eosinophilic and non-eosinophilic variants. The use of anti-IgE therapy would be particularly interesting in IgE-mediated OA, but so far only one small controlled trial has not shown abolition of urticaria, rhinitis and conjunctivitis due to latex allergy [25].

Conclusion

Managing a worker with OA requires an understanding of the mechanism (particularly the distinction between acute irritant-induced asthma and OA due to sensitisation). The basic tools for OA diagnosis; spirometry, serial PEF, specific IgE, non-specific reactivity and specific challenge testing, may all be needed in the management of a worker after the diagnosis has been made to arrive at the best outcome. Leaving a worker unemployed because of medical intervention is a failure of our management; it is the outcome in about a third of all those with OA [7].

References

1 Hudson P, Cartier A, Pineau L, Lafrance M, St Aubin JJ, Dubois JV et al. Follow-up of occupational asthma caused by crab and various agents. *J Allergy Clin Immunol.* 1985; 76: 682–688

2 Park HS, Nahm DH. Prognostic factors for toluene diisocyanate-induced occupational asthma after removal from exposure. *Clin Exp Allergy.* 1997; 27(10): 1145–1150

3 Piirilä PL, Nordman H, Keskinen HM, Luukkonen R, Salo SP, Tuomi T et al. Long-term follow-up of hexamethylene diisocyanate-, diphenylmethane diisocyanate-, and toluene diisocyanate-induced asthma. *Am J Respir Crit Care Med.* 2000; 162(2 Pt 1): 516–522

4 Rosenberg N, Garnier R, Rousselin X, Mertz R, Gervais P. Clinical and socio-professional fate of isocyanate-induced asthma. *Clin Allergy.* 1987; 17: 55–61

5 Ross DJ, McDonald JC. Health and employment after a diagnosis of occupational asthma: a descriptive study. *Occup Med.* 1998; 48: 219–225

6 Tarlo SM, Banks D, Liss G, Broder I. Outcome determinants for isocyanate induced occupational asthma among compensation claimants. *Occup Environ Med.* 1997; 54(10): 756–761

7 Nicholson PJ, Cullinan P, Newman Taylor AJ, Burge PS, Boyle C. Evidence based guidelines for the prevention, identification, and management of occupational asthma. *Occup Environ Med.* 2005; 62: 290–299

8 Burge PS. Non-specific bronchial hyper-reactivity in workers exposed to toluene diisocyanate, diphenyl methane di-isocyanate and colophony. *Eur J Respir Dis* (Suppl). 1982; 123: 91–96

9 Douglas JD, McSharry C, Blaikie L, Morrow T, Miles S, Franklin D. Occupational asthma caused by automated salmon processing. *Lancet.* 1995; 346(8977): 737–740

10 Grammer LC, Shaughnessy MA, Henderson J, Zeiss CR, Kavich DE, Collins MJ et al. A clinical and immunologic study of workers with trimellitic-anhydride-induced immu-

nologic lung disease after transfer to low exposure jobs. *Am Rev Respir Dis.* 1993; 148: 54–57

11 Merget R, Schulte A, Gebler A, Breitstadt R, Kulzer R, Berndt ED et al. Outcome of occupational asthma due to platinum salts after transferral to low-exposure areas. *Int Arch Occup Environ Health* 1999; 72(1): 33–39

12 Pisati G, Baruffini A, Zedda S. Toluene diisocyanate induced asthma: Outcome according to persistence or cessation of exposure. *Br J Ind Med.* 1993; 50: 60–64

13 Beach J, Russell K, Blitz S, Hooton N, Spooner C, Lemiere C et al. A systematic review of the diagnosis of occupational asthma. *Chest.* 2007; 131(2): 569–578

14 Niezborala M, Garnier R. Allergy to complex platinum salts: A historical prospective cohort study. *Occup Environ Med.* 1996; 53(4): 252–257

15 Linnett PJ, Hughes EG. 20 years of medical surveillance on exposure to allergenic and non-allergenic platinum compounds: The importance of chemical speciation. *Occup Environ Med.* 1999; 56: 191–196

16 Rioux JP, Malo JL, L'Archeveque J, Rabhi K, Labrecque M. Workplace-specific challenges as a contribution to the diagnosis of occupational asthma. *Eur Respir J.* 2008; 32: 997–1003

17 Krop E, Doekes G, Stone M, Aalberse R, van der Zee JS. Spreading of occupational allergens: Laboratory animal allergens on hair-covering caps and in mattress dust of laboratory animal workers. *Occup Environ Med.* 2007; 64(4): 267–272

18 Venables KM, Dally MB, Burge PS, Pickering CAC, Newman Taylor AJ. Occupational asthma in a steel coating plant. *Br J Ind Med.* 1985; 42(8): 517–524

19 Tran S, Hoyle J, Niven RM, Francis HC. The paper recycling industry, hydroxylamine and occupational asthma: two case reports. *Thorax.* 2007; 62 suppl 3: A130

20 Cathcart M, Nicholson P, Roberts D, Bazley M, Juniper C, Murray P et al. Enzyme exposure, smoking and lung function in employees in the detergent industry over 20 years. Medical Subcommittee of the UK Soap and Detergent Industry Association. *Occup Med.* 1997; 47(8): 473–478

21 Cullinan P, Harris JM, Newman Taylor AJ, Hole AM, Jones M, Barnes F et al. An outbreak of asthma in a modern detergent factory . *Lancet.* 2000; 356: 1899–1900

22 Hnizdo E, Yu L, Freyder L, Attfield M, Lefante J, Glindmeyer HW. The precision of longitudinal lung function measurements: Monitoring and interpretation. *Occup Environ Med.* 2005; 62(10): 695–701

23 Burge PS, O'Brien IM, Harries MG. Peak flow rate records in the diagnosis of occupational asthma due to colophony. *Thorax.* 1979; 34(3): 308–316

24 Anees W, Huggins V, Pavord I, Robertson AS, Burge PS. Occupational asthma due to low molecular weight agents: Eosinoiphilic and non-eosinophilic variants. *Thorax.* 2002; 57: 231–236

25 Leynadier F, Doudou O, Gaouar H, Le Gros V, Bourdeix I, Guyomarch-Cocco L et al. Effect of omalizumab in health care workers with occupational latex allergy. *J Allergy Clin Immunol.* 2004; 113: 360–361.

Social consequences and quality of life in work-related asthma

Olivier Vandenplas and Vinciane D'Alpaos

Service de Pneumologie, Cliniques de Mont-Godinne, Université Catholique de Louvain, Yvoir, Belgium

Abstract

Work-related asthma can interfere with patient's daily life, including professional, familial, and social activities. Occupational asthma (OA) is associated with a high rate of prolonged work disruption and loss of income. Available information indicates that work-exacerbated asthma has a negative socio-economic impact to the same extent as OA. The socio-economic outcome seems to be predominantly influenced by professional and socio-demographic factors. Adverse professional and economic consequences are more pronounced when workers have to leave their workplace because of reduced possibilities for accommodation in unexposed jobs within the same company or lack of effective retraining programs. The socio-economic outcome is also affected by the age and the level of education of affected workers. There is growing evidence that work-related asthma is associated with a lower quality of life than asthma unrelated to work.

Introduction

The workplace environment can cause the development of asthma through immunological or toxic mechanisms (i.e., occupational asthma, OA) and trigger asthma symptoms in subjects with pre-existing or coincidental asthma (i.e., work-exacerbated asthma, WEA) [1]. There is growing evidence that the various forms of work-related asthma contributes substantially to the global burden of asthma [2–4]. Asthma can cause a physiological defect (i.e., impairment) that may affect daily life activities (i.e., disability), leading to socio-economic consequences and altered quality of life (QoL).

Asthma-related impairment can be quantified based on the degree of airflow limitation, the level of nonspecific bronchial hyperresponsiveness to histamine/methacholine, and medications required to control symptoms, as recommended by the American Thoracic Society [5]. Although airway inflammation is a key feature of asthma, there is little information on the relationship between inflammation and impairment in work-related asthma. Recent studies have shown that airway inflammation may persist in a substantial proportion of subjects with OA several years after avoidance of exposure, even in subjects with normal functional parameters [6].

It remains unknown whether persistent inflammation is associated with higher rates of asthma exacerbation and worse functional outcome.

Assessment of disability is a much more complex process, as it should take into account the global impact that impairment may have on patients' functioning. Translation of physiological impairment into disability is affected by many non-medical variables, including: job conditions, age, gender, socio-economic status, emotional factors, and co-morbidities. In addition, the patient should be compared to himself prior to the disease in terms of daily activities and QoL. The discordance between physiological impairment and disability is probably best illustrated in OA. Affected workers should be considered completely and permanently disabled in terms of occupations that entail exposure to the sensitizing agent that caused OA, even when they demonstrate little physiological impairment without such exposure. Work-related asthma may, therefore, lead predominantly to disability rather than physiological impairment [7].

This section reviews available information pertaining to the impact of work-related asthma on the different components of the socio-economic burden, including health care utilization, work productivity, loss of income, and QoL [8, 9]. The factors that determine the socio-economic outcomes are explored to identify potential targets for interventions aimed at minimizing the adverse consequences of the condition.

Healthcare utilization

An analysis of the Ontario Workers' Compensation Board data found that the rates of hospitalization for respiratory diseases and mortality among subjects compensated for OA were similar to those observed in asthmatic subjects without work-related asthma [10, 11]. However, recent data derived from the Quebec's Public Health Insurance Plan [12] indicated that subjects with work-related asthma visited a physician or an emergency department because of their asthma and were hospitalized more frequently than asthmatic subjects without work-related symptoms. The medical resource utilization decreased after removal from exposure to the causal work environment.

Work productivity

Work disability is a key component for evaluating the consequences of a disease, as it can lead to reduced earning capacity and socio-economic status. Health-related work disability can take different forms, including reduced workforce participation and employment rates, restrictions in job duties or working time, lost work days (i.e., absenteeism), and impaired effectiveness at work (i.e., presenteeism) [7].

Follow-up studies of workers with OA have consistently documented that the condition is associated with a high rate of work disruption (Tab. 1) [13–22], with the lowest rates being reported from Finland (14%) and Quebec, Canada (25%). The reported rates of unemployment among subjects with OA and WEA seem higher than in the general population, although there is a need for further characterization of the specific impact of OA as compared with asthma unrelated to work. Whatever its etiology, asthma may be associated with substantial disability, including reduced workforce participation [23, 24] and impaired work productivity [23, 25–29]. In the only available study that compared OA with non-OA, the rate of unemployment was similar in the two groups, whereas a reduction of income was more frequently reported by subjects with OA (62%) as compared with those with asthma unrelated to work (38%) [16]. These two groups were, however, not matched for the severity of asthma and other relevant socio-demographic variables.

Table 1. Employment and loss of income in workers with occupational asthma

Country	No. of subjects	Duration of follow-up (years)	Rate of unemployment (%)	Loss of income (% of workers)	Reference
UK	112	Median: 1.4	35%	Exposed: 44% Unexposed: 74%	Gannon, 1993 [13]
Canada, BC	128	Mean: 4.8	41%	NA	Marabini, 1993 [14]
Canada, Qc	134	Range: 2–5	25%	NA	Dewitte, 1994 [15]
UK	87	5	39%	55%	Cannon, 1995 [16]
France	209	Mean: 3.1	34%	46%	Ameille, 1997 [17]
USA	55	Mean: 2.6	69%	NA	Gassert, 1998 [18]
UK	770	Range: 1.5–5.5	37%	NA	Ross, 1998 [19]
Belgium	86	Median: 3.3	38%	62%	Larbanois, 2002 [20]
Norway	496	Range: 2–6	49%	51%	Leira, 2005 [21]
Finland	213	Mean: 10	14%	NA	Piirila, 2005 [22]

NA, data not available; BC, British Colombia; Qc, Quebec

The number of work days lost by workers with work-related asthma while they are still employed is unknown. It should be outlined that the time elapsed between the onset of work-related symptoms and the diagnosis of OA is often very long and the economic impact of lost work productivity during this period should not be neglected. Although a substantial proportion of employed asthmatics (9–27%) report a reduction in work performance because of their condition [25, 27, 30], presenteeism has never been specifically assessed in subjects with OA who are working (either exposed or not to the offending agent). It is, however, conceivable that work effectiveness may be more impaired in subjects who experience work-related asthma symptoms than in subjects with asthma unrelated to work [25].

Estimating the financial impact of work-related asthma should also include the cost incurred by employers for hiring and training new workers or for modifying the workplace environment. Up to now, the impact of work-related asthma has never been assessed from the employer perspective.

Earning capacity

A high proportion of workers suffering from OA, ranging from 44% to 74%, report a substantial loss of work-derived income attributed to their condition (Tab. 1) [13, 16, 17, 20, 21].

The socio-economic outcomes of WEA have been explored in a few studies [16, 20, 31]. The rates of unemployment and income loss in subjects with WEA did not differ significantly from those observed in subjects with ascertained OA.

The proportion of subjects with OA who benefit from a financial compensation varies from 17% to 87% in European countries [13, 14, 16, 17, 20–22]. The cost of compensation for OA seems largely unknown. In addition, the effectiveness of compensation systems in minimizing adverse socio-economic consequences of OA has never been evaluated. The disease-related loss of income incurred by workers with OA seems to be offset by the granted compensation in a minority of affected workers (22% of subjects in Belgium [20] and 44% of subjects in France [17]).

Psycho-social and quality-of-life impacts

Health-related QoL refers to the global consequences of asthma and its treatment on physical, emotional, and social aspects of patients' functioning [32]. Malo and co-workers [33] found that subjects with OA, even when removed from exposure, have a slightly but significantly worse QoL than those with non-OA matched for the severity of asthma. More recently, the factors that determine the magnitude of the impact of OA on QoL have been investigated in a large population of subjects with isocyanate-induced OA in Finland [22]. This study found that "satisfaction with life" was related to current employment and higher levels of asthma control. The effects of exposure interventions on QoL have never been assessed prospectively. In a retrospective study of subjects with latex-induced OA, asthma-specific QoL did not differ among subjects who avoided and those who reduced exposure to latex gloves [34]. The impact of OA and WEA on QoL appeared quite similar after removal from exposure to the offending environment [31]. A recent study, conducted among asthmatic member of a US health maintenance organization, compared QoL in subjects with self-reported WEA and those with asthma unrelated to work [35]. Participants with WEA had a lower QoL, especially pertaining to "mood disturbance", "social disruptions", and "health concerns", even after controlling for relevant covariates.

Determinants of adverse socio-economic consequences

Available information indicates that a number of occupational and socio-demographic factors can adversely affect socio-economic outcomes in workers with OA. Financial consequences of OA are consistently more pronounced in workers who avoid further exposure to the causal agent [13, 17, 20, 36]. A loss of income has been more frequently reported by workers who are completely removed from exposure to the causal agent (69–78% of workers) [13, 20, 36] than by those who remain exposed (17–44% of workers) [13, 20, 36]. The median self-reported reduction of income was 54% in workers who were no longer exposed and 35% in workers with persistent exposure [13]. Only one prospective study compared asthma severity, disease-related costs, and work-derived income after cessation or persistence of exposure to various agents causing OA [36]. Complete avoidance of exposure to causal agents resulted in a significant decrease in asthma severity and in health care expenses, but also in work-derived income, as compared with persistence of exposure [36]. This is likely to account for the finding that about one third of workers suffering from OA remains exposed to the causative agent [13, 14, 17, 20, 22, 36], with the notable exception of Quebec where all subjects are removed from exposure with a low rate of unemployment (25%) [15]. There is some suggestion that reducing rather than eliminating exposure to sensitizing agents could be considered a reasonably safe alternative that would be associated with fewer socio-economic consequences. In a retrospective study of 36 subjects with latex-induced OA, respiratory health outcomes improved similarly after reduction or cessation of exposure to airborne latex, whereas reduction of exposure resulted in a substantially lower impact in terms of employment and earnings [34]. Nevertheless, the long-term health effects of reducing exposure to other agents causing OA remain largely uncertain [7].

The loss of income is generally higher in workers who have to change their employer as compared to those who remain employed in the same company [17].

Unfortunately, in European countries, less than 20% of subjects with OA are relocated to unexposed jobs in the same company [13, 17, 20, 22], while this proportion seems somewhat higher (31%) in Quebec [15]. Interestingly, the lowest rates of unemployment (14% and 25%) have been reported in countries (i.e., Finland and Quebec) where a high proportion of workers with OA benefits from effective retraining programs.

Socio-demographic factors that are associated with a worse economic outcome include: unskilled jobs [13, 20], lower levels of education [17, 20], older age [14, 20], younger age [17], a lower number of economically dependent subjects [14], and being employed in small-sized firms [17]. Worth noting is the fact that the severity of asthma does not appear to be an important determinant of employment status in subjects with OA [13–17, 20, 36, 37], with the exception of Finland. In the Finnish survey of workers with isocyanate-induced OA [22], employment was mainly affected by the severity of asthma. These data suggest that the role of disease severity may become apparent only when socio-demographic factors are appropriately minimized.

Conclusion

OA is associated with a substantial impact on employment, earning capacity, and QoL. Interestingly, work disability is affected predominantly by socio-demographic factors, while the severity of asthma plays only a minimal role. Accordingly, interventions aimed at reducing the psycho-social consequences of work-related asthma should focus on retraining and accommodating affected workers to unexposed jobs. However, cost-benefit analysis of preventive interventions would require more precise and quantified data on the relevant cost components [38].

Acknowledgement

This work has been supported in part by the Actions de Recherche Concertées de la Communauté Française de Belgique and the Fonds Scientifique CESI.

References

1 Vandenplas O, Malo JL. Definitions and types of work-related asthma: A nosological approach. *Eur Respir J* 2003; 21: 706–12

2 Leigh JP, Romano PS, Schenker MB, Kreiss K. Costs of occupational COPD and asthma. *Chest* 2002; 121: 264–72

3 Balmes J, Becklake M, Blanc P, Henneberger P, Kreiss K, Mapp C, et al. American Thoracic Society Statement: Occupational contribution to the burden of airway disease. *Am J Respir Crit Care Med* 2003; 167: 787–97
4 Driscoll T, Nelson DI, Steenland K, Leigh J, Concha-Barrientos M, Fingerhut M, et al. The global burden of non-malignant respiratory disease due to occupational airborne exposures. *Am J Ind Med* 2005; 48: 432–45
5 American Thoracic Society. Guidelines for the evaluation of impairment/disability in patients with asthma. *Am Rev Respir Dis* 1993; 147: 1056–61
6 Yacoub MR, Lavoie K, Lacoste G, Daigle S, L'Archeveque J, Ghezzo H, et al. Assessment of impairment/disability due to occupational asthma through a multidimensional approach. *Eur Respir J* 2007; 29: 889–896
7 Vandenplas O, Toren K, Blanc PD. Health and socioeconomic impact of work-related asthma. *Eur Respir J* 2003; 22: 689–97
8 Weiss KB, Sullivan SD. The health economics of asthma and rhinitis. I. Assessing the economic impact. *J Allergy Clin Immunol* 2001; 107: 3–8
9 Sullivan SD, Weiss KB. Health economics of asthma and rhinitis. II. Assessing the value of interventions. *J Allergy Clin Immunol* 2001; 107: 203–10
10 Liss GM, Tarlo SM, Banks D, Yeung KS, Schweigert M. Preliminary report of mortality among workers compensated for work- related asthma. *Am J Ind Med* 1999; 35: 465–71
11 Liss GM, Tarlo SM, Macfarlane Y, Yeung KS. Hospitalization among workers compensated for occupational asthma. *Am J Respir Crit Care Med* 2000; 162: 112–8
12 Lemiere C, Forget A, Dufour MH, Boulet LP, Blais L. Characteristics and medical resource use of asthmatic subjects with and without work-related asthma. *J Allergy Clin Immunol* 2007; 120: 1354–9
13 Gannon PF, Weir DC, Robertson AS, Burge PS. Health, employment, and financial outcomes in workers with occupational asthma. *Br J Ind Med* 1993; 50: 491–6
14 Marabini A, Dimich-Ward H, Kwan SY, Kennedy SM, Waxler-Morrison N, Chan-Yeung M. Clinical and socioeconomic features of subjects with red cedar asthma. A follow-up study. *Chest* 1993; 104: 821–4
15 Dewitte JD, Chan-Yeung M, Malo JL. Medicolegal and compensation aspects of occupational asthma. *Eur Respir J* 1994; 7: 969–80
16 Cannon J, Cullinan P, Newman Taylor A. Consequences of occupational asthma. *BMJ* 1995; 311: 602–3
17 Ameille J, Pairon JC, Bayeux MC, Brochard P, Choudat D, Conso F, et al. Consequences of occupational asthma on employment and financial status: A follow-up study. *Eur Respir J* 1997; 10: 55–8
18 Gassert TH, Hu H, Kelsey KT, Christiani DC. Long-term health and employment outcomes of occupational asthma and their determinants. *J Occup Environ Med* 1998; 40: 481–91
19 Ross DJ, McDonald JC. Health and employment after a diagnosis of occupational asthma: A descriptive study. *Occup Med* (Lond) 1998; 48: 219–25

20 Larbanois A, Jamart J, Delwiche JP, Vandenplas O. Socio-economic outcome of subjects experiencing asthma symptoms at work. *Eur Respir J* 2002; 19: 1107–13

21 Leira HL, Bratt U, Slastad S. Notified cases of occupational asthma in Norway: Exposure and consequences for health and income. *Am J Ind Med* 2005; 48: 359–64

22 Piirila PL, Keskinen HM, Luukkonen R, Salo SP, Tuppurainen M, Nordman H. Work, unemployment and life satisfaction among patients with diisocyanate induced asthma – A prospective study. *J Occup Health* 2005; 47: 112–8

23 Blanc PD, Cisternas M, Smith S, Yelin EH. Asthma, employment status, and disability among adults treated by pulmonary and allergy specialists. *Chest* 1996; 109: 688–96

24 Yelin E, Henke J, Katz PP, Eisner MD, Blanc PD. Work dynamics of adults with asthma. *Am J Ind Med* 1999; 35: 472–80

25 Balder B, Lindholm NB, Lowhagen O, Palmqvist M, Plaschke P, Tunsater A, et al. Predictors of self-assessed work ability among subjects with recent-onset asthma. *Respir Med* 1998; 92: 729–34

26 Blanc PD, Ellbjar S, Janson C, Norback D, Norrman E, Plaschke P, et al. Asthma-related work disability in Sweden. The impact of workplace exposures. *Am J Respir Crit Care Med* 1999; 160: 2028–33

27 Blanc PD, Trupin L, Eisner M, Earnest G, Katz PP, Israel L, et al. The work impact of asthma and rhinitis: Findings from a population-based survey. *J Clin Epidemiol* 2001; 54: 610–8

28 Sauni R, Oksa P, Vattulainen K, Uitti J, Palmroos P, Roto P. The effects of asthma on the quality of life and employment of construction workers. *Occup Med* (Lond) 2001; 51: 163–7

29 Birnbaum HG, Berger WE, Greenberg PE, Holland M, Auerbach R, Atkins KM, et al. Direct and indirect costs of asthma to an employer. *J Allergy Clin Immunol* 2002; 109: 264–70

30 McClellan VE, Garrett JE. Asthma and the employment experience. *N Z Med J* 1990; 103: 399–401

31 Lemiere C, Pelissier S, Chaboillez S, Teolis L. Outcome of subjects diagnosed with occupational asthma and work-aggravated asthma after removal from exposure. *J Occup Environ Med* 2006; 48: 656–9

32 Baiardini I, Braido F, Brandi S, Canonica GW. Allergic diseases and their impact on quality of life. *Ann Allergy Asthma Immunol* 2006; 97: 419–28; quiz 429–30, 476

33 Malo JL, Boulet LP, Dewitte JD, Cartier A, L'Archeveque J, Côté J, et al. Quality of life of subjects with occupational asthma. *J Allergy Clin Immunol* 1993; 91: 1121–7

34 Vandenplas O, Jamart J, Delwiche JP, Evrard G, Larbanois A. Occupational asthma caused by natural rubber latex: Outcome according to cessation or reduction of exposure. *J Allergy Clin Immunol* 2002; 109: 125–30

35 Lowery EP, Henneberger PK, Rosiello R, Sama SR, Preusse P, Milton DK. Quality of life of adults with workplace exacerbation of asthma. *Qual Life Res* 2007; 16: 1605–13

36 Moscato G, Dellabianca A, Perfetti L, Brame B, Galdi E, Niniano R, et al. Occupational

asthma: A longitudinal study on the clinical and socioeconomic outcome after diagnosis. *Chest* 1999; 115: 249–56

37 Venables KM, Davison AG, Newman Taylor AJ. Consequences of occupational asthma. *Respir Med* 1989; 83: 437–40

38 Wild DM, Redlich CA, Paltiel AD. Surveillance for isocyanate asthma: A model based cost effectiveness analysis. *Occup Environ Med* 2005; 62: 743–9.

Prevention of work-related asthma seen from the workplace and the public health perspective

Vivi Schlünssen[1], *Evert Meijer*[2] *and Paul K. Henneberger*[3]

[1]School of Public Health, Department of Environmental and Occupational Medicine, Aarhus University, 8000 Århus C, Denmark
[2]IRAS, Institute for Risk Assessment Sciences, Division Environmental and Occupational Health, Utrecht University, 3508 TD, Utrecht, The Netherlands
[3]Division of Respiratory Disease Studies, National Institute for Occupational Safety and Health, Centers for Disease Control and Prevention, Morgantown, WV 26505-2888, USA

Abstract

Work-related asthma (WRA) includes occupational asthma and work-exacerbated asthma. WRA is by definition preventable. This chapter discusses available tools for prevention of WRA, divided into primary and secondary prevention. For each tool, the available evidence for the effectiveness of the tool is summarized, and examples are provided. Primary prevention addresses healthy workers or persons with asthma due to causes unrelated to work. The principal tool is control of occupational exposure, reached by elimination or reduction in exposure, but vocational guidance and pre-employment screening are also regarded as primary prevention tools. Secondary prevention addresses early detection of work-related sensitization or WRA to prevent further progression. The principal tool for secondary prevention is medical surveillance. Prediction models represent a promising new tool in medical surveillance; this tool is described here in general and by an example. To set priorities for the prevention of WRA, the monitoring of occurrence in populations as well as in specific industries is crucial, and this chapter therefore briefly describes different sources for surveillance data including sentinel reporting systems, population studies, and occupational disease registers. In the future, focus should be on well-conducted intervention studies, improved exposure assessment, improved medical surveillance (e.g., using prediction models) and good quality national surveillance programs.

Introduction

Work-related asthma (WRA) includes occupational asthma (OA) and work-exacerbated asthma (WEA) [1]. OA, or asthma caused by work, is the most common occupational lung disease in developed countries [2]. In addition, WEA, or pre-existing or concurrent/coincident asthma worsened by work factors, is probably even more prevalent and deserves increasing awareness due to the increase in asthma per se during the last 20 years [3]. Concurrent or coincident asthma has onset during employment but is not caused by conditions at work.

Occupational Asthma, edited by Torben Sigsgaard and Dick Heederik

WRA is by definition preventable. The following chapter discusses available tools for prevention of WRA, divided into primary (prevention of development) and secondary (prevention of progression) prevention. Tertiary prevention, or management of WRA, is dealt with in a separate chapter.

Suggestions for evidenced-based guidelines for prevention and management have recently become available for OA [4, 5]. For each tool, the available evidence for the effectiveness of the tool is summarized, and examples are provided.

Prevention of OA and WEA is in general covered together. With regard to primary and secondary prevention, tools for preventing OA and WEA are in principle identical. In order to set priorities for the prevention of WRA, the monitoring of occurrence in populations as well as in specific industries is crucial. This chapter therefore briefly describes different sources for surveillance data including sentinel reporting systems, population studies, and occupational disease registers.

Primary prevention

Here primary prevention addresses healthy workers or persons with asthma caused by reasons other than work. The aim of primary prevention is to prevent development of work-related sensitization and, most importantly, WRA. The principal tool for primary prevention is control of occupational exposure, reached by elimination or reduction in exposure.

As we consider prevention of both OA and WEA as primary prevention, vocational guidance and pre-employment screening are also described in this section.

Control of occupational exposure

According to Nicholson et al. [5], evidence based on well-conducted case-control or cohort studies suggests that reducing airborne exposure reduces the number of workers who become sensitized and who develop OA. In Table 1, different ways of controlling exposure are given focusing on source, room, or person, in decreasing order of preference.

In some industries comprehensive knowledge about determinants of exposure is available. A classic example from healthcare is substitution of low-protein powder-free natural rubber latex (NRL) gloves or non-NRL gloves for powdered NRL gloves. A well-conducted prospective cross-over trial in an operation room found that the mean aeroallergen level was decreased from 13.7 to 1.1 ng/m^3 on days where low-allergen gloves were used [6]. Other examples are studies in bakeries [7–9], wood industries [10–13], and hair dressing saloons [14], where for instance work task, cleaning procedures, quality of ventilation systems, and work routines determine the level of the exposure of interest.

Table 1. Different ways of controlling exposure

The source	- Substitution for the harmful agent - Enclosure, automation, or modification of the process
The room	- Ventilation - Avoiding resuspension of the harmful agent (e.g., cleaning procedures, work practices)
The person	- Personal respirators - Administrative initiatives (reduce number of workers or duration of work time close to the harmful agent)

Several epidemiological studies have documented dose-response relations between high-molecular-weight (HMW) and low-molecular-weight (LMW) allergens and the occurrence of WRA or sensitization, e.g., in bakeries and flour mills [15–18], lab animal workers [19–22], wood workers [23, 24], and isocyanate workers [25–27], strongly suggesting that control of occupational exposure is effective in prevention of WRA.

Only a few studies have directly explored the effect of preventive measures on the occurrence of WRA or sensitization. NRL is the single most common agent addressed in primary preventive intervention studies, as reviewed by Lamontagne et al. [28]. The NRL studies all explored the effect of changing from high-protein powdered gloves to low-protein powder-free NRL or non-NRL gloves, upon either the occurrence of NRL sensitization [29–31] or the occurrence of NRL asthma or NRL-related symptoms [31, 32]. None of the studies fulfilled strict criteria for good quality intervention studies, i.e., they were observational studies without a randomized design and without a control group, but taken together they support assertions that substitution of NRL greatly reduces NRL sensitization and the occurrence of NRL-related asthma.

Smith [33] describes an attempt to prevent bakers' asthma in a UK food company. The intervention was a 5-year health surveillance program, and by no means a strict intervention study. Among other methods, they aimed at decreasing the general total dust level to < 10 mg/m^3, and the bread improver exposures to < 1 mg/m^3, to diminish exposure to mainly fungal amylases. They focused on information and training, installation of local exhaust ventilation, and wearing of respirators during handling of powdered bread improvers. During the 10 years following 1993, they found a decrease in the annual incidence rates of symptomatic sensitization (mostly flour and fungal amylase) from 2085 per million to 405 per million employees per year from the first 5 to the second 5 years. They did not measure the possible decrease in exposure from 1993 to 2003.

An ambitious intervention study was started in the Netherlands in the flour processing sector [9]. More than 900 personal measurements from four flour processing plants together with a thorough collection of control measures were used to model the baseline exposure level and to rule out significant determinants of exposure. The Dutch government and the flour processing sector association agreed to participate in reducing exposure to flour dust. Dust reducing control measures were implemented in the different sectors along with monitoring of trends in exposure as well as sensitization and symptoms in the sector-wide health surveillance system.

In Ontario, the Ministry of Labour introduced a preventive program for diisocyanates in 1983, consisting of a mandatory 0.005 ppm airborne exposure limit for diisocyanates together with a medical surveillance program. Tarlo et al. [34] assessed retrospectively workers compensation data from 1980 to 1993. They showed an initial increase in compensation claims, which was attributed to increased case finding due to the medical surveillance program. The 50% decrease in accepted claims from 1991 to 1992–1993 was attributed to a combination of primary and secondary prevention measures. When measured levels of diisocyanate were compared among companies who had compensated claims for OA with companies without accepted claims, the former were more likely to have had measured levels of diisocyanates >0.005 ppm [35].

In the detergent industry, the occurrence of sensitization among employees apparently decreased dramatically from the late 1960s to the mid-1980s [36]. During this period the detergent industry association had published work practices, and at the same time medical surveillance programs were introduced. Two publications sponsored by major manufacturing companies described significant reductions in the prevalence of OA after introducing granulated proteases [37, 38]. Unfortunately neither study reported incidence rates. A Danish retrospective follow-up study reports decreasing incidence rates from the 1970s to 1990s for sensitization (0.2 to 0.06 per person year), but not for allergic diseases (0.03 to 0.02 per person year) among 1207 enzyme plant workers followed the first 3 year of their employment [39]. Cullinan et al. [40] reported an outbreak of asthma in a modern detergent factory that exclusively used encapsulated enzymes. As many as 90 (26%) of the workers were sensitized to a least one detergent enzyme, and 7% had a confirmed diagnosis of OA. Sensitization rate was clearly related to exposure level. This study indicates that the use of encapsulated enzymes is insufficient to control exposure and prevent enzyme-induced OA.

Case reports on OA caused by newly introduced enzymes [41, 42] highlight the importance of careful surveillance after introduction of new agents in the workplace. In addition, exposure to enzymes has increasingly shifted from the detergent industry to intermediate industries, e.g., the baking industry, where people are exposed to enzymes in low-technology environments [15].

In the US, a major pharmaceutical company introduced a preventive program for laboratory animal allergy (LAA) [43]. The program included education, engineering controls, administrative controls, use of respirators and medical surveillance. During a 5-year period, the incidence rate of asthma decreased from 10% to 0%. In the same period, the percent of workers using respirators increased from 86% to 100%

(workers with LAA) and from 50% to 81% (workers without LAA). No data on other specific preventive measures were available.

In the UK, Botham et al. [44] studied a retrospectively assembled cohort of new employees working with laboratory animals. In 1981, an education program for persons working with laboratory animals was introduced. From 1980 to 1984, the annual cumulative incidence proportion of symptoms consistent with LAA decreased from 44% to 16%, and this effect was at least partly attributed to the educational program.

Use of respiratory protective equipment

There is only limited evidence, based on mainly two non-analytical studies, to support a reduction in the incidence of OA through the use of respiratory protective equipment (RPE). Grammer et al. [45] investigated the effect of introducing RPE devices among 66 newly hired workers in an epoxy resin producing factory using acid anhydrides. Only 4 of the 66 workers did not use RPE. From 1993 to 1999 the incidence rate of acid anhydride sensitization combined with respiratory symptoms decreased from 10% to 2%.

In a new wood plant that uses diisocyanate, Petsonk et al. [46] prospectively estimated respiratory health and work practices over a 2-year period. Workers who indicated that they had briefly removed respiratory protection had a five times higher prevalence of new-onset asthma-like symptoms, compared to individuals who reported never doing this (25% *versus* 5%).

Vocational guidance and pre-employment screening

The main purpose of vocational guidance before job choice, and pre-employment screening, is to avoid persons at risk being exposed to sensitizers or irritant work exposures to prevent OA and WEA. According to Nicholson et al. [4] some evidence supports the claim that screening criteria do an inadequate job of identifying potentially susceptible individuals.

Knowledge of the effect of vocational guidance on career choice among teenagers is sparse. In some countries, e.g., Germany, Denmark and Sweden, vocational guidance is a well-established practice in primary schools, but only a few evaluations of the effects have been performed. In 1992 in Sweden, Bremberg et al. [47] evaluated whether medical vocational guidance among chronically ill preliminary school students (including asthma) had any impact on their choice of career. Only 5 of 235 students stated that vocational information from physicians and school nurses had been important for their choice of career, and the distribution of job choices among the chronically ill students did not differ from the job choices among all students. A German study [48] and a Swedish Study [49] longitudinally elucidated career choices among asthmatics. They found self selection into low risk jobs to play a minor role in teenagers with asthma or allergy. This could indicate that vocational guidance among teenagers has a limited impact or has not been given. Knowledge about the quality and nature of vocational guidance and the impact on career choices is not available.

The effectiveness of using personal risk factors in pre-employment screening is low [21, 50–53], which has been very well illustrated by Sorgdrager et al. [54]. They used data on personal risk factors (atopic history, eosinophil count, lung function) and incidence of pot room asthma from a nested case-control study to estimate indicators of effectiveness of pre-employment screening. They calculated the positive predictive value (PPV), number needed to test and number needed to reject on a simulated population of 10 000 persons with high incidence rates (40 cases/1000 person-year) and 10 000 with low incidence (5 cases/1000 person-year) of pot room asthma. The atopic history prevalence was 6–12 times higher among asthmatics compared to controls depending on the incidence rate of asthma. In general, atopic history was the most effective indicator. The PPV was 20% at high incidence rates, and an even lower 7% at low incidence rates. At high incidence rates it was necessary to test 138 persons to prevent one case of OA, and for each prevented case of OA 5 persons were rejected from the job. They concluded that the personal risk factors were far from effective as a selection instrument.

There is an increasing focus on genetic testing for screening out susceptible subjects. Theoretically, genetic testing could be used for pre-employment screening of OA. So far associations between particular mutations and asthma occurrence are modest with low odds ratios. Thus, prediction of future occurrence is unlikely to be effective. Furthermore, asthma is caused by multiple genetic and environmental factors, and information obtained by a single gene test is limited for both diagnostic and preventive causes. Taken together, genetic testing is currently not useful for identifying susceptible subjects in pre-employment screening [55, 56]

In conclusion, screening out susceptible individuals for asthma seems to be inefficient, and it might discourage efforts to reduce risks and prevent diseases in the general working population. Vocational guidance and pre-employment screening should not be used to discriminate who should or should not get a job, but may be valuable tools to give persons at risk, e.g., atopic persons, an informed view of their chance of developing OA or work-aggravated symptoms.

Secondary prevention

Secondary prevention addresses early detection of work-related sensitization or WRA in order to prevent further progression. The principal tool for secondary prevention is medical surveillance.

Medical surveillance of work-related asthma

Individuals with high exposure levels to aeroallergens are more likely to have serious respiratory complaints and disability than workers exposed at lower levels. Even at very low levels a residual sensitization risk remains. Studies also suggest that the risk for work-related respiratory diseases cannot be avoided completely by exposure reduction [57, 58]. Although elimination of airborne allergens from the workplace is the ideal approach, it may not be possible in many workplaces such as bakeries, and animal care facilities. Even if a reduction of exposure has been shown feasible, there is no known no-effect level, other than zero, that will prevent sensitization in all exposed workers. As an example, the experience with NRL, involving the substitution of powdered gloves with "powder-free" gloves, has shown a dramatic reduction of new cases of contact urticaria among health care workers. However, allergic symptoms and asthma remained, although at lower prevalences, after this intervention [32, 59, 60].

The duration of symptoms while working was studied in Canada [60, 61]; the results showed a significant period of time between symptom onset and diagnosis of OA. The reported median time to the first suspicion of WRA by a physician was 1 year for WEA and 2 years for OA patients. The median time to a final diagnosis of OA after the onset of work-related symptoms was 4 years. Patients with OA waited on average 8 months (median 3 months) before discussing their symptoms with a physician. Lower education level and household income were significantly associated with an increased time to diagnosis.

Although exposure reduction may markedly reduce the incidence of OA, the ongoing high rates of work-related allergic diseases and the long time to diagnosis of WRA reinforces the need for secondary prevention by medical surveillance. Therefore, parallel to exposure reduction and exposure control, medical surveillance of the entire workforce should be conducted to detect early evidence of all work-related allergic and respiratory diseases.

However, different problems limit the successful use of medical surveillance programs for the identification of WRA, because asthma is characteristically a disease with exacerbations and remissions, and WRA may, therefore, be unnoticed. Self-reported symptoms and use of medication failed to identify WRA exacerbations as determined by serial peak exploratory flow measurements [62]. Routine surveillance programs in bakery workers showed that the use of questionnaire-reported respiratory symptoms could not discriminate bakery workers with and without clinical diagnosed asthma or specific IgE for baker-related allergens [51, 63]. In addition, disease outcomes are not identical in different workplace circumstances with different allergen exposures. In the case of low-molecular-weight sensitizers such as diisocyanates, the immunological mechanism and the respiratory health outcome are less clear.

Most of the evidence mentioned in the "Guideline for the prevention, identification, and management of occupational asthma" is, however, derived from (clinical) case-control studies. The estimates of sensitivity and specificity are, therefore, biased by preferential referral of patients and distort the determination of predictive accuracies [64]. Besides, the predictive value of a test varies not only across different populations but also within a particular study population, and consequently may have different sensitivities and specificities [40, 65]. So, a generalized conclusion that a medical questionnaire is not a sensitive instrument for diagnosing OA can hardly be drawn.

The diagnosis of WRA is a phased and complex process that requires both the diagnosis of asthma and establishment of the relationship with work. It can only be made at an individual level in a clinical setting [1]. Medical surveillance programs should, therefore, not focus on clinically established allergic respiratory diseases, but on highly associated preliminary characteristics to identify workers at risk of having a work-related (allergic) disease. Sensitization to occupational allergens is one of these strongly related outcomes linked to OA and often the most appropriate preliminary characteristic that can easily be investigated. For occupations characterized by HMW allergens, a logical approach is therefore to identify sensitized workers first, followed by sequential diagnostic investigations only in these workers. Usually, sensitized workers are detected when they present themselves to the occupational physician with symptoms. However, for patients with WRA, only 6% consulted the company doctor first [66]. So, to find all sensitized workers, the whole population must be evaluated by a specific skin prick test (SPT) or IgE serology, which is less efficient and will result in high expenses for occupational health services.

Traditionally, "standardized" respiratory questionnaires used in epidemiological studies and medical surveillance programs contain questions about general and work-related respiratory symptoms, allergy, and asthma. Every answer to a simple question, such as "do you wheeze", can be considered as a test result. However, different questions often provide the same information because they are all associated with the same underlying disorder, and thus mutually correlated. For the occupational physician it is relevant to know which questions are redundant and which have true, independent additional predictive value for the presence or absence of, for instance, sensitization. Assessing the results of a particular test in view of other test results may even diminish its diagnostic contribution, simply because the information provided by that test is already provided by the other tests.

So far, none of the medical surveillance programs have made use of prediction research-derived diagnostic models in which personal and work-related characteristics are applied to estimate the individual probability of the presence (diagnostic) or occurrence (prognostic) of an outcome that is closely related to the disease(s) of interest. After detecting workers with an elevated risk, sequential diagnostic investigations are only necessary in these workers. So, by using a questionnaire as a first phase instrument, the probability of the occurrence of sensitization can be calculated and subsequently be followed by more advanced tests in the clinical evaluation.

Prediction research and risk stratification

A diagnosis of a disease is the consequence of interpretations by individual medical doctors of consecutive test results, estimating the probability of the presence of a disease or other outcome of interest. As many test results generate more or less identical information it is important to evaluate the independent and additional predictive value of a test given the presence of earlier information. Prediction research offers a solution for this by using a multivariate approach that accounts for mutual dependence between different test results. The information of every item is translated into a predicted probability of the chosen outcome. This technique provides estimations of the probability of an outcome at present (diagnosis) or in the future (prognosis). Prediction models applied in occupational health practice may therefore enable occupational physicians to deal with uncertainties in considering workers at risk of having occupational diseases. The main goal is to optimize risk estimation at low costs, and may be the first step in the clinical evaluation and management of WRA [67, 68]. The models may initiate counseling and interventions, and are thus useful for identification of specific groups at risk. In Figure 1, a flow chart of medical surveillance of WRA using scores is outlined.

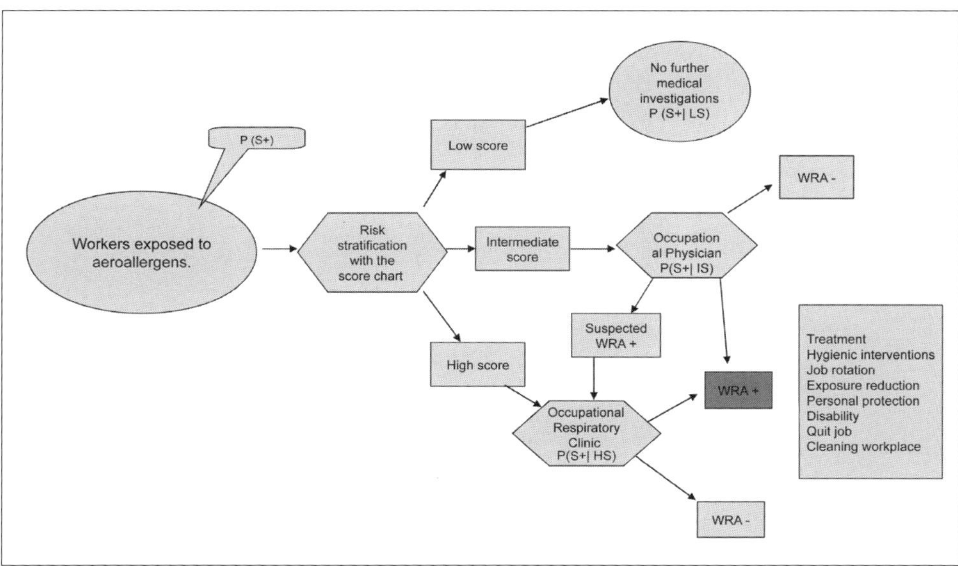

Figure 1.
Medical surveillance of work related asthma (WRA). P (S+), prior probability of sensitization to aeroallergens; P(S+|LS), probability of sensitization conditionally a low score; OAD, occupational allergic disease.

An example of a prediction model in occupational health practice

Models to predict IgE sensitization have only recently been developed for workers such as bakers and laboratory animal workers who are exposed to HMW allergens [67–69]. The models were transformed into scoring rules with a restricted number of questionnaire items with different weighing factors. In a medical surveillance program among 5325 bakers in the Netherlands, a short questionnaire, containing 19 questions with four predictors for sensitization to wheat and/or fungal α-amylase allergens, was used as a decision tool in considering workers at risk of WRA. The results of the questionnaire were transformed into sum scores to predict the presence of sensitization in every individual worker as shown in Table 2.

Table 2. Predictors and Predicted probability for sensitization (wheat and or α-amylase) among bakers

Score chart		
Predictors	**Answer**	**Score**
"Have you ever had asthma in the past 12 months?"	If yes	2
"Have you ever had allergic rhinitis including hay-fever?"	If yes	2
"Have you ever had itchy and/or red eyes in the past 12 months?"	If yes	1
"Do you experience more of the following symptoms during work: shortness of breath, chest tightness, itchy eyes, itchy nose, and/or sneezing?"	If yes	1.5
Sum scores	Max	6.5

Sum score	**0**	**1**	**2**	**3.5**	**4.5**	**5.5**	**6.5**
Predicted probability (%)	9	14	20	31	42	53	64

The scores were used to split bakery workers into three groups with different sensitization risk: a high-risk group in which detailed clinical investigations were required to set a diagnosis of WRA and other work-related allergies more accurately, an intermediate group in which medical follow-up by occupational physicians was essential for diagnosis and health protection, and a low-risk group comprising about 60% of the population in which medical investigations could be held back. The results are shown in Table 3.

Table 3. General characteristics and questionnaire responses across low-, intermediate and high-score groups

	Low score (≤1.0)	Intermediate score (1.5–3.0)	High score (≥3.5)	Total
Participants, *n* (%)	3059 (57.4)	1282 (24.1)	984 (18.5)	5325
Work duration, mean years (SE)	13.8 (0.2)	11.7 (0.3)	12.9 (0.3)	13.1 (0.14)
Upper or lower respiratory tract symptoms to common allergens (at least 1 positive answer), *n* (%)	209 (6.8)	448 (35.2)	642 (65.8)	1299 (24.5)
Symptoms suggestive for NSBHR (at least 2 positive answers), *n* (%)	24 (.8)	52 (4.1)	144 (14.9)	220 (4.2)
Use of medication to improve respiratory complaints in the last 12 months (e.g. inhalants), *n* (%)	74 (2.4)	186 (14.6)	468 (48.1)	728 (13.7)
Doctor visit for allergic complaints in the last 12 months, *n* (%)	134 (4.4)	197 (15.5)	379 (38.7)	710 (13.4)
Absenteeism due to allergic symptoms in the last 12 months, *n* (%)	6 (0.2)	34 (2.7)	79 (8.2)	119 (2.2)
Change of function or task due to respiratory symptoms, *n* (%)	16 (0.5)	19 (1.5)	83 (8.5)	118 (2.2)

The predicted probability of sensitization can be calculated as:

$$= 1 / \{1 + \mathrm{EXP}[- (-2.32 + 0.92 \times \text{asthma} + 0.90 \times \text{rhinitis} + 0.46 \times \text{conjunctivitis} + 0.62 \times \text{during work symptom})]\}.$$

Workers with high scores showed the highest IgE sensitization rate to wheat and/or α-amylase, and the highest rates in medication use, absenteeism, and doctor's visits.

This example illustrates that by using a score chart to predict the sensitization risk in workers exposed to HMW workplace allergens, a diagnosis of WRA can be considered more effectively and efficiently in the initial phase of a medical surveillance program performed by occupational physicians at the worksite. Prediction models based on IgE-mediated sensitization is not useful for LMW workplace allergens. To our knowledge no prediction models for LMW-related OA has been developed, but models based on bronchial hyperresponsiveness (BHR) could potentially be useful.

Use of public health surveillance data to stimulate, guide, and document prevention of work-related asthma

Public health surveillance comprises more than the identification and counting of cases. It is "the ongoing systematic collection, analysis, and interpretation of health data essential to the planning, implementation, and evaluation of public health practices, closely integrated with the timely dissemination of these data to those who need to know." [70]. This section highlights examples of how public health surveillance has contributed to the prevention of WRA. While the examples are drawn from experience in the United States and Canada, this does not mean that similar surveillance activities are lacking in other countries.

Investigations of reported cases have identified the measures needed to prevent the onset and/exacerbation of asthma in specific workplaces, benefiting the index case, co-workers, and the employer. The Sentinel Event Notification System for Occupational Risks (SENSOR) is a state-based surveillance program for occupational diseases that is coordinated by the National Institute for Occupational Safety and Health in the United States. The SENSOR program in the state of Michigan registered 446 cases of WRA from 416 different workplaces during 1993–1995 [71]. Inspections were conducted at 185 (44.5%) of these workplaces, and air sampling for known agents were conducted at 123 (29.6%). Many recommendations or citations were issued as a result of the inspections: 60 for medical monitoring, 80 for engineering controls, 63 for air monitoring, 126 for hazard communication program, and 71 for respiratory protection program [71]. These figures suggest that workplace inspections stimulated by WRA case reports frequently identified deficiencies that inhibited prevention.

Ongoing surveillance programs facilitate the identification of and response to an increase in the number or severity of asthma cases. Deaths due to work-related diseases are powerful warnings for workers with similar exposures. The Fatality Assessment and Control Evaluation (FACE) program identifies and investigates work-related deaths in several states in the United States. The Michigan FACE (MIFACE) program reported a worker who died after he sprayed an isocyanate-containing coating inside a van [72]. This surface coating is normally sprayed onto the open cargo beds of trucks, but in this case was applied onto the floor and up the walls of an enclosed van. The MIFACE investigation revealed deficiencies in several factors that contributed to this unfortunate occurrence: product stewardship by the manufacturer of the materials used by the case, engineering controls, company health and safety program, and health care provider recognition that the asthma was work-related. The Michigan Occupational Safety and Health Administration (MIOSHA) issued 11 citations to the company. Also, MIOSHA initiated contact with over 100 other companies in Michigan that applied spray-on truck bedliners and provided educational and technical assistance. The surveillance program's expeditious investigation and dissemination of the findings likely had a positive impact on asthma morbidity and mortality.

Surveillance data can also be used to document the impact of preventive interventions. In the province of Ontario in Canada, legislation was passed in 1983 that required workplace monitoring of diisocyanate levels to maintain exposures within acceptable limits, as well as medical monitoring of exposed workers. The impact of this legislation was tracked using worker compensation data. The number of diisocyanate OA cases began to increase during the early 1980s, probably due to the increased medical screening of exposed workers [34]. The number of claims peaked in 1988–1990 and began to decline after that. Also, the cases were less severe as the number declined [34]. This decline in the number and severity of diisocyanate WRA cases was likely the result of many activities, including better control of exposures at work, and increased and earlier recognition of disease.

Future developments

Most intervention studies are best characterized as "complex intervention studies" consisting of several intervention components, where the actual change in exposure is seldom monitored. It is therefore not realistic to assume that most future studies will fulfill strict criteria for good quality single intervention studies. However, it is desirable to put more effort into ongoing monitoring of changes in exposure. Many companies and organizations do collect data continuously on exposure, exposure determinants, and health outcomes. The use and extension of this valuable data source could be improved by establishing a closer cooperation between companies and experts in exposure assessment and occupational lung diseases.

There is still a need for development of more effective medical surveillance programs, and predictions models are a promising attempt to achieve that goal. A major future challenge will be to develop effective prediction models for LMW asthma.

Collection of surveillance data is essential in planning, implementation, and evaluation of the prevention of WRA. In the future it will be crucial to maintain resources for ongoing surveillance programs, and it will be of equal importance to initiate surveillance programs in countries where no surveillance data currently exist.

Finally, an increased focus on education of workers and health professionals is crucial to increase the possibilities for prevention of WRA.

References

1 Tarlo SM, Balmes J, Balkissoon R, Beach J, Beckett W, Bernstein D et al (2008) Diagnosis and management of work-related asthma: American College Of Chest Physicians Consensus Statement. *Chest* 134 (3 Suppl): 1S–41S

2 Venables KM, Chan-Yeung M (1997) Occupational asthma. *Lancet* 349: 1465–1469
3 Pearce N, Douwes J, Beasley R (2000) The rise and rise of asthma: A new paradigm for the new millennium. *J Epidemiol Biostat* 5: 5–16
4 Nicholson PJ, Cullinan P, Taylor AJ, Burge PS, Boyle C (2005) Evidence based guidelines for the prevention, identification, and management of occupational asthma. *Occup Environ Med* 62: 290–299
5 Beach J, Rowe BH, Blitz S, Crumley E, Hooton N, Russel K et al (2005) Diagnosis and Management of Work-Related Asthma. Agency for Health Care and Quality, Rockville, MD, AHRQ publication No. 06–E003–2
6 Heilman DK, Jones RT, Swanson MC, Yunginger JW (1996) A prospective, controlled study showing that rubber gloves are the major contributor to latex aeroallergen levels in the operating room. *J Allergy Clin Immunol* 98: 325–330
7 Burdorf A, Lillienberg L, Brisman J (1994) Characterization of exposure to inhalable flour dust in Swedish bakeries. *Ann Occup Hyg* 38: 67–78
8 Bulat P, Myny K, Braeckman L, van Sprundel M, Kusters E, Doekes G et al (2004) Exposure to inhalable dust, wheat flour and alpha-amylase allergens in industrial and traditional bakeries. *Ann Occup Hyg* 48: 57–63
9 Meijster T, Tielemans E, de PN, Heederik D (2007) Modelling exposure in flour processing sectors in the Netherlands: A baseline measurement in the context of an intervention program. *Ann Occup Hyg* 51: 293–304
10 Schlünssen V, Jacobsen G, Erlandsen M, Mikkelsen AB, Schaumburg I, Sigsgaard T (2008) Determinants of wood dust exposure in the Danish furniture industry – Results from two cross-sectional studies 6 years apart. *Ann Occup Hyg* 52: 227–238
11 Scheeper B, Kromhout H, Boleij JS (1995) Wood-dust exposure during wood-working processes. *Ann Occup Hyg* 39: 141–154
12 Alwis U, Mandryk J, Hocking AD, Lee J, Mayhew T, Baker W (1999) Dust exposures in the wood processing industry. *Am Ind Hyg Assoc J* 60: 641–6
13 Friesen MC, Davies HW, Teschke K, Marion S, Demers PA (2005) Predicting historical dust and wood dust exposure in sawmills: Model development and validation. *J Occup Environ Hyg* 2: 650–658
14 Hollund BE, Moen BE (1998) Chemical exposure in hairdresser salons. Effect of local exhaust ventilation. *Ann Occup Hyg* 42: 277–282
15 Houba R, Heederik DJJ, Doekes G, van Run PEM (1995) Exposure-sensitization relationship for α-amylase allergens in the baking industry. *Am J Respir Crit Care Med* 154: 130–136
16 Houba R, Heederik D, Doekes G (1998) Wheat sensitization and work-related symptoms in the baking industry are preventable. An epidemiologic study. *Am J Respir Crit Care Med* 158: 1499–1503
17 Peretz C, de Pater N, de Monchy J, Oostenbrink J, Heederik D (2005) Assessment of exposure to wheat flour and the shape of its relationship with specific sensitization. *Scand J Work Environ Health* 31: 65–74
18 Nieuwenhuijsen MJ, Heederik D, Doekes G, Venables KM, Newman Taylor AJ (1999)

Exposure-response relations of alpha-amylase sensitisation in British bakeries and flour mills. *Occup Environ Med* 56: 197–201

19 Kruize H, Post W, Heederik D, Martens B, Hollander A, van der BE (1997) Respiratory allergy in laboratory animal workers: A retrospective cohort study using pre-employment screening data. *Occup Environ Med* 54: 830–835

20 Cullinan P, Cook A, Gordon S, Nieuwenhuijsen MJ, Tee RD, Venables KM et al (1999) Allergen exposure, atopy and smoking as determinants of allergy to rats in a cohort of laboratory employees. *Eur Respir J* 13: 1139–1143

21 Nieuwenhuijsen MJ, Putcha V, Gordon S, Heederik D, Venables KM, Cullinan P et al (2003). Exposure-response relations among laboratory animal workers exposed to rats. *Occup Environ Med* 60: 104–108

22 Heederik D, Venables KM, Malmberg P, Hollander A, Karlsson AS, Renstrom A et al (1999) Exposure-response relationships for work-related sensitization in workers exposed to rat urinary allergens: Results from a pooled study. *J Allergy Clin Immunol* 103: 678–684

23 Brooks SM, Edwards JJJ, Apol A, Edwards FH (1981) An epidemiologic study of workers exposed to western red cedar and other wood dusts. *Chest* 80: 30–32

24 Schlünssen V, Schaumburg I, Heederik D, Taudorf E, Sigsgaard T (2004) Indices of asthma among atopic and non-atopic woodworkers. *Occup Environ Med* 61: 504–511

25 Pronk A, Preller L, Raulf-Heimsoth M, Jonkers IC, Lammers JW, Wouters IM et al (2007) Respiratory symptoms, sensitization, and exposure response relationships in spray painters exposed to isocyanates. *Am J Respir Crit Care Med* 176: 1090–1097

26 Ott MG (2002) Occupational asthma, lung function decrement, and toluene diisocyanate (TDI) exposure: A critical review of exposure-response relationships. *Appl Occup Environ Hyg* 17: 891–901

27 Meredith SK, Bugler J, Clark RL (2000) Isocyanate exposure and occupational asthma: A case-referent study. *Occup Environ Med* 57: 830–836

28 LaMontagne AD, Radi S, Elder DS, Abramson MJ, Sim M (2006) Primary prevention of latex related sensitisation and occupational asthma: A systematic review. *Occup Environ Med* 63: 359–364

29 Jones KP, Rolf S, Stingl C, Edmunds D, Davies BH (2004) Longitudinal study of sensitization to natural rubber latex among dental school students using powder-free gloves. *Ann Occup Hyg* 48: 455–457

30 Levy D, Allouache S, Chabane MH, Leynadier F, Burney P (1999). Powder-free protein-poor natural rubber latex gloves and latex sensitization. *JAMA* 281: 988

31 Saary MJ, Kanani A, Alghadeer H, Holness DL, Tarlo SM (2002) Changes in rates of natural rubber latex sensitivity among dental school students and staff members after changes in latex gloves. *J Allergy Clin Immunol* 109: 131–135

32 Schlünssen V, Ebbehøj NE, Sherson D, Skadhauge L (2004) Erhvervsvejledning af børn og unge med astma og høfeber. *Månedsskrift Prakt Lægegern* 82: 257–267 [In Danish]

33 Smith TA (2004) Preventing baker's asthma: An alternative strategy. *Occup Med* 54: 21–27

34 Tarlo SM, Liss GM, Yeung KS (2002) Changes in rates and severity of compensation claims for asthma due to diisocyanates: A possible effect of medical surveillance measures. *Occup Environ Med* 59: 58–62

35 Tarlo SM, Liss GM, Dias C, Banks DE (2000) Assessment of the relationship between isocyanate exposure levels and occupational asthma. *Am J Ind Med* 32: 517–521

36 Schweigert MK, Mackenzie DP, Sarlo K (2000) Occupational asthma and allergy associated with the use of enzymes in the detergent industry – A review of the epidemiology, toxicology and methods of prevention. *Clin Exp Allergy* 30: 1511–1518

37 Juniper CP, Roberts DM (1984) Enzyme asthma: Fourteen years' clinical experience of a recently prescribed disease. *J Soc Occup Med* 34: 127–132

38 Cathcart M, Nicholson P, Roberts D, Bazley M, Juniper C, Murray P et al (1997) Enzyme exposure, smoking and lung function in employees in the detergent industry over 20 years. Medical Subcommittee of the UK Soap and Detergent Industry Association. *Occup Med* 47: 473–478

39 Larsen AI, Johnsen CR, Frickmann J, Mikkelsen S (2007) Incidence of respiratory sensitisation and allergy to enzymes among employees in an enzyme producing plant and the relation to exposure and host factors. *Occup Environ Med* 64: 763–768

40 Feinstein AR (2002) Misguided efforts and future challenges for research on "diagnostic tests". *J Epidemiol Community Health* 56: 330–332

41 Brant A, Hole A, Cannon J, Helm J, Swales C, Welch J et al (2004) Occupational asthma caused by cellulase and lipase in the detergent industry. *Occup Environ Med* 61: 793–795

42 Hole AM, Draper A, Jolliffe G, Cullinan P, Jones M, Taylor AJ (2000) Occupational asthma caused by bacillary amylase used in the detergent industry. *Occup Environ Med* 57: 840–842

43 Fisher R, Saunders WB, Murray SJ, Stave GM (1998) Prevention of laboratory animal allergy. *J Occup Environ Med* 40: 609–613

44 Botham PA, Davies GE, Teasdale EL (1987) Allergy to laboratory animals: A prospective study of its incidence and of the influence of atopy on its development. *Br J Ind Med* 44: 627–632

45 Grammer LC, Harris KE, Yarnold PR (2002) Effect of respiratory protective devices on development of antibody and occupational asthma to an acid anhydride. *Chest* 121: 1317–1322

46 Petsonk EL, Wang ML, Lewis DM, Siegel PD, Husberg BJ (2000) Asthma-like symptoms in wood product plant workers exposed to methylene diphenyl diisocyanate. *Chest* 118: 1183–1193

47 Bremberg S, Andersson R (1992) Medical vocational guidance for adolescents – Is it effective? *Acta Paediatr* 81: 253–256

48 Radon K, Huemmer S, Dressel H, Windstetter D, Weinmayr G, Weiland S et al (2006) Do respiratory symptoms predict job choices in teenagers? *Eur Respir J* 27: 774–778

49 Wiebert P, Svartengren M, Lindberg M, Hemmingsson T, Lundberg I, Nise G (2008)

Mortality, morbidity and occupational exposure to airway-irritating agents among men with a respiratory diagnosis in adolescence. *Occup Environ Med* 65: 120–125
50 Slovak AJ, Hill RN (1987) Does atopy have any predictive value for laboratory animal allergy? A comparison of different concepts of atopy. *Br J Ind Med* 44: 129–132
51 Gordon SB, Curran AD, Murphy J, Sillitoe C, Lee G, Wiley K et al (1997) Screening questionnaires for bakers' asthma – Are they worth the effort? *Occup Med* 47: 361–316
52 Cockcroft A, Edwards J, McCarthy P, Andersson N (1981) Allergy in laboratory animal workers. *Lancet* 11: 827–830
53 Walusiak J, Palczynski C, Hanke W, Wittczak T, Krakowiak A, Gorski P (2002) The risk factors of occupational hypersensitivity in apprentice bakers – The predictive value of atopy markers. *Int Arch Occup Environ Health* 75 (Suppl): S117–S121
54 Sorgdrager B, Hulshof CT, van Dijk FJ (2004) Evaluation of the effectiveness of pre-employment screening. *Int Arch Occup Environ Health* 77: 271–266
55 Mapp CE (2003) The role of genetic factors in occupational asthma. *Eur Respir J* 22: 173– 178
56 Mapp CE (2009) What is the role of genetics in occupational asthma? *Eur Respir J* 33: 459–460
57 Liss GM, Tarlo SM (2001) Natural rubber latex-related occupational asthma: Association with interventions and glove changes over time. *Am J Ind Med* 40: 347–353
58 Filon FL, Radman G (2006) Latex allergy: A follow up study of 1040 healthcare workers. *Occup Environ Med* 63: 121–125
59 Mapp CE, Boschetto P, Maestrelli P, Fabbri LM (2005) Occupational asthma. *Am J Respir Crit Care Med* 172: 280–305
60 Heederik D, Houba R (2001) An exploratory quantitative risk assessment for high molecular weight sensitizers: Wheat flour. *Ann Occup Hyg* 45: 175–185
61 Poonai N, van DS, Bharatha A, Manduch M, Deklaj T, Tarlo SM (2005) Barriers to diagnosis of occupational asthma in Ontario. *Can J Public Health* 96: 230–233
62 Bolen AR, Henneberger PK, Liang X, Sama SR, Preusse PA, Rosiello RA et al (2007) The validation of work-related self-reported asthma exacerbation. *Occup Environ Med* 64: 343–348
63 Brant A, Nightingale S, Berriman J, Sharp C, Welch J, Newman Taylor AJ et al (2005) Supermarket baker's asthma: How accurate is routine health surveillance? *Occup Environ Med* 62: 395–399
64 Diamond GA (1993) "Work-up bias". *J Clin Epidemiol* 46: 207–209
65 Moons KG, Harrell FE (2003) Sensitivity and specificity should be de-emphasized in diagnostic accuracy studies. *Acad Radiol* 10: 670–672
66 Santos MS, Jung H, Peyrovi J, Lou W, Liss GM, Tarlo SM (2007) Occupational asthma and work-exacerbated asthma: Factors associated with time to diagnostic steps. *Chest* 131: 1768–1775
67 Meijer E, Grobbee DE, Heederik D (2002) Detection of workers sensitised to high

molecular weight allergens: A diagnostic study in laboratory animal workers. *Occup Environ Med* 59: 189–195

68 Suarthana E, Vergouwe Y, Moons C, de Monchy J, Grobbee DE, Heederik D, Meijer E (2010) A diagnostic model for the detection of sensitization to wheat allergens was developed and validated in bakery workers. *J Clin Epidemiol, in press*

69 Meijer E, Grobbee DE, Heederik D (2004) A strategy for health surveillance in laboratory animal workers exposed to high molecular weight allergens. *Occup Environ Med* 61: 831–837

70 DHHS (2001) Tracking occupational injuries, illnesses, and hazards: The NIOSH surveillance strategic plan. Cincinnati: Government Printing Office. Report No. DHHS-2001–118

71 Jajosky RA, Harrison R, Reinisch F, Flattery J, Chan J, Tumpowsky C et al (1999) Surveillance of work-related asthma in selected U.S. states using surveillance guidelines for state health departments – California, Massachusetts, Michigan, and New Jersey 1993–1995. *MMWR CDC Surveill Summ* 48: 1–20

72 Chester DA, Hanna EA, Pickelman BG, Rosenman KD (2005) Asthma death after spraying polyurethane truck bedliner. *Am J Ind Med* 48: 78–84

Prevention and regulatory aspects of exposure to asthmagens in the workplace

Henrik Nordman

Finnish Institute of Occupational Health, Topeliuksenkatu 41 aA, 00250 Helsinki, Finland

Abstract

The consequences of occupational asthma (OA) in terms of health, quality of life and costs incurred for the individual as well as society are considerable and make prevention worthwhile. The majority of cases are caused by comparatively few major asthmagens, such as flour dust, animal epithelium, natural rubber latex, and diisocyanates. A substantial reduction of these exposures is a realistic objective. It is important that preventive strategies are undertaken as concerted actions by all actors involved, i.e. regulatory authorities, branch organisations and worker unions. However, many asthmagens only cause occasional cases. Understandably, the prevention of these will rarely be highly prioritised. Aggravation of any asthma by non-specific exposures at work (work-exacerbated asthma, WEA) has turned out to be as important as OA. The costs incurred by WEA as well as the effects on quality of life equal or surpass those of OA. So far, our understanding of the nature of WEA as compared with OA is poor and far too meagre for scientifically based preventive strategies. Future research needs to focus on practically all aspects of WEA.

Introduction

From the preventive point of view, the full relationship between asthma and work environment exposures is of interest. It is generally recognised that some 15% of adult-onset asthma is attributable to work [1]. Population-based incidence studies indicate even higher figures [2, 3]. The high figures include all forms of work-related asthma, occupational asthma (OA) as well as work-exacerbated asthma (WEA). They are likely to reflect also the multifactorial nature of asthma, with the work environment as one of several interacting etiological genetic and environmental factors.

During the last, almost four decades, the vast majority of research efforts have focused on asthma with a latency period, specifically induced by sensitisation following inhalation of an asthmagen at work. The level of understanding achieved about occurrence and mechanisms of this "classical" OA is rather high and should be sufficient for preventive measures to be taken [4, 5]. However, the more than 250 identified specific inducers of OA, most of which having a low attack rate, explain

Occupational Asthma, edited by Torben Sigsgaard and Dick Heederik

why a realistic aim of prevention is currently to attain a substantial reduction of OA. The nature of OA, its resemblance to the much more prevalent non-OA, and the comparatively benign prognosis are factors explaining why prevention of OA has been disappointing. These and other factors influencing the prevention of OA have been listed by Cullinan and his colleagues [4] (Tab. 1). Fortunately, the vast majority of OA is caused by only a few major asthmagens, such as animal dander, flour dusts, diisocyanates and natural latex rubber.

It has been argued that exacerbation of pre-existing asthma, non-OA at work should be included when considering preventive strategies [6]. During the last decade it has become increasingly evident that the prevention of WEA will eventually be at least as important as the prevention of classical OA [7–9]. The high prevalence of asthma, especially among children and adolescents, makes the well-being of this sub-group of sensitive future workers a high priority issue.

The chapter gives emphasis to the primary and secondary prevention of the various types of OA. Some examples of successful preventive strategies are described. Although acute irritant-induced asthma fulfils the criteria of OA, the condition is almost exclusively caused by accidental exposure to high concentrations of a respiratory irritant. Preventive measures are, therefore, technical and hygienic, including worker education, and are not further dealt with in the chapter. [5]. The

Table 1. Factors influencing the prevention of occupational disease [4]

Influences	
Societal	Frequency of the disease Nature of the disease Perception of the disease Individual and societal costs of the disease
Technical	Strength of epidemiological or clinical evidence of cause/effect Identification of risk factors amenable to manipulation Availability of efficacious technical or organisational means of reducing important risk factors Availability of effective methods of secondary prevention
Business	Frequency of the disease Impact on consumers Public reputation Economic costs of the disease Efficiency and effectiveness of technical or organisational means of reducing important risk factors Effects on competitiveness Influence of employee or consumer organisations

need for preventive strategies for WEA is recognised but, so far, there is a paucity of scientific data on practically every aspect of the condition. Therefore, prevention of WEA can only be addressed in a state-of-the-art manner. Tertiary prevention aims at limiting impairment of OA in workers who are already ill. It is, by and large, synonymous with "management of cases", which is the topic of the chapter by S. Burge in this book [10].

The most important elements of the prevention of OA have been listed in Table 2.

Primary prevention

Primary prevention aims at the avoidance of exposure to agents causing OA and at the prevention of any such pathophysiological changes that may increase the

Table 2. Measures to prevent occupational asthma

Primary prevention

Measures of regulatory authorities
- legislation
- setting of occupational exposure limits
- labelling of sensitising substances
- making recommendations on the use of sensitisers
- guidance on safe working practices
- labour inspection activities

Screening of products before introduction into the market

Identification of highly susceptible individuals
- vocational guidance
- pre-employment health examinations

Pre-placement education of workers

Control of exposure
- substitution of harmful agents with less harmful
- automation or enclosure of processes
- modification of process or agent to reduce risk of sensitisation
- improvement of ventilation
- working practices to reduce dust concentrations

Administrative measures to reduce numbers of exposed and time of exposure

Personal protective equipment

Secondary prevention

Medical surveillance of workers

risk of developing the disease. The main measures for assessing and controlling the exposure in work environments associated with sensitisers were reviewed by Corn in 1983 [11].

Although rarely practicable, elimination of a sensitiser from the work environment, or to never introduce it into a process is ideal. However, there are many typical high risk work environments, where elimination is impracticable, e.g. the baking industry, farming, and laboratory animal handling. In such work environments, the prevention aims at the reduction of the exposure to a minimum [12, 13]. Sufficient ventilation, healthy work practices and housekeeping are central measures of exposure control in all work environments. Although seemingly self-evident, these are often found inadequate and grossly neglected. The extent of ignorance and, at least partly, negligence was registered in a recent survey of bakeries; few were aware of the existence of an exposure limit for flour, nor of recommended work practices in bakeries [14]. Intensive education of workers at risk is a prerequisite for a high-level awareness of risks at the workplace. Investing in education and training programmes should be in the interest of all parties involved.

Testing of products before they are introduced into the market is commendable. It is also to some extent being done, although the impact of testing has so far been modest. Most screening is concerned with skin sensitising potency. For instance, methods such as local lymph node tests in animals probably do not predict the respiratory sensitisation potency with any greater reliability. Cytokine fingerprinting is considered a more promising method of assessing respiratory sensitising properties [4]. Elimination of a sensitiser is desirable, but it has rarely been feasible. The change of natural rubber latex gloves to non-rubber gloves or to powder-free gloves with a low allergen content is an example of a successful intervention (see below), reducing exposure as well as the number of exposed, e.g. users of sensitising gloves. The attempt to substitute a sensitiser may also fail, due in part to the lack of reliable methods for testing substances before introduction. An example of failure often quoted, is the substitution of toluene diisocyanate (TDI) with the less volatile methylene diisocyanate (MDI), which, however, turned out to be just another respiratory sensitiser [4, 5].

There are many ways to achieve a reduction of either exposure or numbers of exposed. In the prevention of OA, the modification of a process or an agent to reduce the risk of sensitisation has been successfully applied and documented in the detergent enzyme industry. It was achieved by encapsulating enzymes in powder form and, at least partly, by isolation of processes [16, 17]. It is also an example reminding us that prevention programmes cannot be "parachuting operations"; continuous surveillance of the work environment and the workers' health is needed. In this particular case, over the years new enzymes were introduced into the detergent production processes with unexpected new outbursts of OA [18, 19]. Complete isolation and enclosure are effective means of exposure control used, for instance, in the handling of complex platinum salts and in many processes involving organic acid anhydrides.

Control of exposure is also exerted by various administrative decisions. The numbers of workers exposed and the duration of exposure can be restricted by job rotation, rest periods, shift or location changes where fewer people are working with sensitisers or irritant exposures [5].

Role of regulatory authorities

In reviews on prevention of OA, the role of regulatory authorities is rarely addressed. However, regulatory authorities may have a decisive influence on both the primary and secondary prevention of OA. Preventive measures of the regulatory authorities include legislation, collecting information (e.g. by registers), the setting of occupational exposure limits (OELs), and supervision by labour inspection.

Laws and statutes define occupational diseases and the level of diagnostic probability, list compensable diseases and causes of disease and determine modes of compensation.

All these differ from country to country affecting accordingly comparisons of national statistics [20]. A liberal legislation including compensation for disability, loss of income inflicted by occupational diseases, and re-education serve as incentives for workers to come forward with complaints of work-related symptoms. The Finnish legislation on occupational disease and occupational safety and health (OSH) may serve as an example. Insurance policies for all employees are mandatory, voluntary for self-employed. Access to occupational health services is mandatory for all workplaces. Physicians are obliged to report occupational diseases. The modes and level of compensation is fairly high. As there is little reason to believe that the true incidence of OA differs from other industrialised countries, the comparatively liberal legislation is likely to explain the consistently far higher incidence of reported cases of OA in Finland than in the UK, Sweden and the USA [20].

By setting OELs, regulatory authorities may influence the prevention of occupational diseases in several ways. Most OELs are set as 8-hour time-weighted averages (TWA). If critical effects, such as irritation or sensitisation, are expected following brief exposure to high concentrations, a short-term exposure limit (STEL) can be set. STELs are normally recommended for a 15-minute reference period. OELs are meant to protect workers from detrimental health effects of exposure by inhalation over a working life. Health-based OELs are normally set for substances for which studies on dose-response relationships show either a threshold, i.e. a no-observed-effect level (NOEL), or a lowest-observed-effect level (LOEL). For respiratory sensitisers, like genotoxic and carcinogenic substances, NOELs or LOELs are rarely identified. In such cases it is assumed that any level of exposure might carry some risk. The recommended OELs for these substances are established pragmatically. Exposure-response data are used in the setting of these final statutory exposure limits, which include socio-economic as well as technical considerations of practicability [21, 22].

The setting of OELs are rarely, if ever, enough for the prevention of OA. However, OELs direct the attention of workers, employers and OSH personnel towards exposure levels and thereby increase the awareness of risks and safe exposure levels. They may, ideally, be used in the design of new plants and processes to ensure that exposures will be safe [22].

As full dose-response curves are rarely available for respiratory sensitisers, the approach may be to provide decision makers with quantitative risk data at different exposure levels. The final pragmatic recommendation will include socio-economic considerations and may vary substantially between countries. Flour dust is a good example. Although distinct exposure-response relationships between exposure to flour dust and wheat allergen and sensitisation with nasal and asthma symptoms exist [23–26], there seems to be no identifiable threshold for these effects [27]. Basically the same data on exposure-response relationships have been used for the setting of OELs, which, however, display a huge range between the health-based OEL of 0.5 mg/m^3 by the American Conference of Governmental Industrial Hygienists (ACGIH) [28] and a maximum exposure limit (MEL) of 10 mg/m^3 set by the Health and Safety Executive in the UK [29]. In this case, it demonstrates the differences between a health-based assessment and a tripartite compromise. Yet another approach was adopted by the Dutch Expert Committee on Occupational Standards [30]. Based on advanced analysis of the studies by Houba and colleagues [25, 26], the excess risk of sensitisation for workers over a working life of 40 years was calculated. An excess risk of sensitisation of 1% and 10% was calculated at exposure levels of 0.12 and 1.2 mg/m^3, respectively. The excess risk at various levels of exposure will eventually have to be weighted against feasibility issues [30].

In many countries, regulatory authorities have made health surveillance mandatory in all work environments associated with health risks. In a preventive programme launched by the Ministry of Labour in Ontario to reduce diisocyanate-induced asthma (see below), medical health surveillance was one of several elements [31]. In the evaluation of the programme, it was concluded that the decrease of asthma claims may have been due to several causes, one of which was medical surveillance. It was stated that medical surveillance may act in several ways. Apart from early identification of cases, it may improve worker education and general awareness of hazardous exposures, intensify the use of personal protection and, in general, working practices [31].

The formal appointment of safety representatives and industrial safety commissions at workplaces are likely to have a favourable preventive impact. The provision of training and knowledge of the regulations pertaining to bakeries was assessed in 55 bakeries in the UK following the setting of the statutory MEL of 10 mg/m^3 and a 15-min STEL of 30 mg/m^3. The study revealed that only a quarter of the bakeries were aware of the existence of a MEL or a STEL. A copy of a booklet on guidance on dust control and health surveillance in bakeries, produced by Health and Safety in Bakeries Liaison Committee [15], was found only in 28% of bakeries. However, companies with an appointed safety representative were much more likely to be aware of the exposure limits and of the sensitising properties of flour dust, to have a written risk-assessment and to have provided some training on flour dust work [14].

Compensation modes and levels may act as incentives for both workers and employers, i.e. for workers to come forward with their work-related complaints without fearing to loose their income, and for employers to continuously pay attention to safety issues at work. The responsibility of authorities is to ensure that workers receive a satisfactory income replacement indemnity, indemnity for possible permanent disability and rehabilitation. The compensation systems vary between countries, the majority being administered by national or regional agencies and insurance companies. In most countries OA is compensated as an occupational disease [32, 33]. In countries were agents eligible for compensation are listed, e.g. UK and France, the continuous up-dating of lists is essential. It is also important that workers claims for disease caused by agents outside the list are compensated in alternative ways, for instance by national health insurance [4].

In most industrialised countries the employer is assumed to cover the costs of an occupational disease [33]. However, few countries have studied the actual partition of costs. Recently, the distribution of costs of OA in the UK was reported. The study revealed that as much as 49% of the total costs are borne by the diseased worker, 47% by tax payers and only 4% by the employer [34]. As the authors pointed out, on one hand it is understandable if workers under such circumstances hesitate to have their symptoms investigated. On the other, there is little incentive for employers to invest in improvements to reduce exposures.

Finally, data collecting pertaining to OA is an important source of information and affords a basis for preventive strategies. Data can be collected as sentinel events (e.g. USA), occupational disease registers (e.g. Finland) and compensation statistics. Although all these sources of information are known to grossly underestimate the true incidence of occupational disease, they generate useful information and may reveal important trends [5].

Pre-employment screening

Health examinations at the pre-employment stage are customary and also commendable as an instrument to protect the health of workers. Inevitably, applicants may be found unsuitable for a particular work on health-based grounds. This makes it all the more important that exclusion criteria are clearly defined and based on scientific evidence. Reasons for exclusion are comparatively few. Probably the only incontestable reason for exclusion is an applicant with an earlier confirmed OA caused by an agent to which exposure would occur in the new job. If the causative agent is totally unrelated to exposures occurring in the new job, there is little scientific justification for exclusion [4]. Job applicants suffering from non-OA ("community" asthma) constitute a challenging category. As can be expected when there is a lack of solid scientific data for precisely formulated guidelines, the practise varies considerably and often to the disadvantages of the asthmatics [4, 35]. The assessments need to take into account the severity of asthma. Although scientifically ungrounded, it may seem justified not to subject persons with severe or moderately severe asthma to a risk of developing additional respiratory impairment [4].

Although host factors increase susceptibility to OA, screening for and applying such factors for pre-employment selection is a questionable issue. One reason is that screening for susceptible individuals may lead to the selection of workers that are thought to tolerate a work environment associated with harmful levels of exposures, whereas the preventive approach should be to make the work environment tolerable to workers despite such host factors [4, 5]. Another reason is the fact that no single marker of susceptibility has been identified having a predictive value that would justify its use for pre-employment screening [4]. Atopy undoubtedly increases the risk of sensitisation to high-molecular-weight allergens. However, the predictive value of atopy is generally accepted to be too low, even in workplaces associated with a high risk of IgE-mediated sensitisation, such as laboratory animal handling, to be used for screening purposes; a substantial number of those excluded from work would never become sensitised. Apart from a low predictive value, the prevalence of atopy in some 30–40% of young adults is common in industrialised countries and the exclusion of such a number of otherwise health individuals cannot be justified for socio-economic reasons [4, 5]. Although smoking is a risk factor in certain work environments such as laboratory animal work, and in association with exposure to platinum salts and some acid anhydrides, in practice, smoking has not been considered useful in pre-employment screening, Still, it is appropriate to inform smokers of the increased risk of sensitisation they may carry in some work environments due to their smoking habits [5].

Genetic polymorphism and susceptibility to, especially small-molecular-weight occupational agents has attracted some research interest. In particular, studies on the human leucocyte antigen (HLAs) have shown some interesting associations with OA. The HLA-DQB-0501 has repeatedly been shown to positively correlate with diisocyanate asthma, whereas HLA-DQB-503 has displayed an inverse correlation. HLA associations also exist with platinum salts and beryllium. The polymorphic occurrence of glutathione S-transferase (GSTs) and *N*-acetyl transferase (NAT) has been used for similar studies of associations with OA and sensitisation. Both GSTM1 null and NAT 1 and NAT 2 slow acetylator genotypes correlate with susceptibility to diisocyanate asthma. However, the predictive values of the so-far-identified polymorphic genes are not even remotely high enough for pre-employment selection purposes. Considering the multifactorial nature of OA, it is not to be expected that a single polymorphic gene would determine the disease, although it may well increase individual susceptibility or resistance to disease. Irrespective of demonstrated associations with OA, genetic testing, let alone the application of individual genetic profiles for screening purposes, remains both ethically and legally a strongly contentious issue [36].

The widely accepted view is that pre-employment examinations are only meant to establish a base for periodic health surveillance. Due to low predictive values, they should not be used for screening of potentially susceptible individuals on such ground as atopy, smoking, or genetic disposition [4, 5, 37, 38].

Secondary prevention

The term 'secondary prevention' implies that primary prevention has, in one way or another, failed. Thus, the purpose of secondary prevention measures is either to detect occupational disease as early as possible to improve the prognosis of the disease, or, ideally, to detect predictive markers of disease to prevent the development of clinical disease. Another objective is to prevent further cases from developing in the same, or similar work environment. The principal means of secondary prevention is regular medical surveillance of employees. There is sufficient evidence showing that duration of exposure after onset of symptoms, as well as continuance of exposure after onset of asthma, are important prognostic factors, whereas cessation of exposure is associated with various degrees of recovery [39–41]. It is, therefore, generally accepted that we can improve the prognosis of OA by early detection of the disease and by avoidance of further exposure to the causative agent. A consensus statement by the American College of Chest Physicians (ACCP) recommends routine surveillance of all workers exposed to agents known to cause OA [42].

The main tool of health surveillance is the questionnaire on respiratory symptoms. Questionnaires are normally administered at regular intervals of 6–12 months in accordance with latencies of particular sensitisers [43]. Although, the first 2 years of exposure appears to be the most important period, surveillance mostly continues indefinitely as sensitisation and the onset of OA may occur at a much later time if exposure continues [4]. Questionnaires have rarely been validated and their sensitivity and specificity are mostly unknown. Workers' compliance with regularly administered questionnaires has mostly not been assessed. It has been postulated that the threshold for admitting to work-related symptoms is lower in large companies with good possibilities to relocate workers, than in small enterprises [4]. The interest in answering truthfully is likely to vary considerably with expected consequences of coming forward with complaints. Fear for loosing the job without trusting the compensation systems for being equitably compensated for possible incurred income loss and disability are poor incentives for participation.

Objective means of surveillance include occasional workplace spirometry and measurement of bronchial hyperreactivity. Regularly performed spirometry is not a sensitive tool to detect OA and probably does not add much to a questionnaire [44].

Unspecific bronchial hyperresponsiveness is a feature of asthma that develops as a consequence of sensitisation. As a mean of health surveillance, it does not predict OA [45]. It is also often absent in cases of OA [37].

A new and simple approach has been tested in the Netherlands [46]. A national surveillance scheme involving the Dutch government, branch organisations and unions designed to reduce the exposure to flour dust and related allergens was assessed in the bakery, mill and baking product manufacturing industry in the Netherlands. The central tool was a diagnostic questionnaire developed using the experience gained in a previous study on laboratory animals, to estimate the probability of sensitisation to wheat and/or α-amylase allergens. The participating 5546 workers were divided into three categories of probability of developing sensitisation (low 57.4%, intermediate 24.1%, high 18.5%). In the second phase of the programme, the intermediate-probability group will be evaluated further by occupational physicians and the high-probability group will be referred to an occupational respiratory clinic. The low-probability group will be enrolled in the next surveillance cycle. The preliminary results indicate that the simple two-page questionnaire comprising only 19 questions can capture workers with different risks of sensitisation. The approach is thought to be applicable in small and medium-size enterprises [46].

The regular testing for specific IgE antibody, as rule by skin testing, with workplace allergens has been useful in some work environments. During work with complex platinum salts, the positive skin test has a high predictive value for the development of OA [47]. In the production and use of enzyme, e.g. the detergent industry, skin testing is common. It may, in combination with questionnaires, guide decision making. It is also used as a kind of biological monitoring of the successfulness of exposure control [48, 49].

Rhinoconjunctivitis is known to precede the development of symptoms from the lower respiratory tract. It has been shown to precede development of asthma, although the predictive value was low [50]. This pertains to high-molecular-weight allergens, whereas rhinoconjunctivitis is less frequent in exposure to low-molecular-weight agents [50, 51]. Although rhinoconjunctivitis is a rather poor predictor of OA, the condition in itself is an occupational disease that ought to be prevented.

Examples of preventive approaches in specific work environments

There are only a few successful preventive programmes that have been both evaluated and published. The study designs have been rather crude, and control groups have regularly been lacking. There are a number of reasons for the low number of published studies, most of which pertain to the nature of OA and the low public profile of the condition (Tab. 1) [4]. Formal assessment of the successfulness of preventive programmes can be expected only in large industries or in certain branches, for instances bakeries. Only a handful of agents, such as flour dust, animal epithelium and dander cause exposure of great numbers of workers and are, therefore, good environments for interventions [4].

Enzymes

A classical example of primary prevention by alteration of processes and working practices was carried out in the detergent industry in the early 1970s. Asthma symptoms were described in a detergent factory in the course of the first year of employment. The symptomatic workers (primarily respiratory) were sensitised to protease products [52]. Clusters of enzyme allergy in such plants were shown to be caused by *Bacillus subtilis* proteases. This resulted in primary preventions measures to control the exposure. The enzymes were encapsulated to prevent dusting, enclosure of processes was undertaken and the use of protective respiratory equipment was introduced. A major reduction of sensitisation and symptoms was consequently reported [16, 17, 53]. Thus, enzyme allergy abated and cases of enzyme-induced asthma in the detergent industry were rare during the 1990s [48, 54].

However, despite encapsulation of enzyme preparations, the risk of enzyme sensitisation and respiratory allergy still exists in the detergent industry. The use of enzymes has increased and new enzymes such as cellulase, amylase and lipase have been introduced into the washing powder production. Some 25 years after the outbreaks described above, an epidemic of asthma was revealed in a detergent producing plant in the UK with a prevalence of enzyme sensitisation of 26% and work-related lower-respiratory symptoms in 16% of exposed workers [18]. In a Finnish detergent plant having no recognised health problem, a survey disclosed a prevalence of sensitisation among exposed workers of 22%, either to protease, lipase or cellulase compared with unexposed office workers (0%). When interviewed, all sensitised workers reported work-related respiratory symptoms [19]. These incidences emphasise the continuous need of monitoring of exposure, and education of workers, combined with secondary preventive measures such as health surveillance.

The enzyme using industry is aware of the minute amounts (nanogram levels) of enzyme needed to sensitise and have adopted guidelines as low as 15 ng/m^3 for proteases [48]. Health surveillance schemes have been suggested. They include the periodic skin testing of workers as a secondary preventive measure [49].

Natural rubber latex

Primary prevention by substitution of an allergen is ideal, although not very often practicable. The interventions applied to decrease latex allergies, including OA, serves as a rare example of this strategy. In the late 1980s and 1990s, powdered gloves with a high protein content was recognised as the cause of high prevalences of sensitisation to latex and latex-induced allergies including OA among hospital personnel [55–57]. Interventions at an institution level including replacement of powdered gloves having a high protein content with non-powdered, low-protein gloves have been reported to be successful, leading to cessation or significant decrease in sensitisation rate. Moreover, already sensitised and even asthmatic workers have been able to continue working avoiding the use of latex products [58–60].

In 1996, the Ontario Workplace Safety and Insurance Board recommended the reduction of aerosols of latex proteins and encouraged hospitals to use powder-free, low-protein or non-latex gloves. At various points of time, hospitals introduced latex policies including education and medical surveillance. The latex strategies were temporally associated with a decline in claims for latex-induced asthma [61]. In Germany, a nationwide interdisciplinary information campaign was carried out in 1997–1998. The campaign was accompanied by a revision of the technical regulations for dangerous substances, demanding only powder-free, low-allergen latex gloves to be used in institutions providing health-care services. An insurance company covering 60% of hospitals in Germany made financial resources available for the information campaign. The preventive programme was evaluated by monitoring compensation claims before and after the campaign, as well as by assessing changes in glove-wearing behaviour. A temporal association, with a 2-year delay, was registered between the amount of purchased powdered gloves by acute care hospitals and the fall in reported cases of OA (Fig. 1). The use of powdered gloves decreased by 50% and the use of non-powered gloves doubled [58, 62]. After recognising that latex allergy is caused by the inhalation of latex allergen that, adhered to the starch powder, becomes airborne, the preventive strategies have proven successful in reducing latex allergy. Unfortunately, the possibility of removal of a sensitising agent or substitution of it with a non-sensitising is a rare occasion.

Laboratory animal allergy

Due to the nature of some working environments, total avoidance of exposure cannot be achieved.

Typical for such environments are animal laboratory work, farming, veterinary work, bakeries and mills. Laboratory animal handling is associated with a well-recognised risk of sensitisation and respiratory allergies. In a prospective study of a cohort of laboratory animal workers, the incidence of allergic symptoms was as high as 37% in 1979–1980. In 1982–1983 there was a decrease to 10–12%. The drop in incidence coincided with the introduction of a site order and code of working practice together with an education programme to increase awareness of the problem. For instance, the use of personal protective equipment became mandatory [63]. A further follow-up of employees recruited in 1987–1990 revealed that

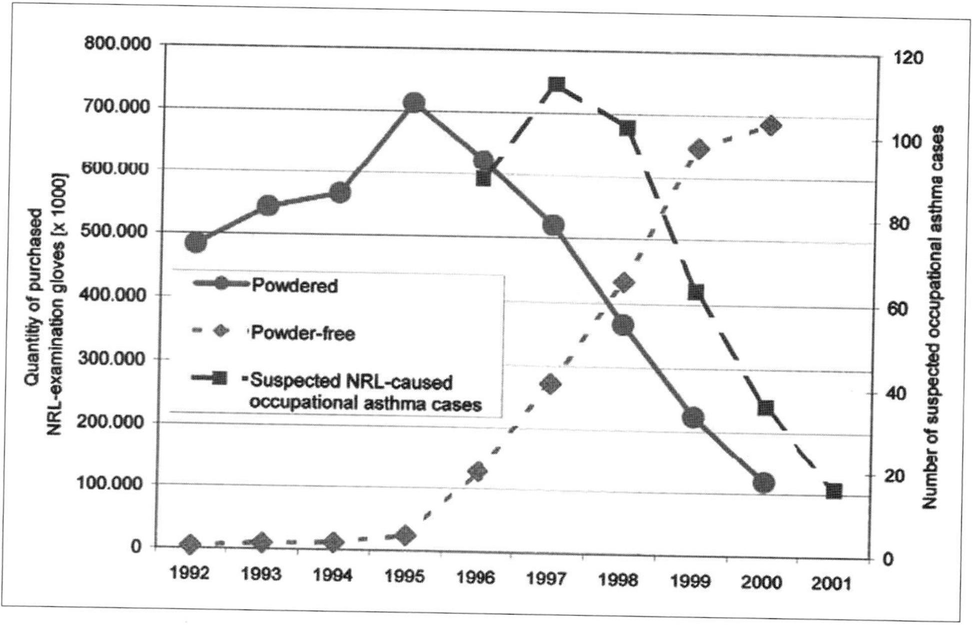

Figure 1.
Reported cases of latex-induced occupational asthma (OA) in relation to purchases of gloves 1992–2001 [58].

the incidence of laboratory animal allergy had remained at the same level of about 10%. The predictive value of atopy and sensitisation to laboratory animal during this 2-year follow-up was 66% and 87%, respectively [64]. The studies by Botham and colleagues show that primary preventive measures aiming at the reduction of exposure do reduce the incidence of animal-induced allergic symptoms, and may make it possible for already sensitised individuals to continue working with laboratory animals.

Flour dust

Considering the size of the exposed population and the high prevalence of sensitisation, the prevention of baker's asthma appears highly meaningful. Sensitisation to flour dust may occur in more than 20% of those exposed, and asthma may be prevalent in 10% [25]. The exposure levels have remained high in the baking industry in general and, contrary to expectations, levels have been even higher in modern medium and large size bakeries than in small enterprises [14]. Primary prevention is difficult due to several circumstances, e.g. the great number of sensitisers including a number of antigens such as various flours, storage mites, enzymes and other so-called dough improvers present in the baking industry. The background sensitisation to wheat of 2–4% of the unexposed population makes a total avoidance of sensitisation impossible. As prevention cannot aim at a total avoidance of exposure, exposure has to be controlled in other ways.

Setting OELs is a way of directing focus on exposure levels. Despite access to solid data, most countries have set pragmatic exposure limits far too high for protection. Regulatory authorities have access to better exposure-response data on wheat flour and α-amylase than for any other occupational sensitisers [23, 24, 27, 65]. It appears that the risk of asthma in a previously un-sensitised population starts at about 3 mg/m^3 and rhinitis at about 1 mg/m^3 [23]. Reviews of the scientific evidence agree that, although no distinct threshold for symptoms or sensitisation can be identified, the risk of both end-points below 1 mg/m^3 would be small and symptoms would most likely be mild [30].

From the point of view of sensitisation, frequent peak exposures in the baking process are recognised as an important problem. The scientific basis for recommending a 15-min STEL is, however, lacking. On the other hand, peaks are related to some specific tasks such as weighing/sieving, mixing, and cleaning. Exposure levels can be significantly reduced by ensuring sufficient exhaust ventilation and by applying good working practices such as the use of dredgers instead of hand throwing and vacuum cleaning instead of brushing. A study on 55 UK bakeries revealed a poor knowledge of elementary working practices for reducing dust levels; only 27% of bakeries were aware of the existence of an OEL, the MEL or a STEL. Less than one third possessed a copy of a booklet on guidance to reduce exposures released by the Health and Safety in Bakeries Liaison Committee [14, 15].

Secondary prevention measures to reduce morbidity by early detection of OA or sensitisation are common in the baking industry [4]. They comprise pre-placement evaluations followed by periodic questionnaires on respiratory symptoms and frequent periodic spirometry, sometimes combined with skin testing. Preventive programmes have rarely been evaluated. The rationale for carrying out medical surveillance has been questioned [44]. The accuracy of such a surveillance programme was tested by Brant and colleagues [66]. They carried out a study on 324 supermarket in-store bakeries using a health surveillance programme focusing on work-related chest symptoms together with specific IgE either to wheat flour or fungal α-amylase as a surrogate for OA [66]. The surveillance included three stages starting with a short questionnaire on respiratory symptoms (stage 1), a further questionnaire on work-relatedness of symptoms, if any, (stage 2) and, finally an IgE-analysis of a serum samples (stage 3). To assess the accuracy, a cross-sectional survey was undertaken in 20 bakeries. The surveillance system resulted in a quarter of those with symptoms reporting that symptoms were work-related; 61% of those with work-related chest symptoms had specific IgE antibodies to wheat or fungal α-amylase, which corresponded to 1% of the bakers. However, the cross-sectional survey arrived at a prevalence of 4%. Thus, the surveillance system underestimated the presence of disease and the conclusion was that a more efficient method of surveillance in bakeries is needed [66].

Much remains to be done to prevent asthma and other allergies in the baking industry. The setting of health-based OELs will necessarily include socio-economic consideration of practicability and will not protect the entire workforce. It is obvious that a successful reduction of OA in the baking industry needs a closer co-operation between regulatory authorities, branch organisations, unions and OSH personnel. It should be in the interest of all parties involved to ensure that recommendations and guidance reaches the workplaces and are actively implemented.

Diisocyanates

An example showing how regulatory authorities can exert preventive strategies is afforded by a Canadian legislation initiative for the prevention of diisocyanate-induced asthma. In 1983 the Ontario Ministry of Labour introduced a preventive programme consisting of two components.

As a primary prevention measure, employers had to ensure that the time-weighted average of diisocyanate exposure did not exceed 0.005 ppm. The second component was a mandatory medical surveillance including pre-employment respiratory questionnaires and spirometry. The questionnaires were repeated every 6 months and spirometry at least every second year. Respiratory symptoms and/or changes in spirometry were followed by an assessment by a physician as to the safety of continuing work [31].

The programme was retrospectively assessed from workers' compensation statistics. Following the introduction of the programme, there was an increase in annual compensation claims, which reflected a more efficient case finding. Starting in 1991, the claims decreased, whereas claims of OA of other causes remained at an earlier level. The time from onset of symptoms to diagnosis decreased from 2.7 to 1.7 years and cases had milder asthma. Companies with claims were more likely to have exceeded the exposure level of ≥0.5 ppb. The conclusion was that one or more component of the programme had a beneficial effect. There was a comparatively long time lag before the decrease of claims became discernible (Fig. 2). It is possible that the programme *per se* has initiated a series of favourable measures undertaken by separate companies following the introduction of the mandatory programme. These may have included technical improvements to reduce exposures, more active education of workers, supervision of working practices including the use of protective equipment, etc. [31].

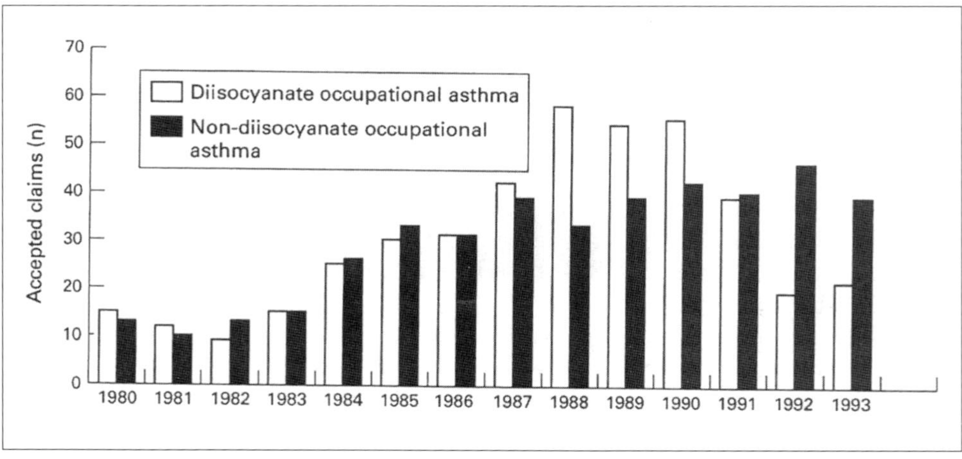

Figure 2.
Accepted workers claims of diisocyanate-induced OA and OA induced by other causes in Ontario [71].

Work-exacerbated asthma

Non-OA, being an increasingly common disease and getting worse because of the vast number of various irritant exposures in the workplace, has attracted more and more attention over the last few years. A definition of WEA was suggested in 1995 by the American College of Chest Physicians (ACCP) as concurrent asthma worsened by non-toxic irritants or physical stimuli in the workplace. The suggested medical case definition requires a diagnosis of asthma and an association between symptoms of asthma and work, provided that the subject has had symptoms or medication before, and experiences an increase of symptoms or needs more medication after entering a new occupational setting [43]. Because of the obvious need for preventive strategies concerning work-related aggravation of non-OA, Wagner and Wegman [6] in an editorial suggested that work-aggravated asthma should be included into the definition of OA. The proposal, although not uniformly accepted as such by the scientific society [67], led to the now generally adopted, broader concept of 'work-related asthma' covering both OA and WEA [68]. WEA indicates 'aggravation of pre-existing or coincident adult new-onset asthma because of workplace environmental exposure' [68, 69].

The need to prevent work-related worsening of any asthma is becoming widely recognised, but the scientific knowledge about the condition is still scanty. From the point of view of prevention, it is interesting to note that WEA is associated with a similar impact on work productivity and loss of income as OA. Some studies indicate that WEA may be associated with higher rates of symptoms and exacerbations than asthma unrelated to work exposures [9].

Preventive strategies including guidelines as to the health surveillance of WEA require that the condition can be separated from OA. However, the differentiation between WEA and OA is still a diagnostic challenge and not always possible. Negative specific inhalation challenge tests, when available, often exclude OA. In cases where inhalation challenges are not practicable, serial peak-flow (PEF) recordings are normally used; however, they do not necessarily discriminate between WEA and OA [70].

Regrettably little is so far known about the frequency of WEA and, especially, what aggravation of symptoms means in terms of health. In the few reports available, the frequency of WEA varies depending on differences in information collection and definition. Focusing on studies including employed adults with asthma, the prevalence estimates have been in the range of 8–25% [71, 72]. A prevalence as high as 52% has been reported [8]. The frequency of symptom aggravation was included in an interview study with 969 asthmatics, where 21% reported work-related aggravation for symptoms at least once a week [73]. These studies comprise self-reported symptoms. Objectively assessed work-related functional changes, e.g. by serial PEF recordings or the monitoring of inflammatory responses, are necessary to assess the health risk involved. Similarly, studies with optimal medication are needed to evaluate how the increased frequency and aggravation of symptoms should be managed without risking permanent health implications, but also to avoid unnecessary discrimination of workers with asthma or bronchial hyperreactivity.

Asthma symptoms may be aggravated by a number of factors such as irritant agents, dusts, fumes, physical exercise, changes in temperature and strong odours. When such exposures occur in the workplace, the prevention of choice is to reduce exposures. However, it is rarely known to what extent the exposure ought to be reduced to protect asthmatics from aggravation of symptoms. For most substances exposure-response data are lacking. Solid data on nitrogen dioxide (NO_2), a typical respiratory irritant, show that asthmatics and hyperreactive individuals are far more sensitive to the irritant effects of NO_2 than healthy individuals [74]. Safe exposure levels for asthmatics appear to be as low as 0.2–0.4 ppm, which may make asthmatics unsuitable for tunnelling and under-ground mining work, where such low exposure limits may be impracticable. A risk assessment on similar dose-response data for another irritant, sulphur dioxide (SO_2), likewise found a higher vulnerability of asthmatics to SO_2 at or even below current OELs [75]. However, the assumption that asthmatics are invariably more sensitive to all irritants may lead to discrimination of asthmatics, similarly to the ungrounded weeding out of atopics in the 1980s. Exposure-response data are needed for preventive strategies. A more active use of exposure assessments have been suggested as a routine means of prevention [76].

The implementation of scientific-based preventive strategies requires more information on all aspects of WEA. There is a need for clinical assessments of WEA to obtain objective data, in addition to the self-reported data, on inflammatory responses and on the effect of continuing exposure on the underlying condition with or without treatment. It is also important to have exposure assessments to better understand what levels of exposures are hazardous to asthmatics. Such data are needed for the production of guidelines to primary health care, and occupational health personnel. The awareness of WEA should be improved among physicians working in respiratory clinics.

Asthma attributable to work

A significant proportion of asthma is attributable to work. In a review of available literature, the authors arrived at a median of 9% for the attributable risk, whereas inclusion of the 12 studies of the highest quality resulted in a median of 15% [1]. Similar estimates have subsequently been reported in a study on physician-diagnosed asthma in Beijing residents [77] and are even higher for asthma including wheezing [78].

Only a few population-based incidence studies have been conducted. In one such study a cohort of 79 204 health maintenance organisation members was followed for 3 months registering new-onset asthma, re-activation of previous asthma and exacerbation of asthma. Criteria for onset of asthma attributable to work exposures were met by 21% [2]. In another large study covering the entire employed Finnish population aged 25–59 years, the cohort was followed from 1986 to 1998. Combining a register on asthmatics entitled to reimbursement of medication costs and the census data of 1985, 1990 and 1995 classified according to occupation, relative risks of the 49 575 incident cases of asthma were estimated. The attributable fraction of occupation for men was 29% and for women 17% [3].

From the preventive point of view, it is interesting that studies, despite different designs, report increased risks of asthma in work environments associated with irritant chemical agents and dusts [2, 3, 77–80]. An increased risk of OA among cleaners has been reported repeatedly [79, 81, 82]. In a study on identical twins discordant for asthma, solvent were found to significantly increase the risk of contracting asthma [83]. Similar exposures may explain an increased risk among shoemakers [79]. Moulds in water-damaged buildings have been suggested as a possible explanation for an increased risk of asthma among educators [84]. This receives some support by a meta-analysis on the associations between water-damaged buildings and respiratory outcomes [85].

Population-based studies on attributable risk consistently show risks that are several times higher than can be estimated from reporting programmes, surveillance schemes and disease registers [5]. The risk of asthma is frequently associated with exposures not previously recognised as being sensitising. Several possibilities are conceivable. To some extent the differences may reflect a failure in finding, or at least reporting, cases of OA. This is supported by the subsequent analysis by Karjalainen and co-workers [79] of their population cohort. When all registered cases of OA were deleted from the analysis, an increased relative risk of asthma remained in the typical high-risk occupations baking 2.13 (95% CI 1.74–2.83) and farming 1.76 (95% CI 1.64–1.89). Both environments are known to cause IgE-mediated OA without posing diagnostic difficulties.

However, the excess risk of asthma in workers exposed to dusts, gas, and chemical fumes, i.e. irritants, may be due to other reasons. For one thing, diagnostics of OA has focused on specific sensitisers previously recognised as inducers of OA. Other unknown and less frequent inducers may have been overlooked. A probably more important explanation is the complex aetiology of asthma. Various host factors are likely to interact with environmental exposures including occupational sensitisers, irritant chemicals, dusts, viruses and other microbes. The occupational exposures are not necessarily the main inducers of disease. However, the attributable factor by definition signifies the fraction of disease in the population that would not have occurred if exposure to the risk factor had not taken place. Thus, learning more about the associations between asthma and the work environment will eventually afford strategies for the prevention of the induction of adult-onset asthma [5, 6, 61].

Is prevention feasible and worthwhile?

Feasibility issues

OA should to a large extent be preventable. What makes prevention difficult are the manifold causative agents and the low attack rate in single workplaces together with a comparatively low public profile [4] (Tab. 1). An evidence-based assessment of preventive measures concluded that a reduction of exposure leads to a decrease in the number of workers who become sensitised and who develop asthma [37]. Health surveillance is generally considered an effective way of detecting OA at an early stage and the prognosis of disease is better in workers who have participated in health surveillance programmes [4, 5, 37]. Still, few studies have evaluated the efficacy in terms of reduced morbidity [4, 37].

Some preventive programmes conducted in specific working environments have included evaluations of the impact. The preventive programmes on natural rubber latex [58, 59], diiscoyanates [31] and flour dust [46] represent strategies in which authorities, the industry and unions have joined forces. The programme directed against diisocyanate exposure was successful in reducing the number of claims, although the design of the programme did not allow the assessment of the effectiveness of separate components of the programme [31]. The successful preventive programmes on natural rubber latex [31, 58, 59] also represent before and after comparisons.

The prevention of WEA is a fairly new domain. The knowledge about associations between adult-onset asthma and occupational exposures are still too fragmented for science-based preventive initiatives. Asthma-outcomes have mostly been based on self-reported symptoms without objective assessments of functional disturbances as a consequence of exposures, and exposure-response relationships have not been studied. Thus, strategies for prevention of work exacerbation of asthma are confined to vocational guidance and education of OSH personnel as to health surveillance of asthmatics in work environments associated with dusts and irritants.

Is prevention worthwhile?

Many countries report OA as the most common cause of occupational respiratory occupational disease [20]. Ethically, occupational disease is unacceptable, and all reasonable means available should be used to prevent it. However, only a few attempts have been made to assess the costs of OA and possible saved costs as a result of successful interventions. In one recent study commissioned by the Health and Safety Executive in the United Kingdom, the true costs of OA were calculated [34]. The total lifetime costs were derived from both direct costs (e.g. use of health care resources, treat and rehabilitation costs), and indirect costs (e.g. costs from sickness absence, labour turnover, compensation and insurance). OA caused on an average 3.5–4.5 days of absence from work per year. The total lifetime cost incurred by reported new cases (631 cases) of OA in 2003 was estimated at £ 36–78 millions. Taking into account that OA is probably under-reported by up to one third, the costs increase substantially [34].

The cost effectiveness of specific preventive programmes has rarely been calculated. In the successful German preventive programme directed against natural rubber latex (see above), the number of claims decreased drastically with a time lag of a few years, the use of latex gloves was halved and that of latex-free gloves doubled. The saved costs of professional training were calculated to exceed those invested by some ten times [62].

Recent assessments of the socio-economic implications of WEA have arrived at the conclusion that WEA inflicts considerable costs to employers and the community. Assuming that 15% of asthma can be attributed to work exposures, the annual costs of WEA in the United states could be as high as US$ 1.6 billion [9]. WEA may be associated with higher rates of symptoms and exacerbations as asthma unrelated to work. The effect of WEA on the work productivity and earning capacity is similar to those of specifically induced OA [9]. It is obvious that more attention has to be paid to the prevention of WEA in the coming years.

Future developments

A shift in priorities of research related to the complex associations between asthma and the work environment is discernible. With respect to "classical" OA with a latency period, the level of understanding of causation of OA is already sufficient for the implementation of preventive strategies. Preventive programmes should focus primarily on exposure control and worker education. In the design of such programmes, there is a need for a more scientific approach; for instance, the design should include measurable parameters allowing a quantitative evaluation of programmes. It is important that evaluations of interventions, also smaller ones conducted in single enterprises and institutions, are reported. Also secondary preventive measures need to be refined. Considering the present extensive routine use of secondary preventive measures, it should be easy to plan, evaluate and report the impact of such activities. Further research on markers predictive of OA seems necessary for secondary preventive purposes as well as for the discrimination between OA and WEA.

WEA has become increasingly important. Epidemiological studies indicate that WEA is a common problem. It seems to have a similar socio-economic impact as OA. When allocating resources, it seems advisable to invest in the research of WEA. The current level of knowledge and understanding of WEA is modest. Although work-related aggravation of asthma is encountered by occupational physicians at least as often as OA, the exposures, mechanisms, extent and consequences in term of the worker's health are largely unknown. From a preventive point of view, WEA will be an important issue owing to the still increasing prevalence of asthma and asthma-like conditions among children and adolescents. There is a need for science-based information already at the stage of vocational guidance.

Recognising that some 10–30% of adult-onset asthma is attributable to work, there is a need for a more profound understanding of the full phenotype of asthma and, especially, the associations with different work environments. Well-conducted epidemiological studies frequently show an increased risk of asthma in work environments and occupations not formerly known to be associated with specific inducers of OA. In particular, long-term exposure to a broad range of irritants seems to be important. A full understanding of the role of work exposures in the development of asthma may eventually lead to new preventive insights.

References

1 Blanc PD, Toren K (1999) How much adult asthma can be attributed to occupational factors? *Am J Med* 107: 580–587

2 Milton DK, Solomon GM, Rosiello RA, Herrick RP (1998) Risk and incidence of

asthma attributable to occupational exposure among HMO members. *Am J Ind Med* 33: 1–10

3 Karjalainen A, Kurppa K, Martikainen R, Klaukka T, Karjalainen J (2001) Work is related to a substantial portion of adult-onset asthma incidence in the Finnish population. *Am J Respir Crit Care Med* 164: 565–568

4 Cullinan P, Tarlo S, Nemery B (2003) The prevention of occupational asthma. *Eur Respir J* 22: 853–860

5 Liss GM, Nordman H, Tarlo S, Bernstein DI (2006) In: IL Bernstein, M Chan-Yeung, J-L Malo, DI Bernstein (eds): *Asthma in the Workplace*, Taylor & Francis Group, New York, 353–375

6 Wagner GR, Wegman DH (1998) Occupational asthma: prevention by definition. *Am J Ind Med* 33: 427–429

7 Malo J-L (2005) Future advances in work-related asthma and the impact on occupational health. *Occup Med* 55: 606–611

8 Henneberger PK (2007) Work-exacerbated asthma. *Curr Opin Allergy Clin Immunol* 7: 146–151

9 Vandenplas O, Henneberger PK (2007) Socioeconomic outcomes in work-exacerbated asthma. *Curr Opinion Allergy Clin Immunol* 7: 236–241

10 Tarlo S, Liss G (2005) Prevention of occupational asthma-practical implications for occupational physicians. *Occup Med* 55: 588–594

11 Corn M (1983) Assessment and control of environmental exposure. *J Allergy Clin Immunol* 72: 231–241

12 Baur X (2003) Are we closer to developing threshold limit values for allergens in the workplace? *Ann Allergy Asthma Immunol* 90 (Suppl 2): 153–163

13 Bush RK, Stave GM (2003) Laboratory animal allergy. Un up-date. *ILAR J* 44: 114–122

14 Elms J, Robinson E, Rahman S, Garrod A (2005) Exposure to Flour Dust in UK Bakeries: Current Use of Control measures. *Ann Occup Hyg* 49: 2005

15 Health and Safety in Bakeries Liaison Committee (1998) *Guidance on dust control and health surveillance in bakeries*. London, HSBLC 1998

16 Juniper CP, How MJ, Goodwin BF, Kinshott AK (1977) *Bacillus subtilis* enzymes: A 7–year clinical, epidemiological and immunological study of an industrial allergen. *J Soc Occup Med* 27: 3–12

17 Cathcart M, Nicholson P, Roberts D, et al (1997) Enzyme exposure, smoking and lung function in employees in the detergent industry over 20 years. Medical Subcommittee of the UK Soap and Detergent Industry Association. *Occup Med* Lond 47: 473–478

18 Cullinan P, Harris JM, Newman Taylor AJ, et al (2000) An outbreak of asthma in a modern detergent factory. *Lancet* 356: 1899–1900

19 Vanhanen M, Tiikkainen U, Tupasela O, Voutilainen R, Nordman H (2000) Risk of enzyme allergy in the detergent industry. *Occup Environ Med* 57: 121–125

20 Meredith S, Nordman H (1996) Occupational asthma – Measures of frequency from four countries. *Thorax* 51: 435–440

21 Topping M (2001) Industry's perception and use of occupational exposure limits. *Ann Occup Hyg* 42: 357–366

22 Scientific Committee on Occupational Exposure Limits (SCOEL) (1998) *Methodology for the Derivation of Occupational Exposure Limits: Key Documentation*. European Commission, Directorate-General V, Luxembourg, December 1998

23 Brisman J, Järvholm B, Lillienberg L (2000) Exposure-response relations for self reported asthma and rhinitis in bakers. *Occup Environ Med* 57: 335–340

24 Cullinan P, Lowson D, Nieuwenhuijsen MJ, Sandiford C, Tee RD, Venables KM, McDonald JC, Newman Taylor AJ (1994) Work related symptoms, sensitisation, and estimated exposure in workers not previously exposed to flour. *Occup Environ Med* 51: 579–583

25 Houba R (1996) *Occupational respiratory allergy in bakery workers – Relationships with wheat and fungal alpha-amylase aeroallergen exposure*. Doctoral Thesis. Wageningen, The Netherlands: Agricultural University Wageningen, Department of Occupational and Environmental Health, Wageningen, 1996

26 Houba R, Heederik D, Doekes G (1998) Wheat sensitisation and work related symptoms in the baking industry are preventable: An epidemiological study. *Am J Respir Crit Care Med* 158: 1499–1503

27 Heederik D, Houba R (2001) An explorative quantitative risk assessment for high molecular weight sensitizers: Wheat flour. *Ann Occup Hyg* 45: 175–185

28 American Conference of Governmental Industrial Hygienists. Document on Flour Dust. ACGIH, Cincinnati, 1999

29 Health and Safety Executive (2002) *Occupational exposure limits 2002*. EH40/2002). London, HSE Books

30 DECOS (2004) *Wheat and other cereal flour dusts. An approach for evaluating health effects from occupational exposure*. Dutch Expert Committee on Occupational Standards. No. 2004/020SH, The Hague, August 10, 2004

31 Tarlo S (2007) Prevention of occupational asthma in Ontario. *Can J Physiol Pharmacol* 85: 167–172

32 Dewitte J.D, Chan-Yeung M, Malo J-L (1994) Medicolegal and compensation aspects of occupational asthma. *Eur Respir J* 7: 969–980

33 Bernstein IL, Keskinen H, Chan-Yeung M, Malo J-L (2006) Medicolegal aspects, compensation aspects and evaluation of impairment/disability. In: IL Bernstein, M Chan-Yeung, J-L Malo, DI Bernstein (eds): *Asthma in the Workplace*, 3rd edn. Taylor & Francis, New York, 319–351

34 Boyd R, Cowie H, Hurley F, Ayres J (2006) *The true cost of occupational asthma in Great Britain*. Health and Safety Executive HSE Books, research Report 474/2006

35 De Zotti R, Molinari S, Larese F, Bovenzi M (1995) Pre-employment screening among trainee bakers. *Occup Environ Med* 52: 279–283

36 Newman Taylor AJ, Yucesoy B. Genetics and Occupational Asthma (2006) In: IL Bernstein, M Chan-Yeung, J-L Malo, DI Bernstein (eds): *Asthma in the Workplace*. Taylor & Francis Group, New York, 89–108

37 BOHRF Guidelines for Occupational asthma (2004) The British Occupational Health Research Foundation. www.bohrf.org.uk

38 Newman Taylor AJ, Nicholson PJ, Cullinan P (2004) *Guidelines for the prevention, identification and management of occupational asthma: Evidence review and recommendations*. London, British Occupational Health Research Foundation (BOHFR), 2004

39 Coté J, Kennedy S, Chan-Yeung M (1990) Outcome of patients with cedar asthma with continuous exposure. *Ann Rev Respir Dis* 141: 373–376

40 Perfetti L, Cartier A, Ghezzo H, Gautrin D, Malo JL (1998) Follow-up of occupational asthma after removal from or diminution of exposure to the responsible agent. *Chest* 114: 398–403

41 Malo JL, Cartier A, Ghezzo H, Lafrance M, McCants M, Lehrer SB (1988) Patterns of improvement of spirometry, bronchial hyperresponsiveness and specific IgE antibody levels after cessation of exposure in occupational asthma caused by snow-crab processing. *Am Rev Respir Dis* 138: 807–812

42 Chan-Yeung M (1977) Assessment of asthma in the workplace. ACCP consensus statement. American College of Chest Physicians. *Chest* 11: 922–928

43 Chan-Yeung M (1995) Fate of occupational asthma. A follow-up study of patients with occupational asthma due to western red cedar (*Thuja plicata*). *Am Rev Respir Dis* 1077: 116: 1023–1029

44 Gordon SB, Curran AD, Murphy J, et al (1997) Screening questionnaires for baker's asthma – Are they worth the effort. *Occup Med Lond* 47: 361–366

45 Burge PS, Moscato G, Johnson A, Chan-Yeung M (2006) Physiological Assessment: Serial measurements of lung function and bronchial responsiveness. In: IL Bernstein, M Chan-Yeung, J-L Malo, DI Bernstein (eds): *Asthma in the Workplace*. Taylor & Francis Group, New York, 199–226

46 Suarthana E (2008) *Predicting occupational lung diseases*. Utrecht University, Institute for Risk Assessment Sciences and Julius Center for Health Sciences and Primary Care of the University Medical Center Utrecht, The Netherlands, 2008. ISBN 9789039347867

47 Merget R, Caspari C, Dierkes-Globisch A, Kulzer R, Breitstadt R, Kniffka A, Degens P, Schultze-Werninghaus G (2001) Effectiveness of a medical surveillance program for the prevention of occupational asthma caused by platinum salts: A nested case-control study. *J Allergy Clin Immunol* 107: 707–712

48 Schweigert MK, MacKenzie DP, Sarlo K (2000) Occupational asthma and allergy associated with the use of enzymes in the detergent industry – A review of the epidemiology, toxicology and methods of prevention. *Clin Exp Allergy* 30: 1511–1518

49 Nicholson PJ, Newman Taylor AJ, Oliver P, et al (2001) Current best practice for the health surveillance of enzyme workers in the detergent industry. *Occup Med* (Lond) 51: 81–92

50 Gautrin D, Newman-Taylor AJ, Nordman H, Malo J-L (2003) Controversies in epidemiology of occupational asthma. *Eur Respir J* 22: 551–559

51 Malo J-L, Lemière C, Desjardins A, Cartier A (1997) Prevalence and intensity of rhinconjunctivitis in subjects with occupational asthma. *Eur Respir J* 10: 1513–1515

52 Flindt MLH (1969) Pulmonary disease due to inhalation of derivatives of *Bacillus subtilis* containing proteolytic enzymes. *Lancet* 1: 1177–1181

53 Juniper CP, Roberts DM (1984) Enzyme asthma: Fourteen years' clinical experience of a recently prescribed disease. *J Soc Occup Med* 34: 127–132

54 Sarlo K ((2003) Control of occupational asthma and allergy in the detergent industry. *Ann Allergy Asthma Immunol* 90 (Suppl 5): 32–34

55 Turjanmaa K, Kanto M, Kautiainen H, Palosuo T (2002) Long-term outcome of 160 adult patients with natural rubber latex allergy. *J Allergy Clin Immunol* 110: S70–74

56 Lagier F, Vervloet D, Lhermet I, Poyen D, Charpin D (1992) Prevalence of latex allergy in operating room nurses. *J Allergy Clin Immunol* 90: 319–322

57 Vandenplas O, Binard-Van Cangh F, Brumagne A, Caroyer JM, Thimpont J, Sohy C, Larbanois A, Jamart J (2001) Occupational asthma in symptomatic workers exposed to natural rubber latex: Evaluation of diagnostic procedures. *J Allergy Clin Immunol* 107: 542–547

58 Allmers H, Schmengler J, Skudlik C (2002) Primary prevention of natural rubber latex allergy in the German health care system through education and intervention. *J Allergy Clin Immunol* 110: 318–323

59 Tarlo S, Easty A, Eubanks K, Parsons CR, Min F, Juvet S, Liss GM (2001) Outcome of a natural rubber latex control program in an Ontario teaching hospital. *J Allergy Clin Immunol* 108: 628–633

60 Saary MJ, Kanani A, Alghadeer H, Holness DL, Tarlo S (2002) Changes in rates of natural rubber latex sensitivity among dental school students and staff members after changes in latex gloves. *J Allergy Clin Immunol* 109: 131–135

61 Liss GM, Tarlo S (2001) Natural rubber latex-related occupational asthma: Association with interventions and glove changes over time. *Am J Ind Med* 40: 347–353

62 Latza U, Haamann F, Baur X (2005) Effectiveness of a nationwide interdisciplinary preventive programme for latex allergy. *Int Arch Occup Environ Health* 78: 394–402

63 Botham PA, Davies GE, Teasdale EL (1987) Allergy to laboratory animals: A prospective study of its incidence and of the influence of atopy on its development. *Br J Ind Med* 44: 627–632

64 Botham PA, Lamb CT, Teasdale EL, Bonner SM, Tomenson JA (1995) Allergy to laboratory animals: A follow up study of its incidence and of the influence of atopy and pre-existing sensitisation on its development. *Occup Environ Med* 52: 129–133

65 Cullinan P, Cook A, Nieuwenhuijsen MJ, Sandiford C, Tee RD, et al (2001) Allergen and dust exposure as determinants of work-related symptoms and sensitization in a cohort of flour-exposed workers; a case-control analysis. *Ann Occup Hyg* 45: 97–103

66 Brant A, Nightingale S, Berriman J, Newman Taylor AJ, Cullinan P (2005) Supermarket baker's asthma: how accurate is routine health surveillance? *Occup Environ Med* 62: 395–399

67 Malo J-L, Chan-Yeung M (1998) Comment on the editorial "Occupational asthma - Prevention by Definition. *Am J Ind Med* 35: 207–208

68 Vandenplas O, Malo JL (2003) Definition and types of work-related asthma: A nosological approach. *Eur Respir J* 21: 706–12

69 Bernstein IL, Chan-Yeung M, Malo JL (2006) Definition and classification of asthma in the workplace. In: IL Bernstein, M Chan-Yeung, J-L Malo, DI Bernstein (eds): *Asthma in the Workplace*, 3rd edn. Taylor & Francis, New York, 1–8

70 Chiry S, Cartier A, Malo J-L, Tarlo S, Lemière C (2007) Comparison of peak expiratory flow variability between workers with work-exacerbated asthma and occupational asthma. *Chest* 132: 483–487

71 Tarlo S, Liss GM, Yeung KS (2002) Changes in rates and severity of compensation claims for asthma due to diisocyanates: A possible effect of medical surveillance measures. *Occup Environ Med* 59: 58–62 s

72 Henneberger P, Deprez RD, Asdigian N, et al (2003) Workplace exacerbation of asthma symptoms: Findings form a population-based study in Maine. *Arch Environ Health* 58: 781–788

73 Saarinen K, Karjalainen A, Martikainen R, Uitti J, Tammilehto L, Klaukka T, Kurppa K (2003) Prevalence of work-aggravated symptoms in clinically established asthma. *Eur Respir J* 22: 305–309

74 Folinsbee LJ (1992) Does nitrogen dioxide exposure increase airways responsiveness? *Toxicol Ind Health* 8: 273–283

75 DECOS (2003) *Sulphur dioxide. Health-based recommended occupation al exposure limit.* Dutch Expert Committee on Occupational Standards No. 2003/08 OSH, The Hague, December 2003

76 Heederik D, van Roy F (2008) Exposure assessments should be integrated in studies on the prevention and management of occupational asthma. *Occup Environ Med* 65: 149–151

77 Xu X, Christiani DC, Dockery DW, Wang L (1992) Exposure-response relationships between occupational exposures and chronic respiratory illness: A community-based study. *Am Rev Respir Dis* 413–418

78 Arif AA, Whitehead LV, Delclos GL, et al (2002) Prevalence and risk factors of work-related asthma by industry among United States workers: Data from the third national Health and Nutrition Examination Survey (1988–1994). *Occup Environ Health* 59: 505–511

79 Karjalainen A, Kurppa K, Martikainen R, Karjalainen J, Klaukka T (2002) Exploration of asthma risk by occupation – Extended analysis of an incidence study of the Finnish population. *Scand J Work Environ Health* 28: 49–57

80 Ng TP, Hong CY, Wong ML, Koh KT, Ling SL (1994) Risks of asthma associated with occupations in a community-based case-control study. *Am J Ind Med* 25: 709–718

81 Kogevinas M, Anto JM, Sunyer J, et al (1999) The European Community Respiratory Health Survey Study Group. Occupational asthma in Europe and other industrialized areas: A population-based study. *Lancet* 353: 1750–1754

82 Zock JP, Kogevinas M, Sunyer J, Jarvis D, Torén K, Antó JM for the European Community Respiratory Health Survey (2002) Asthma characteristics in cleaning workers, workers in other risk jobs and office workers. *Eur Respir J* 20: 679–685

83 Antti-Poika M, Nordman H, Koskenvuo M, Kaprio J, Jalava M (1992) Role of exposure to airway irritants in the development of asthma. *Int Arch Occup Environ Health* 64: 195–200

84 Liss G, Tarlo S (2002) Work-related asthma. *Occup Environ Med* 59: 503–504

85 Fisk WJ, Lei-Gomez Q, Mendell MJ (2007) Meta-analyses of the associations of respiratory health effects with dampness and mold in homes. *Indoor Air* 17: 284–296

Design, conduct and analysis of surveys on work-related asthma

Kathleen Kreiss[1] *and Dick Heederik*[2]

[1]National Institute for Occupational Safety and Health, Morgantown, WV 26505, USA
[2]Division of Environmental Epidemiology, Institute for Risk Assessment Sciences, University of Utrecht, Utrecht, The Netherlands

Abstract

Surveys on work-related asthma serve public health investigation, research on exposure-response relations, screening for pre-clinical disease, and demonstrations of effectiveness of interventions. Hypotheses dictate survey design, which include cross-sectional, case-control, cohort, and intervention studies. Tools for characterizing medical risk factors and outcomes include questionnaires, spirometry, tests of bronchial hyperreactivity, exhaled indices, induced sputum, immunological tests, and nasal inflammatory indices. An important component of surveys is exposure assessment to compare a population to existing literature and other surveys with attention to exposure level, range, and variability among workers. Allergen exposures are challenging to characterize with respect to peak exposures and evolving immunochemical measurement methods. Exposure assessment strategies are developing rapidly for analysis of exposure-response relationships, whether for sensitization to allergens or for respiratory symptoms or diagnoses. Power calculations should guide decisions about whether to implement surveys. Research needs include surveys of populations with irritant or neutrophilic asthma and populations in damp buildings. The relevance of dermal exposure to sensitizers requires examination as a risk factor for asthma. New causes of work-related asthma may be identified by surveying industries with excess asthma in population-based studies that do not have recognized causes of asthma.

Introduction

Our knowledge of new asthmagens, risk factors, and primary prevention of occupational asthma (OA) depends largely on epidemiological surveys of workforces and populations. Such surveys complement clinical investigation for diagnoses in individuals, laboratory investigation for mechanisms, and animal experiments for assessing biological plausibility. We consider surveys as a research tool when sentinel cases in a workforce prompt public health investigation; when primary prevention requires understanding of exposure-response relations or work and worker risk factors; and when secondary prevention requires attempts to identify pre-clinical disease. In addition, population surveys can be used in medical surveillance to show trends and the effectiveness of interventions.

Occupational Asthma, edited by Torben Sigsgaard and Dick Heederik

These motivations for research surveys dictate the research questions. In the case of sentinel-event follow-back to workplace populations, the questions may be whether an excess of respiratory disease consistent with asthma exists and, if so, whether an occupational cause is apparent. In the case of primary prevention research, work-related risk factors, such as process and exposures, are examined for their relations to respiratory health and disease prevalence or incidence. In the case of secondary prevention studies, worker attributes, such as biomarkers of immunological responses, are examined for their relations to exposures or clinical outcomes either in cross-sectional or longitudinal designs. Medical surveillance for intervention effectiveness is often considered a public health endeavor, rather than research, since comparison groups are rarely feasible or even ethical. Nonetheless, intervention outcome can be powerful evidence of causality when changing a particular exposure results in lessening of asthma incidence or prevalence.

In turn, research questions dictate survey design, along with feasibility of implementation (Tab. 1). Regardless of survey design, it is important to capture exposure status at the time of disease onset. The simplest and cheapest studies are commonly cross-sectional surveys of a workforce, but the findings are limited to associations, which may or may not be causal. To answer the questions of whether excess asthma is present requires a comparison group. External comparisons might be another workforce or population-based estimates. In large workforces, internal comparisons may be possible if the workforce has a range of exposure to implicated processes or agents. If the workforce suspected of having an asthma risk is large and has many affected workers, case-control studies may be efficient in determining potential risk factors, but again, only associations are found, and their interpretation depends on biological plausibility, evaluation of potential confounders, attempts to establish work-related patterns, and replication in other exposed populations.

To address questions of incidence in relation to occupational risk, longitudinal cohort studies are advantageous, but are expensive and difficult. Longitudinal studies avoid the temporal confusion of whether environmental conditions precede the

Table 1. Different survey design options and some typical characteristics, assuming appropriate implementation

Design	Frequency of use	Strength of scientific evidence	Costs
Cross-sectional	++++	+	+
Case-control	++	++	+
Cohort	+	+++	+++
Intervention study	+	++++	++++

health outcome. However, employee turnover, particularly with the healthy worker effect commonly found in populations at risk of OA, may preclude obtaining follow-up on affected individuals. Similarly, intervention effectiveness studies are difficult unless subclinical biomarkers of health effect are available, and comparison populations for longitudinal follow-up are seldom feasible or ethical (unless interventions are being compared).

For some diseases, such as cancer, follow-back of time-space clusters in a workplace is inherently limited by power issues and bias. In contrast, work-related symptoms of asthma as an outcome warrant follow-back much of the time. Although asthma is a prevalent disease affecting about 10% of the population, adult-onset asthma has an incidence in the range of 1.2 to 4.0 per thousand person-years [1, 2] based on questionnaire responses. Obtaining incidence density estimates over employment in a workforce can show whether excess incidence is likely, despite neglecting workers who may have left because of asthma before a cross-sectional survey.

Before a study design is chosen

Any survey always starts with a research question, translated into a hypothesis. The research questions can have a wide range of backgrounds. Employers, workers or occupational health specialists may have questions related to health risks. These questions may have been initiated by observations from the scientific literature. The question then arises as to whether observations made "in a population X with exposure to agent Y, with specific health effects Z" are of relevance for another population with a similar exposure pattern. Research questions may also be triggered by sentinel cases or a series of cases occurring in a company (place) or within a narrow time window (time), which require a more thorough survey to establish whether an excess risk exists and whether determinants in the work environment may have played a role. An example is the occurrence of OA in enzyme-exposed workers in the detergent industry in the 1970s. Reports of such cases to the occupational physician were followed by systematic surveys. Sentinel case reporting in the U.S. to state health departments have resulted in new asthmagens being established, such as 3-amino-5-mercapto-1, 2, 4-triazole (AMT) in the pesticide industry [3], and new settings for asthma risk, such as damp buildings [4, 5].

Research questions refer to what epidemiologists call an occurrence relation. An occurrence relation describes disease occurrence in relation to known or suspected determinants. Occurrence relations can be simple and straightforward, as in the case of a respiratory irritant causing the reactive airways dysfunction syndrome. Here, symptoms occur immediately after exposure and the relationship manifests itself easily. In the case of immune-mediated asthma, the natural history is a complex interplay of exposure and sensitization followed by inflammatory responses. These relations are modified by individual susceptibility, and the combination of all relevant variables results in complex time patterns of disease. These elements of the occurrence relation have to be considered when the research question is translated into a study design and practical study plan. The study plan contains the design of the study, what is being measured and how, a power analysis, and a description of the planned data analysis.

Design options

Cross-sectional studies

Two epidemiological designs usually lead to results relatively rapidly: cross-sectional surveys and case-control studies. Many cross-sectional surveys on asthma have been conducted. They consist of measurement of the disease (asthma) prevalence using questionnaires and sometimes medical tests or other measures of disease presence. They give a rapid and relatively cost-effective indication of the presence of asthma, although assessing the work-relatedness of symptoms and signs may require a more thorough clinical evaluation in the individual worker. Relating excess risk in subgroups to particular exposures, processes, or work indices is another approach to determining work-relatedness.

The disadvantage of this design is that cross-sectional surveys are extremely sensitive to the healthy worker effect. A survey by Peretz et al. [6] among bakers and workers from related industries with exposure to flour and α-amylase showed that strong differences existed in the prevalence of atopy (against common allergens) and atopic responses to work-environment allergens. Workers from flour milling industries were less often atopic than bakers. It is most likely that these differences are to some extent associated with differences in health-related selection in and out of the workforce. This type of selection out of the workforce may be associated with flattening of exposure-response relationships between exposure to allergens and sensitization, symptoms, and medication use [6, 7], although development of tolerance may play a role. Few studies exist that have explicitly studied selection out of the workforce for OA, but a range of studies indicate that health selection has taken place. It is expected to operate strongly in the case of immune-mediated OA because affected workers often observe a direct relationship between exposure and their symptoms. Although there is little doubt that this phenomenon plays a crucial role in creating healthier current workforces for cross-sectional studies, its magnitude has yet to be established in most situations. The healthy worker effect leads to biased results from cross-sectional studies. The bias may affect prevalence estimates, as well as measures of association between asthma, sensitization or other outcome, and determinants under study.

Case-control studies

Case-control studies are not as often applied, but they may be used within (nested) a cross-sectional study, based on prevalent cases, as a cost-effective and efficient follow-up design. Usually all cases identified in the cross-sectional survey and a sample of the controls receive a more detailed evaluation. An important role for case-control studies is in the evaluation of potential health clusters of asthma. Prevalent studies are likely to have cases and controls that do not adequately represent either group, and this is especially true for the cases, considering the healthy worker effect. Incident case-control studies can be nested within longitudinal studies.

Cohort and intervention studies

A cohort is a group of persons who are followed or traced over a period of time. The concept of a cohort comes from the Roman Empire where it was common to follow the mortality experience of cohorts (the Latin word '*cohors*' refers to one tenth of a legion) of soldiers over time to keep track of the fighting potential of the army. Cohort studies have been shown to be extremely powerful in OA research.

A simple measure to describe disease occurrence in a cohort is the incidence, the number of cases with disease divided by the number of individuals at risk at the beginning of follow-up. This measure of disease is sensitive to loss to follow-up and competing causes of disease or mortality. A better measure is the incidence rate. An incidence rate is the number of cases who developed the disease of interest during follow-up in a cohort of initially disease-free individuals, divided by the accumulated person-time (usually expressed as person-years). Cohort studies require calculation of person-time of follow-up until development of disease or loss to follow-up. This calculation can be extremely complex when different time-related variables are involved, such as age, birth cohort, and exposure duration, although most studies published so far have been relatively straight forward with regard to these aspects. The Life Table Analysis System software designed by the National Institute for Occupational Safety and Health (NIOSH), which was developed for mortality studies, exists to make these calculations. This software can be used for this type of study as well by manipulating the input structure of the data. An example of a well-conducted study in which this approach was used is the follow-up of laboratory animal workers by Elliot et al. [8]. A total of 603 workers contributed 2527 person-years over a 12.3-year period. The 12-year incidence rates of laboratory animal allergy (LAA) symptoms and LAA for all workers were 2.26 (95% CI 1.61–2.91) and 1.32 (95% CI 0.76–1.87) per 100 person-years, respectively. Higher rate ratios were seen with increasing reported hours of exposure to tasks that required working with animal cages or with many animals at one time. The most common symptoms were related to rhinitis rather than to asthma. If incidence rates are available for an exposed and a control group, incidence rate ratios or relative risks can be calculated as a measure of association between exposure and disease.

Several approaches have been used in the design of cohort studies for OA. Most published cohort studies have been of workforces in one company, one industry, or one job category. Cohort studies among individuals naïve towards their occupational exposure, often among apprentices, have given good insight into the determinants of OA and allergy [9]. Apprentices become exposed to specific agents for the first time in their lives because some occupational exposures may be exceptionally rare in the general environment. This is true for spray painters exposed to isocyanate monomers and oligomers. Domestic or general environmental exposure to these agents is usually absent. Alternatively, some allergens are not exclusively found in the work environment, but exposure in the work environment is orders of magnitude higher than in other environments. This is likely the case for allergens like latex and wheat allergens. Studies of apprentices are extremely powerful, but studies among workers, starting with a cross-sectional survey and following disease-free workers with only a brief exposure history, have comparable potential as demonstrated in studies of the baking industry [10]. Cohort studies for non-allergic asthma in relation to irritant or bioaerosol exposures are in their infancy.

Cohort studies for asthma usually involve an extensive baseline survey and regular follow-up surveys. The incidence rate of development of sensitization is relatively high – between 1 and 10 cases per 100 person years of follow-up – and cases may occur within the first few months of exposure [11–13]. The frequency of follow-up surveys varies in available studies. A reasonable follow-up frequency is one survey per year, although studies of mechanistic aspects of development of sensitization may require more intensive follow-up [14]. Unfortunately, follow-up time in most studies has been relatively short, not more than a few years. Studies with more than 5 years of follow-up [12, 15] show that asthma or sensitization incidence remains high after the first few years of follow-up. This finding is at odds with the suggestion that risk declines rapidly after the first month of exposure. Because most studies have been relatively short, little is known about the predictive value of determinants of asthma and allergy over longer periods of time. Most published cohort studies are prospective, but retrospective studies exist [15]. Retrospective studies make use of information collected earlier, and in the example of Kruize et al. [15], pre-employment testing information was available for a population of laboratory animal workers.

Some cohort studies have not focused on incidence, but considered change in a physiological parameter like lung function over time. Few such studies have been conducted among populations with a high risk for developing OA. The study by Portengen et al. [16] showed that the decline in lung function over a 3-year follow-up period was strongest among sensitized and allergen-exposed individuals compared to non-exposed or non-sensitized individuals. This type of cohort study is often referred to as a longitudinal or repeated measurement study.

Health outcome tools

Questionnaires

Standard questions about respiratory symptoms and physician diagnoses should be selected from validated instruments, with a view to the purpose of the survey [17, 18]. If the aim is to identify possible cases, then questions of high sensitivity are needed. In an analytical epidemiological study of risk factors, questions with high specificity for asthma should be used. In emerging issues, such as asthma among occupants of damp buildings, analytical comparisons can be made with other populations if identical questions are used.

For asthma, the long-standing American Thoracic Society-Division of Lung Disease (ATS/DLD) questions [19], designed for study of chronic bronchitis and emphysema, have largely been replaced with questions used in the European Community Respiratory Health Study (ECRHS), which were derived from the International Union Against Tuberculosis and Lung Disease questionnaire [20]. A combination of symptoms or weighted score can predict airways hyperreactivity, clinical diagnosis by an expert panel, incident asthma, and other asthma outcomes in relation to risk factors for asthma [21–24]. Regardless of questions, symptoms-based definitions of asthma result in classifying a much higher proportion of a worker population as having asthma compared to the self-report of physician-diagnosed asthma. Questions aimed at establishing associations between symptom patterns and work-related exposures are an important issue in questionnaires focused on OA. Work-related symptom patterns include predominance at work, exacerbation during spills, or a delayed immunological response after working hours or during the night. Similarly, symptoms may progress over the work week or improve during holidays or weekends.

In the United States, questions from the Third National Health and Nutrition Examination Survey [25], the National Health Interview Survey [26], or the Behavioral Risk Factor Surveillance Survey [27] allow external comparisons regarding symptom and diagnosed asthma prevalences in a working population in comparison to national or state-based prevalences. In Europe, comparisons of symptom and diagnosis prevalences in workforces can be compared with ECRHS prevalences. Such comparisons can establish that excesses of asthma or chest symptoms exist in working populations suspected of occupational lung disease [5, 28, 29].

Cross-sectional questionnaire analyses can also address asthma incidence in relation to employment or process changes during employment. The ATS/DLD and ECRHS questionnaires ask persons with physician-diagnosed asthma for their age at asthma onset. This information, in conjunction with employment date and current age, allows calculation of incidence density of asthma in adulthood prior to employment, in comparison with incidence after onset of employment, both expressed as asthma diagnoses per person-months at risk. With this rate ratio comparison, employment-related incidence excesses as high as 7.5-fold have been documented in damp buildings with high prevalences of building-related chest symptoms [5, 30]. The healthy worker effect tends to underestimate asthma incidence after employment in cross-sectional studies, so such rate ratio comparisons may be lower than would be found in a longitudinal cohort study.

All strong questionnaires need a work history module, which is usually tailored to the workforce being studied. As mentioned above, dates of employment or entry into job titles with exposure correlates can be used to calculate incidence density of asthma before and after exposure began. Work history can be linked to exposure assessment to calculate cumulative, average, or peak exposure based on job-exposure matrices. In the absence of extensive quantitative exposure assessment, questionnaire indices of exposure, such as process, job title, tasks, history of spill exposure and frequency, duration of exposure, and use of respiratory protection can be associated with respiratory health outcomes. Some exposure risks, such as spills, may never be characterized quantitatively because they are unanticipated and unmeasured events. Nonetheless, these qualitative risks may have considerable public health value in suggesting priorities for intervention and the possible importance of peak exposures. Examples include early studies of the pulp and paper industry, which has a risk of reactive airways dysfunction syndrome [31], and the isocyanate industry, in which spills were associated with asthma cases [32, 33]. In early studies within an industry, such qualitative associations may help prioritize needs for careful exposure assessment, such as in process-related risk.

An evolving area of possible exposure risk that can be partially addressed by questionnaire is dermal exposure to allergens and sensitizers. In a new waferboard factory, incident asthma-like symptoms were associated with affirmative responses to questions about skin and clothing stains from isocyanates [34]. Dermal exposure assessment is in its infancy, with attempts to estimate relative exposures with skin wipes, surface wipes, cotton glove burden of analytes [35], and adhesive tape stripping [36]. In the meantime, questions reflecting the likelihood of skin integrity, use of skin protection, stains where applicable, and dermatitis may push this field forward in relation to asthma prevention measures [37]. For another sensitizing occupational lung disease, beryllium disease, skin exposure may be an important route of sensitization [38]. The parallels with latex asthma, in which latex dermatitis may be a sensitizing event, are intriguing. Considerable animal evidence exists for sensitization *via* the dermal route for latex, beryllium, and isocyanates [39–41].

Socioeconomic implications of OA can be addressed by adding questionnaire modules pertinent to absenteeism due to respiratory disease and quality of life. Examples include SF12 and the Marks' asthma quality of life questionnaires [42, 43].

Spirometry

Although asthma attacks precipitate airways obstruction, the utility of spirometry in surveys of populations at risk of OA is limited. Between asthma attacks, asthmatics usually have normal spirometry. Hence, cross-sectional studies of spirometry at work are seldom sensitive in identifying those with physician-diagnosed asthma or work-related asthma. In workforces at risk for asthma, bronchodilator testing of those with abnormal spirometry of an obstructive nature may differentiate asthmatic workers from those with chronic obstructive lung disease. Cross-shift and cross-week changes of spirometry are labor-intensive and also insensitive. Thus, the serial peak flow or serial spirometry that is of clinical value in documenting work-related decrements over several weeks of measurements [44] is seldom practical in a survey setting [45]. Compliance with several measurements per day on work days and days away from work is rarely obtained on a population basis, even when restricted to those with symptoms, measured bronchial hyperreactivity, or physician-diagnosed asthma.

Long-standing asthma can result in partial irreversible airflow limitation. For longitudinal cohort studies, assessment of average decrements of forced expiratory volume in one second (FEV_1) over periods of time may be of some utility, although such evaluation is more pertinent to chronic obstructive lung disease than asthma. In such studies, the detection of excess declines in FEV_1 in individuals over an interval is dependent on frequency of measurement, spirometry quality, and time of follow-up [46]. Recent NIOSH software for evaluation of longitudinal spirometry makes these analyses much easier [47].

Bronchial hyperreactivity

Methacholine or histamine challenge tests are done in field settings with abbreviated protocols. In those with chest symptoms suggestive of asthma, documented hyper-reactivity is an attractive objective measure of asthma. However, in workforce populations, normal tests are frequently found in those reporting physician-diagnosed asthma. This insensitivity may reflect adequately treated asthma. One approach to objective documentation is to aggregate those with prescription asthma medication with those with documented hyperreactivity and those with bronchodilator responses on spirometry (an alternative test for reversible airways obstruction in those with abnormal spirometry) [5].

Exhaled indices

Exhaled nitric oxide (eNO) has been adopted in clinical settings as a means of monitoring control of allergic asthma. As a marker of eosinophilic inflammation, increased eNO may indicate inadequate medication or compliance. Recently, eNO has been used in general population field studies in the evaluation of asthma [48]. However, the applicability of this test among workers at risk of immunological or irritant OA in surveys of current workers has not been established [49, 50].

Some investigators have examined eNO as a marker of inflammation in relation to workplace irritant or particulate exposures, sometimes excluding known asthmatics [51, 52]. Inconsistent findings have been found for irritant and particulate exposures [53, 54] and also for biomass exposures [55, 56]. A cross-sectional study among farmers demonstrated that eNO levels were positively associated with endotoxin exposure in non-smokers and non-atopics [55]. However, in building-related asthma associated with biomass markers, eNO was not higher in those with either physician-diagnosed asthma or epidemiologically defined asthma based on symptoms [56]; however, the pathophysiology of dampness-associated asthma may not involve immunoglobulin E (IgE) and eosinophilic inflammation [5], which are associated with elevated eNO.

Exhaled breath condensate is currently being investigated in field studies as a means of identifying malondialdehyde as a biomarker of oxidative stress, inflammatory markers such as cytokines, and to establish dose for metals and solvents [57]. In a building-related asthma study, interleukin-8 in exhaled breath condensate was higher in those with physician-diagnosed asthma and with work-related respiratory symptoms compared to controls [56].

Induced sputum indices

Sputum induction for cell differential counts has been investigated in clinical settings evaluating those with OA [49]. Those with IgE-associated asthma usually have increased sputum eosinophilia with exposure. Some evidence exists for sputum neutrophilia in those with isocyanate asthma, irritant exposure as in paper mill workers [58], and microorganism exposure. Induced sputum has also been used for evaluating other inflammatory markers, such as interleukins, matrix metalloprotease-9 activity, and activated basophils by flow cytometry. Induced sputum is difficult for survey participants in field settings, particularly in those without symptoms [59]. Accordingly, survey application has been limited. An investigation of mushroom workers used spontaneous sputum induction in those with cough and no other diagnoses, rather than induced sputum in the entire population [60]. Others have induced sputum in clinical settings [61, 62].

Immunological tests

Atopy is a risk factor for asthma caused by high-molecular-weight agents in the workplace, although its predictive value is not high enough to warrant preplacement screening in the workplace. Exposure level determines the likelihood of developing asthma due to high-molecular-weight sensitizers because specific sensitization is the primary mechanism. Individual susceptibility, such as atopy, is merely a modifying factor for exposure-response relations, but may merit characterization of atopic status in exposure-response studies. The means of assessing atopy are by questionnaire regarding history of hay fever, eczema, and asthma; by total IgE measurement in serum; by antigen-specific IgE levels for a panel of common allergens; or by skin prick tests to a similar panel of common aeroallergens.

In field surveys of populations at risk for asthma, tests of specific immunological reactivity are often an outcome variable or an intermediate variable between allergen exposure and OA. Tests for specific immunological reactivity include specific serum IgE and IgG antibody tests and skin prick tests to specific allergens. Thus, workplace surveys exist that examine reactivity to wheat allergen, α-amylase, soy antigens, rat urinary protein, snow crab antigen, latex antigens, and many others. There is no role in field studies for specific inhalation challenge to assess immunological reactivity to an inhaled allergen, since these tests must be performed in specialty clinical centers and entail risk that is unacceptable outside of a clinical diagnostic context. In other occupational lung diseases, cell-mediated immunological reactivity is an endpoint and intermediate outcome in epidemiological study. The dominant example is testing for beryllium sensitization in beryllium-exposed worker surveillance with the beryllium lymphocyte proliferation test [63]. However, such lymphocyte tests may have a role in field surveys for low-molecular-weight antigens such as isocyanates [64] if shown to play a role in pathophysiology of isocyanate asthma [65].

Nasal inflammatory indices

Work-related nasal disease is common and may be a risk factor for OA [66]. Thus, a variety of tools have been considered for characterizing nasal disease, such as nasal eNO and nasal lavage for inflammatory markers; nasal swabs for cytology; nasal inspiratory peak flow, rhinomanometry, and acoustic rhinometry for nasal resistance; and nasal morphometry. Their application in field studies has been limited because of participant reaction, invasiveness, time, and the need to establish normal values. Murgia et al. [62] demonstrated higher interleukin-6 in nasal lavage of chromium-exposed electroplating workers in comparison to controls.

Exposure assessment in occupational asthma surveys

There are several reasons to include an exposure assessment component in OA surveys. The first and most basic one is for documentation purposes. To allow meaningful comparisons with the existing literature and between different studies, it is useful to have some insight into the level, range, and variability of exposure of workers in a newly conducted survey. Results from a survey are difficult to put in context, especially when there is no background information about the exposure.

Information about specific industries or job titles is usually not sufficient because exposure levels can differ between countries for the same industry and job title. Also, the level of technological development may differ between companies, resulting in exposure differences. A basic impression of the exposure can be obtained simply by monitoring a random sample of workers and taking a limited number of repeated measurements for each worker.

Another reason to monitor exposure is the analysis of exposure-response relationships and to evaluate the effect of interventions. These two aims require more elaborate exposure assessment strategies. The analysis of exposure-response relationships for high-molecular-weight allergens and asthma has a short history and started in the early 1990s. Results from this research have shown that a range of exposure-endpoint relationships exist for OA. These studies have indicated that lowering exposure will most likely reduce the burden of disease, although a residual risk can probably not be avoided completely. There is still very little experience with intervention studies in the field of OA, and the need to improve the methodology and implement exposure studies is clearly present [67]. The most thoroughly described evidence involves latex gloves. Use of powder-free gloves is known to be associated with considerably lower exposure to latex allergens [68]. Follow-up studies in dental school student cohorts have shown that introduction of powder-free gloves is associated with disappearance of latex sensitization and asthma [69]. Some useful references exist that describe some methodological issues for intervention studies in occupational respiratory disease epidemiology. Brosseau et al. [70] describe the exposure assessment component of a pilot study of the Minnesota Wood Dust Study. In this study, an intervention was undertaken in 48 businesses (written recommendations, technical assistance, and worker training). The comparison companies received only written recommendations. Changes from baseline in dust concentration, dust control methods, and worker behavior were compared between the groups 1 year later. Workers in intervention relative to comparison businesses reported greater awareness, increases in stage of readiness, and behavioral changes consistent with dust control. The median dust concentration change in the intervention group from baseline to follow-up was 10.4% lower than the change in comparison businesses [71, 72]. Meijster et al. [73] describe results from a four-year intervention program in the baking and flour processing industry with similarly modest exposure reductions. These changes in exposure were smaller than expected and illustrate that conducting effective rigorous interventions is extremely complex. Such changes can hardly be detected without quantitative exposure measurements.

Occurrence of and variability in allergen exposure

Little information exists about how exposure to allergens in the work environment occurs. A recent study among bakery workers, who are exposed to allergens in particulate form, has shown that workers are exposed to a high number of peaks over a work shift (Fig. 1). These peaks are usually associated with a range of different tasks. Between the peaks, exposure is extremely low. There is hardly any background exposure to particulates. More than 75% of the work shift time-weighted average exposure could be explained by peak exposures during a limited set of well-defined tasks and activities [74].

For some other high-molecular-weight allergens, like latex and rat urinary allergens in lab animal settings, detailed information is lacking, but it is likely that for allergens in particulate form, peaks are equally important. Peak patterns of exposure can easily be explained by the properties of particulates. Earlier studies among bakery workers have shown that most of the particulates are relatively large, >5 μm. Particulates of this size remain airborne for only a short period of time because of gravity. Sedimentation is rapid and occurs often in less than a minute to maximally a few minutes. Thus, exposure occurs only when bags are opened, flour is used for manual dusting of dough, and brooms or pressurized air are used for cleaning.

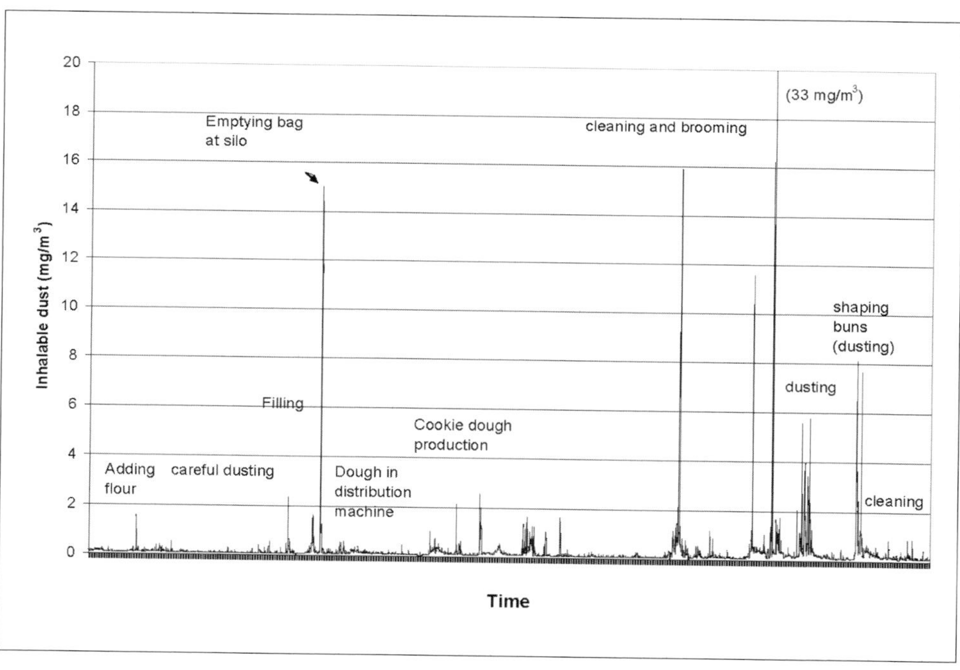

Figure 1.
Typical peak pattern of dust exposure for a bakery worker with some major tasks during the peaks described (from the study described by Meijster et al. [74], figure not published in the original paper, courtesy of the author).

For low-molecular-weight allergens, which are more often gaseous, constant low background exposure may theoretically occur, with peaks superimposed, dependent on the performance of certain tasks. However, the evidence for this is very limited. Recent studies among car spray painters, who are exposed to isocyanate monomers and oligomers in gaseous and solid (particulate) phase suggest that the exposure is often undetectably low, probably because of the presence of rigorous exposure control measures like spray-painting booths and local exhaust ventilation [75, 76]. The exposure is detectable when high exposure tasks are performed and when tasks are performed without exposure control measures: during spraying outside the booth, when spills occur, during preparation of paints, etc. So, also here, exposure occurs as a series of peaks over time.

Exposure to particulates and gases is always extremely dynamic and varies strongly over time and space. Pronk et al. [75] describe results from a large measurement series among car and industrial spray painters. For each worker, repeated measurements were performed (Fig. 2). These results show that car spray painters

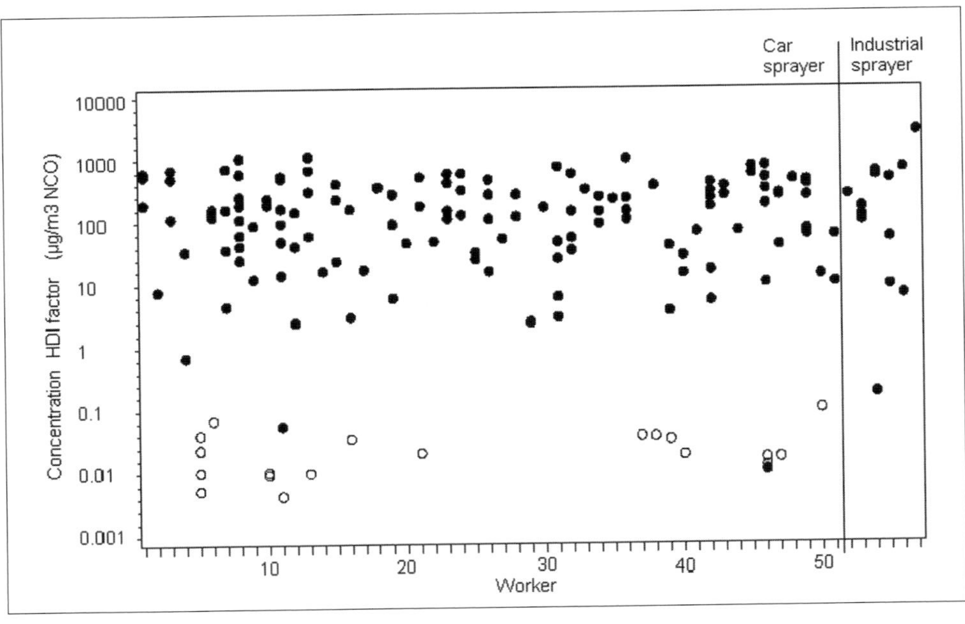

Figure 2.
Variability in isocyanate exposure for each sampled worker and by type of industry (car spray painting and industrial spray painting). Total isocyanate exposure (monomer and different oligomers) is expressed in µg/m³ NCO. Closed circles refer to detectable levels, open circles refer to measurements below the detection limit, which are plotted as 2/3 of the detection limit (Pronk et al. [75], with permission of the publisher).

are exposed to lower concentrations than industrial spray painters, but that the variability within a worker (over time) is large, up to several orders of magnitude. Reliable estimation of exposures for epidemiological study requires a sufficient number of samples and attention to design options for the exposure component.

Sampling for allergen exposure

Good quantitative epidemiological studies with state of the art exposure assessment are as yet lacking for most allergens. An important explanation is the absence of methods to measure the exposure accurately for most sensitizers. Exposure-response modeling for sensitizing agents is also complex. Asthma is a variable condition, and a sensitized individual reacts to levels to which he or she did not react before becoming sensitized. This complicates identification of levels that induce sensitization or that induce asthmatic reactions. However, these issues do not make exposure-response analyses impossible. For many diseases, differences in susceptibility exist between individuals, but exposure-response relationships have been described.

Low-molecular-weight sensitizers are usually gaseous or partially in solid phase and have to be measured using conventional equipment for gaseous or mixed phase (solid and gaseous) pollutants in combination with chromatography and, in some cases, mass spectrometry. High-molecular-weight sensitizers have to be analyzed with immunochemical techniques to measure the allergen content of the dust.

Currently, dust sampling equipment is based on particle size-selective sampling using health-based definitions of particular size fractions, such as respirable dust, thoracic dust, and inhalable dust [77]. Since sensitization and respiratory symptoms can occur in the upper and lower airways (rhinitis and asthma, respectively) inhalable dust, reflecting the dust particles that can penetrate the respiratory system, is the dust fraction that is measured most commonly in modern epidemiological studies. Information on up-to-date equipment can be found in occupational hygiene textbooks [78, 79].

Other dust sampling approaches have also been used, like the nasal sampler [36, 80–82]. The major application is in situations where conventional sampling equipment cannot be used, for instance, behind face masks [82].

In a very large study among wood workers, passive samplers that hold pieces of sticky tape were used to capture particulates from different angles. These samplers can be calibrated against conventional dust sampling equipment. The advantage is that no expensive sampling pumps have to be used. A disadvantage is that very little dust is sampled, often not enough for immunochemical analysis. The group that used these samplers was able to take several thousands of samples over a relatively short time period and related measured dust exposure with asthma occurrence in wood workers [83].

Measuring sensitizers

Immunochemical methods for measurement of high-molecular-weight agents make use of antibodies, specifically directed against the antigen(s) to be measured. These antibodies form measurable antigen-antibody complexes, which can be detected by different labels – isotopes, enzymes, fluorescents or luminescents – in either inhibition or sandwich assays. Enzyme-linked immunosorbent assays (ELISA) with chromogenic substrates are most commonly used. Validation studies for each immunoassay are necessary, and the outcome depends on sensitivity and particularly specificity of the antibodies used. Specificity of antibodies, as well as the properties and purity of calibration standards or other reference preparations, can be assessed by gel electrophoresis and immunoblotting. Sensitivity of inhibition assays depends mainly on the avidity and concentration of the inhibited antibodies in the assay. With high-avidity antibodies, a sensitivity of 10–20 ng/ml for protein allergen molecules of 10–20 kDa can be reached. Sandwich assays can be much more sensitive, depending on the quality of the reagents; if sufficiently specific, the detection system can be markedly amplified by using various secondary reagents, and in some assays, sensitivities in the pg/ml range are possible.

Considering the large number of aeroallergens pertinent to asthma, few studies are available that evaluate the comparability of immunoassays that have been used to measure them [84–89]. The optimal situation for analyzing allergens immunochemically is reached when the allergen has been identified, and purified allergen and monoclonal or polyclonal antibodies against the allergen are available.

Low-molecular-weight sensitizers such as platinum salts, isocyanates and other chemical agents have to be analyzed using standard chemical techniques such as atomic absorption spectrometry and gas and high-pressure liquid chromatography. Many low-molecular-chemical sensitizers are highly reactive and this complicates sampling and analysis.

Exposure assessment strategies

How should the exposure of a population be characterized? Usually several sources of information have to be combined. Two quantitative exposure assessment strategies exist: measurement for each individual in the population, or measurements for so-called homogeneous exposure categories, for instance, on the basis of job titles. Often, exposure assessment on the individual level is considered the gold standard. However, this strategy is most sensitive to variability of the exposure over time. High variability over time is known to lead to potentially strong underestimation of the exposure-response relationship relative to the variability between individuals in the population. Intuitively, this can easily be understood. When the variability is large and few measurements per individual are taken, the average exposure for a certain worker will be estimated poorly and can be overestimated or underestimated. This will occur for each worker, and this misclassification of exposure leads in a regression analysis to underestimation of the exposure-response relationship. This underestimation becomes smaller when more repeated measurements per individual have been taken. Categorization of the population in homogeneous exposure groups and use of the measured average exposure per exposure group in an exposure-response relationship is less sensitive to variability over time. In most cases, this strategy is known to lead to unbiased relationships between exposure and response. However, differences within an exposure category are associated with unexplained differences in health risk. This leads to a reduction of power of this strategy in comparison with the individual exposure assessment strategy. Despite the lower power, homogenous exposure groups are the most commonly used strategy. Alternative strategies used in respiratory epidemiology, which have the same properties as the grouping strategy, are estimation on the basis of determinants of exposure [90] and strategies, which consist of combining categorical structures, and individual exposure data [6, 91].

Exposure assessment in epidemiology has developed into a discipline on its own and covers issues such as categorizing the population into exposure categories, allocation of sampling effort over these categories to obtain accurate estimates of the average exposure, use of exposure modeling approaches to estimate the exposure, and evaluation of different exposure assessment strategies as part of an optimization process. These issues have received little attention so far in the field of allergen exposure, since the emphasis has been on instrumental issues, such as developing assays and monitoring techniques. However, more and more examples have been published in which these principles have been applied.

Analysis of exposure-response relationships

In epidemiological studies, exposure-response relationships are usually evaluated with dichotomous outcomes, even when based on a measurement on a continuous scale, for example, IgE titer. The most evaluated exposure-response relationships in allergic respiratory disease are exposure-sensitization and exposure-symptom relationships. However, examples exist in which time to sensitization has been evaluated [15].

Exposure leads to sensitization, and sensitization in conjunction with further exposure may lead to an inflammatory airways response that is accompanied by symptoms, bronchial hyperresponsiveness, airflow variability, etc. For both steps, risk modifying variables have been identified. Atopic workers have higher risk of sensitization against high-molecular-weight sensitizers. Smoking and gender might modify the sensitization risk as well, but the evidence for their roles is weak and depends on the sensitizing agent. In the case of the low-molecular-weight sensitizer, platinum salts, smokers are at higher risk, and atopy is not a risk modifier for most low-molecular-weight sensitizers. The consequences of these observations are that the exposure-response relationship is potentially modified by these factors, and that the slope of the relationship may differ for different sub-categories of workers. Recent papers have evaluated these variables in epidemiological analysis of quantitative exposure-response relationships for several high-molecular-weight sensitizers, such as wheat allergens, fungal α-amylase, and rat urinary proteins [92–96]. In all cases, the slope of the exposure-response relationship was steeper for atopics compared to non-atopics. In some cases, there was a suggestion that an elevated sensitization risk only occurred in non-atopics among the highly exposed, and the exposure-response relationship was also shifted somewhat to the right.

When one is interested in the relationship between exposure to allergens and work-related symptoms, all modifiers on the causal pathway between exposure and symptoms have to be considered. Workers with work-related sensitization are at higher risk for having or developing symptoms, but atopic workers without work-related sensitization may also have high symptom rates, as may smokers and older workers. Despite the fact that Becklake recognized this problem some time ago [97], most studies have not addressed these modifiers explicitly in their analytical strategies by careful stratification by all potential modifiers.

Power and biological relevance

It is simple to make power calculations in the design phase of a study. Several textbook and internet sites give guidance for specific types of endpoints for a range of designs (see for instance: http://www.cs.uiowa.edu/~rlenth/Power/). Power calculations help optimize the study design and give insight into what can be expected from a study of a given size. Power calculations are extremely useful in situations where major constraints exist in terms of potential number of individuals who can be included. For instance, study of a disease cluster in a company or section of a company is usually limited to a fixed number of workers. If low numbers lead to an extremely low power to detect a biologically relevant increase in disease risk, one might decide not to study a cluster in greater detail at all, or to use completely different approaches such as risk assessment based on literature reviews and exposure assessment studies. Studying clusters in a situation where the power to detect an excess risk is extremely low can be misleading. With large surveys it is possible to detect small differences in prevalence or incidence between populations or in continuous endpoint variables like lung function or inflammatory markers such as eNO (Tab. 2). For instance, a survey including several thousand individuals can detect differences between exposed and non-exposed that are lower than 1%, and such small changes may defy biological interpretation.

These changes are usually not considered relevant on the level of one individual and are smaller than the measurement error found on one occasion and the intra-

Table 2. Required population size for exposed and controls to be able to detect a difference in FEV_1 between these two populations (2xN) with α=0.05 and β=0.20 and a population standard deviation of 0.5 l (after Berry [100]).

Δ (liter/second)	N
0.030	4356
0.060	1089
0.090	484
0.120	272
0.150	174
0.180	121
0.210	89
0.240	68
0.270	54
0.300	44

individual variation in lung function assessed over a period of a few weeks. The major question does not refer to statistical significance, but to biological relevance of small changes in respiratory function. Several considerations exist:

- It is known that FEV_1 reductions of several hundred milliliters can be associated with an approximate doubling of the number of individuals with abnormal lung function when the whole distribution has been shifted [98].
- Similarly small lung function reductions are also associated with an elevated mortality for respiratory diseases and total mortality, underpinning the importance of small changes in lung function on the population level.

What may put this in perspective is to consider the effect of smoking on lung function. In population studies, usually differences between (ex)-smokers and non-smokers are between 100 and 300 mL. While such effects are small in the clinical context, a strong population level determinant like smoking is associated with a relatively small change in function. This epidemiological paragraph has been extensively discussed by Rose et al. [99]. Lung function is one of the parameters for which a considerable amount of evidence exists to place small changes in a broader context. For many recent inflammatory markers, such contextual information is usually not present, making it more difficult to interpret findings from surveys, which are usually smaller than effects seen in clinical cases.

In large longitudinal population studies, the frequency of follow-up measurements and the time between surveys determine the power to a great extent [100].

Very frequent measurement is not useful with long follow-up. Schlesselman [101, 102] has given exact formulas to calculate the population size based on the standard deviations and different combinations of α, β, Δ, measurement frequency, and follow-up duration.

Cross-shift studies are a special case of longitudinal studies with an extremely short follow-up time (8 hours or less). Even when measurements can be performed with very small analytical errors (< 1–3%), the signal-to-noise ratio of these studies is usually not very good, because the expected changes over the work shift on the population level may be relatively small and, therefore, difficult to detect. Peak expiratory flow (PEF) monitoring in OA cases is effective because the changes seen in PEF may be as large as 30–50%.

Research needs

Although much progress is being made on eosinophilic OA, less survey work exists for irritant asthma or asthma with neutrophilic inflammation. The recent recognition that the latter phenotypic group may account for half of asthma cases [103] is particularly pertinent to work-related asthma. Neutrophilic airway inflammation may be triggered by bacterial endotoxin, particulate air pollution, solvents, cleaners, and ozone. Surveys of agricultural workers and office workers in damp indoor spaces are now associating bioaerosol exposures, such as endotoxin and fungal biomass markers, with work-related asthma symptoms [104]. The approaches to exposure assessment in non-industrial damp spaces differ from that for allergen exposure, in that settled dust biomass measurements have a role, whereas air sampling has generally not been associated with work-related respiratory symptoms. In principle, the techniques for surveys examining asthma symptoms in relation to exposures for low level irritant or biomass exposures should be similar to those for eosinophilic asthma, with the exception of examining immune health outcomes or intermediates, such as sensitization. Target industries for such surveys will likely be motivated by population-based studies that indicate asthma excess that has not been clinically recognized.

References

1 Rudd RA, Moorman JE (2007) Asthma incidence: Data from the National Health Interview Survey, 1980–1996. *J Asthma* 44: 65–70

2 Kogevinas M, Zock JP, Jarvis D, Kromhout H, Lillienberg L, Plana E, Radon K, Torén K, Alliksoo A, Benke G, et al (2007) Exposure to substances in the workplace and new-onset asthma: An international prospective population-based study (ECRHS-II). *Lancet* 370: 336–341

3 Hnizdo E, Sylvain D, Lewis DM, Pechter E, Kreiss K (2004) New-onset asthma associated with exposure to 3-amino-5-mercapto-1, 2, 4-triazole. *J Occup Environ Med* 46: 1246–1252

4 Hoffman RE, Wood RC, Kreiss K (1993) Building-related asthma in Denver office workers. *Am J Public Health* 83: 89–93

5 Cox-Ganser JM, White SK, Jones R, Hilsbos K, Storey E, Enright PL, Rao CY, Kreiss K (2005) Respiratory morbidity in office workers in a water-damaged building. *Environ Health Perspect* 113: 485–490

6 Peretz C, de Pater N, de Monchy J, Oostenbrink J, Heederik D (2005) Assessment of exposure to wheat flour and the shape of its relationship with specific sensitization. *Scand J Work Environ Health* 31: 65–74

7 Jacobs JH, Meijster T, Meijer E, Suarthana E, Heederik D (2008) Wheat allergen exposure and the prevalence of work-related sensitization and allergy in bakery workers. *Allergy* 63: 1597–604

8 Elliott L, Heederik D, Marshall S, Peden D, Loomis D (2005) Incidence of allergy and allergy symptoms among workers exposed to laboratory animals. *Occup Environ Med* 62: 766–771

9 Gautrin D, Ghezzo H, Infante-Rivard C, Magnan M, L'archevêque J, Suarthana E, Malo JL (2008) Long-term outcomes in a prospective cohort of apprentices exposed to high-molecular-weight agents. *Am J Respir Crit Care Med* 177: 871–879

10 Cullinan P, Lowson D, Nieuwenhuijsen MJ, Sandiford C, Tee RD, Venables KM, McDonald JC, Newman Taylor AJ (1994) Work related symptoms, sensitisation, and estimated exposure in workers not previously exposed to flour. *Occup Environ Med* 51: 579–583

11 Cullinan P, Acquilla SD, Dhara VR (1996) Long-term morbidity in survivors of the 1984 Bhopal gas leak. *Natl Med J India* 9: 5–10

12 Elliot L, Heederik D, Marshall S, Peden D, Loomis D (2005) Progression of self-reported symptoms in laboratory animal allergy. *J Allergy Clin Immunol* 116: 127–132

13 Gautrin D, Ghezzo H, Infante-Rivard C, Malo JL (2001) Natural history of sensitization, symptoms and occupational diseases in apprentices exposed to laboratory animals. *Eur Respir J* 17: 904–908

14 Krop EJM, Heederik D, Lutter R, Meer G, Aalberse RC, Jansen HM, van der Zee JM (2009) Association between pre-employment immunologic and airway mucosal factors and the development of occupational allergy. *J Allergy Clin Immunol* 123: 694–700

15 Kruize H, Post W, Heederik D, Martens B, Hollander A, van der Beek E (1997) Respiratory allergy in laboratory animal workers: A retrospective cohort study using pre-employment screening data. *Occup Environ Med* 54: 830–835

16 Portengen L, Hollander A, Doekes G, de Meer G, Heederik D (2003) Lung function decline in laboratory animal workers: The role of sensitisation and exposure. *Occup Environ Med* 60: 870–875

17 Toren K, Brisman J, Jarvholm B (1993) Asthma and asthma-like symptoms in adults assessed by questionnaire. A literature review. *Chest* 104: 600–608

18 Pekkanen J, Pearce N (1999) Defining asthma in epidemiologic studies. *Eur Respir J* 14: 951–957

19 Ferris BG (1978) Epidemiology standardization project (American Thoracic Society). *Am Rev Respir Dis* 118: 1–120

20 Burney P, Chinn S (1987) Developing a new questionnaire for measuring the prevalence and distribution of asthma. *Chest* 91 (Suppl. 6): 79s–83s

21 Pekkanen J, Sunyer J, Anto JM, Burney P, on behalf of the European Community Respiratory Health Study (ECRHS) (2005) Operational definitions of asthma in studies on its aetiology. *Eur Respir J* 26: 28–35

22 Venables KM, Farrer N, Sharp L, Graneek BJ, Newman AJ (1993) Respiratory symptoms questionnaire for asthma epidemiology: Validity and reproducibility. *Thorax* 48: 214–219

23 Sunyer J, Pekkanen J, Garcia-Esteban R, Svanes C, Kunzli N, Janson C, de Marco R, Anto J, Burney P (2007) Asthma score: Predictive ability and risk factors. *Allergy* 62: 142–148

24 Grassi M, Rezzani C, Biino G, Marinoni A (2003) Asthma-like symptoms assessment through ECRHS screening questionnaire scoring. *J Clin Epidemiol* 56: 238–247

25 Centers for Disease Control and Prevention (CDC) (1996) *Third National Health and Nutrition Examination Survey, 1988–1994, NHANES III Examination Survey*. Hyattsville, MD: U.S. Department of Health and Human Services, Public Health Service, Centers for Disease Control and Prevention. (Public use data file documentation No. 76300.)

26 National Center for Health Statistics (2002) *Data File Documentation, National Health Interview Survey, 2002 (machine readable data file and documentation)*. National Center for Health Statistics, Centers for Disease Control and Prevention, Hyattsville, MD

27 Centers for Disease Control and Prevention (CDC) (2008) *Behavioral Risk Factor Surveillance System Survey Questionnaire*. Atlanta, GA: U.S. Department of Health and Human Services, Centers for Disease Control and Prevention

28 van Rooy FG, Smit LA, Houba R, Zaat VA, Rooyackers JM, Heederik DJ (2009) A cross-sectional study on lung function and respiratory symptoms among chemical workers producing diacetyl for food flavorings. *Occup Environ Med* 66: 105–110

29 Sahakian N, White S, Park J-H, Cox-Ganser J, Kreiss K (2008) Identification of mold and dampness-associated respiratory morbidity in two schools: Comparison of questionnaire survey responses to national data. *J Sch Health* 78: 32–37

30 Laney AS, Cragin LA, Blevins LZ, Sumner AD, Cox-Ganser JM, Kreiss K, Moffatt SG, Lohff CJ (2009) Sarcoidosis, asthma, and asthma-like symptoms among occupants of a historically water-damaged office building. *Indoor Air* 19: 83–90

31 Henneberger PK, Olin AC, Andersson E, Hagberg S, Toren K (2005) The incidence of respiratory symptoms and diseases among pulp mill workers with peak exposures to ozone and other irritant gases. *Chest* 128: 3028–3037

32 Ott MG, Klees JE, Poche SL (2000) Respiratory health surveillance in a toluene di-

isocyanate production unit, 1967–97: Clinical observations and lung function analyses. *Occup Environ Med* 57: 43–52
33 Leroyer C, Perfetti L, Cartier A, Malo J-L (1998) Can reactive airways dysfunction syndrome (RADS) transform into occupational asthma due to "sensitization" to isocyanates? *Thorax* 53: 152–153
34 Petsonk EL, Wang ML, Lewis DM, Siegel PD, Husberg BJ (2000) Asthma-like symptoms in wood product plant workers exposed to methylene diphenyl diisocyanate. *Chest* 118: 1183–1193
35 Day GA, Stefaniak AB, Schuler CR, Stanton ML, Miller WE, Kreiss K, Hoover MD (2007) Exposure pathway assessment at a copper-beryllium alloy facility. *Ann Occup Hyg* 51: 67–80
36 Poulos LM, O'Meara TJ, Hamilton RG, Tovey ER (2002) Inhaled latex allergen (Hevb1). *J Allergy Clin Immunol* 109: 701–706
37 Redlich CA, Herrick CA (2008) Lung/skin connections in occupational lung disease. *Curr Opin Allergy Clin Immunol* 8: 115–119
38 Cummings K, Day G, Henneberger P, Kitt M, Kreiss K, Schuler C (2007) Enhanced preventive program at a beryllium oxide ceramics facility reduces beryllium sensitization among new workers. *Occup Environ Med* 64: 134–140
39 Woolhiser MR, Munson AE, Meade BJ (2000) Immunological responses of mice following administration of natural rubber latex proteins by different routes of exposure. *Toxicol Sci* 55: 343–351
40 Tinkle SS, Antonini JM, Rich BA, Roberts JR, Salmen R, DePree K, Adkins EJ (2003) Skin as a route of exposure and sensitization in chronic beryllium disease. *Environ Health Perspect* 111: 1202–1208
41 Bello D, Herrick CA, Smith TJ, Woskie SR, Steicher RP, Cullen MR, Liu Y, Redlich CA (2007) Skin exposure to isocyanates: Reasons for concern. *Environ Health Perspect* 115: 328–335
42 Marks GB, Sunn SM, Woolcock AJ (1992) A scale for the measurement of quality of life in adults with asthma. *J Clin Epidemiol* 45: 461–472
43 Ware J Jr, Kosinski M, Keller SD (1996) A 12-item short-form health survey: Construction of scales and preliminary tests of reliability and validity. *Med Care* 34: 220–233
44 Gannon GF, Burge, S (1997) Serial peak expiratory flow measurement in the diagnosis of occupational asthma. *Eur Respir J* 24: 57s-63s
45 Hollander A, Heederik D, Brunekreef B (1998) Work-related changes in peak expiratory flow among laboratory animal workers. *Eur Respir J* 11: 929–936
46 Hnizdo E, Yan T, Sircar K, Harber P, Fleming J, Glindmeyer HW (2007) Limits of longitudinal decline for the interpretation of annual changes in FEV1 in individuals. *Occup Environ Med* 64: 701–707
47 Longitudinal Data Analysis (SPIROLA) software available at: http: //www.cdc.gov/niosh/topics/spirometry/spirola.html (accessed 10 October 2008)
48 Bommarito L, Migliore E, Bugiani M, Heffler E, Guida G, Bucca C, de Marco R, Rolla

G on behalf of ECHRS Turin, Italy Study Group (2008) Exhaled nitric oxide in a population sample of adults. *Respiration* 75: 386–392
49 Lemiere C (2007) Induced sputum and exhaled nitric oxide as noninvasive markers of airway inflammation from work exposures. *Curr Opin Allergy Clin Immunol* 7: 133–137
50 Lund MB, Oksne PI, Hamre R, Kongerud J (2000) Increased nitric oxide in exhaled air: An early marker of asthma in non-smoking aluminum potroom workers? *Occup Environ Med* 57: 274–278
51 Maniscalco M, Grieco L, Galdi A, Lundberg JO, Sofia M (2004) Increase in exhaled nitric oxide in shoe and leather workers at the end of the work-shift. *Occup Med (Lond)* 54: 404–407
52 Ulvestad B, Lund MB, Bakke B, Djupesland PG, Kongerud J, Boe J (2001) Gas and dust exposure in underground construction is associated with signs of airway inflammation. *Eur Respir J* 17: 416–421
53 Kim JY, Wand MP, Hauser R, Mukherjee S, Herrick RF, Christiani DC (2003) The association of expired nitric oxide with occupational particulate metal exposure. *Environ Health Perspect* 111: 676–680
54 Sundblad BM, Larsson BM, Palmberg L, Larsson K (2002) Exhaled nitric oxide and bronchial responsiveness in healthy subjects exposed to organic dust. *Eur Respir J* 20: 426–431
55 Smit LA, Heederik D, Doekes G, Wouters IM (2009) Exhaled nitric oxide in endotoxin-exposed adults: Effect modification by smoking and atopy. *Occup Environ Med* 66: 251–255
56 Akpinar-Elci M, Siegel PD, Cox-Ganser JM, Stemple KJ, White SK, Hilsbos K, Weissman DN (2008) Respiratory inflammatory responses among occupants of a water-damaged office building. *Indoor Air* 18: 125–130
57 Goldoni M, Catalani S, De Palma G, Manini P, Acampa O, Corradi M, Bergonzi R, Apostoli P, Mutti A (2004) Exhaled breath condensate as a suitable matrix to assess lung dose and effects in workers exposed to cobalt and tungsten. *Environ Health Perspect* 112: 1293–1298
58 Sikkeland LIB, Haug T, Strangeland AM, Flatberg G, Søstrand P, Halvorsen B, Kongerud J (2007) Airway inflammation in paper mill workers. *J Occup Environ Med* 49: 1135–1142
59 Adelroth E, Hedlund U, Blomberg A, Helleday R, Ledin MC, Levin JO, Pourazar J, Sandström T, Järvholm B (2006) Airway inflammation in iron ore miners exposed to dust and diesel exhaust. *Eur Respir J* 27: 714–719
60 Tanaka H, Saikai T, Sugawara H, Takeya I, Tsunematsu K, Matsuura A, Abe S (2002) Workplace-related chronic cough on a mushroom farm. *Chest* 122: 1080–1085
61 Heldal KK, Halstensen AS, Thorn J, Eduard W, Halstensen TS (2003) Airway inflammation in waste handlers exposed to bioaerosols assessed by induced sputum. *Eur Respir J* 21: 641–645
62 Murgia N, Muzi G, Dell'Omo M, Montuschi P, Melchiorri D, Ciabattoni G, Abbritti EP,

Orazi N, Sapia IE, Abbritti G (2006) Induced sputum, exhaled breath condensate and nasal lavage fluid in electroplating workers exposed to chromium. *Int J Immunopathol Pharmacol* 19: 67–71

63 Kreiss K, Day G, Schuler C (2007) Beryllium: A modern industrial hazard. *Annu Rev Public Health* 28: 259–277

64 Redlich CA, Stowe MH, Wisnewski AV, Eisen EA, Karol MH, Lemus R, Holm CT, Chung JS, Sparer J, Liu Y, Woskie SR et al (2001) Subclinical immunologic and physiologic responses in hexamethylene diisocyanate-exposed auto body shop workers. *Am J Ind Med* 39: 587–597

65 Wisnewski AV, Herrick CA, Liu Q, Chen L, Bottomly K, Redlich CA (2003) Human gamma/delta T cell proliferation and IFN-gamma production induced by hexamethylene diisocyanate. *J Allergy Clin Immunol* 112: 538–546

66 Shaaban R, Zureik M, Soussan D, Neukirch C, Heinrich J, Sunyer J, Wjst M, Cerveri I, Pin I, Bousquet J et al (2008) Rhinitis and onset of asthma: A longitudinal population-based study. *Lancet* 372: 1049–1057

67 Heederik D, van Rooy F (2008) Exposure assessment should be integrated in studies on the prevention and management of occupational asthma. *Occup Environ Med* 65: 149–150

68 Allmers HR, Brehler Z, Chen M, Raulf-Heimsoth H, Fels X, Baur X (1998) Reduction of latex aeroallergens and latex-specific IgE antibodies in sensitized workers after removal of powdered natural rubber latex gloves in a hospital. *J Allergy Clin Immunol* 102: 841–846

69 Jones KP, Rolf S, Stingl C, Edmunds D, Davies BH (2004) Longitudinal study of sensitization to natural rubber latex among dental school students using powder-free gloves. *Ann Occup Hyg* 48: 455–457

70 Brosseau LM, Parker DL, Lazovich D, Milton T, Dugan S (2002) Designing intervention effectiveness studies for occupational health and safety: The Minnesota Wood Dust Study. *Am J Ind Med* 41: 54–61

71 Lazovich D, Murray DM, Brosseau LM, Parker DL, Milton FT, Dugan SK (2002) Sample size considerations for studies of intervention efficacy in the occupational setting. *Ann Occup Hyg* 46: 219–227

72 Lazovich D, Parker DL, Brosseau LM, Milton FT, Dugan SK, Pan W, Hock L (2002) Effectiveness of a worksite intervention to reduce an occupational exposure: The Minnesota Wood Dust Study. *Am J Public Health* 92: 1498–1505

73 Meijster T, Warren N, Heederik, D, Tielemans E (2009) Comparison of the effect of different intervention strategies for occupational asthma on the burden of disease in bakers. *Occup Environ Med* 66: 810–817

74 Meijster T, Tielemans E, Schinkel J, Heederik D (2008) Evaluation of peak exposures in the Dutch flour processing industry: Implications for intervention strategies. *Ann Occup Hyg* 52: 587–596

75 Pronk A, Tielemans E, Skarping G, Bobeldijk I, Van Hemmen J, Heederik D, Preller L

(2006) Inhalation exposure to isocyanates of car body repair shop workers and industrial spray painters. *Ann Occup Hyg* 50: 1–14

76 Sparer J, Stowe MH, Bello D, Liu Y, Gore RJ, Youngs F, Cullen MR, Redlich CA, Woskie SR (2004) Isocyanate exposures in autobody shop work: The SPRAY study. *J Occup Environ Hyg* 9: 570–581

77 International Standardization Organization (1992) *Air quality – particle size fraction definitions for health related sampling.* ISO/CD 7708 International Standardization Organization, Geneva, Switzerland

78 Perkins JL (Editor) (1997) *Modern industrial hygiene:* Vol. I *Recognition, evaluation of chemical agents.* American Conference of Governmental Industrial Hygienists, Cincinnati, OH, USA

79 Perkins JL (Editor) (2002) *Modern Industrial Hygiene:* Vol. II *Biological Aspects.* American Conference of Governmental Industrial Hygienists, Cincinnati, OH, USA

80 O'Meara TJ, DeLucca S, Sporik R, Graham A, Tovey E (1998) Detection of inhaled cat allergen. *Lancet* 351: 1488–1489

81 Graham JA, Pavlicek PK, Sercombe JK, Xavier ML, Tovey ER (2000) The nasal air sampler: A device for sampling inhaled aeroallergens. *Ann Allergy Asthma Immunol* 84: 599–604

82 Renström A, Karlsson AS, Tovey E (2002) Nasal air sampling used for the assessment of occupational allergen exposure and the efficacy of respiratory protection. *Clin Exp Allergy* 32: 1769–1775

83 Schlünssen V, Sigsgaard T, Schaumburg I, Kromhout H (2004) Cross-shift changes in FEV_1 in relation to wood dust exposure: The implications of different exposure assessment methods. *Occup Environ Med* 61: 824–830

84 Gordon S, Tee RD, Lowson D, Newman Taylor AJ (1992) Comparison and optimization of filter elution methods for the measurement of airborne allergens. *Ann Occup Hyg* 36: 575–587

85 Hollander A, Gordon S, Renström A, Thissen J, Doekes G, Larsson PH, Malmberg P, Venables KM, Heederik D (1999) Comparison of methods to assess airborne rat and mouse allergen levels I. Analysis of air samples. *Allergy* 54: 142–149

86 Renström A, Gordon S, Larsson PH, Tee RD, Newman Taylor AJ, Malmberg P (1997) Comparison of a radioallergosorbent (RAST) inhibition method and a monoclonal enzyme-linked immunosorbent assay (ELISA) for aeroallergen measurement. *Clin Exp Allergy* 27: 1314–1321

87 Renström A, Hollander A, Gordon S, Thissen J, Doekes G, Larsson P, Venables K, Malmberg P, Heederik D (1999) Comparison of methods to assess airborne rat or mouse allergen levels II. Factors influencing antigen detection. *Allergy* 54: 150–157

88 Zock JP, Hollander A, Doekes G, Heederik D (1996) The influence of different filter elution methods on the measurement of airborne potato antigens. *Am Ind Hyg Assoc J* 57: 567–570

89 Lillienberg L, Baur X, Doekes G, Belin L, Raulf-Heimsoth M, Sander I, Ståhl A, Thissen

J, Heedrik D (2000) Comparison of four methods to assess fungal α-amylase in flour dust. *Ann Occup Hyg* 44: 427–433
90 Preller L, Heederik D, Kromhout H, Boleij JS, Tielen MJ (1995) Determinants of dust and endotoxin exposure of pig farmers: Development of a control strategy using empirical modeling. *Ann Occup Hyg* 39: 545–557
91 Seixas NS, Sheppard L (1996) Maximizing accuracy and precision using individual and grouped exposure assessments. *Scand J Work Environ Health* 22: 94–101
92 Houba R, Heederik DJ, Doekes G, van Run PE (1996) Exposure-sensitization relationship for α-amylase allergens in the baking industry. *Am J Respir Crit Care Med* 154: 130–136
93 Houba R, Heederik D, Doekes G (1998) Wheat sensitization and work related symptoms in the baking industry are preventable: An epidemiological study. *Am J Respir Crit Care Med* 158: 1499–1503
94 Heederik D, Venables KM, Malmberg P, Hollander A, Karlsson AS, Renström A, Doekes G, Nieuwenhijsen M, Gordon S (1999) Exposure-response relationships for work-related sensitization in workers exposed to rat urinary allergens: Results from a pooled study. *J Allergy Clin Immunol* 103: 678–684
95 Hollander A, Heederik D, Doekes G (1997) Respiratory allergy to rats: Exposure-response relationships in laboratory animal workers. *Am J Respir Crit Care Med* 155: 562–567
96 Nieuwenhuijsen MJ, Putcha V, Gordon S, Heederik D, Venables KM, Cullinan P, Newman-Taylor AJ (2003) Exposure-response relations among laboratory animal workers exposed to rats. *Occup Environ Med* 60: 104–108
97 Becklake M (1999) Epidemiological approaches in occupational asthma. In: IL Bernstein, M Chan-Yeung, JL Malo, DI Bernstein (eds): *Asthma in the Workplace*, 2nd edn. Marcel Dekker, New York
98 Marine WM, Gurr D, Jacobsen M (1988) Clinically important respiratory effects of dust exposure and smoking in British coal miners. *Am Rev Respir Dis* 137: 106–112
99 Rose G (1981) Strategy of prevention: Lessons from cardiovascular disease. *Br Med J* (Clin Res Ed) 282: 1847–1851
100 Berry G (1974) Longitudinal observations, their usefulness and limitations with special reference to the forced expiratory volume. *Bull Physiopathol Respir* 10: 643–655
101 Schlesselman JJ (1973) Planning a longitudinal study. I. Sample size determination. *J Chronic Dis* 26: 553–560
102 Schlesselman JJ (1973) Planning a longitudinal study. II. Frequency of measurement and study duration. *J Chronic Dis* 26: 561–570
103 Douwes J, Gibson P, Pekkanen J, Pearce N (2002) Non-eosinophilic asthma: Importance and possible mechanisms. *Thorax* 57: 643–648
104 Park JH, Cox-Ganser J, Kreiss K, White S, Rao C (2008) Hydrophilic fungi and ergosterol associated with respiratory illness in a water-damaged building. *Environ Health Perspect* 116: 45–50

Index